Frontiers in Clinical Drug Research: HIV
(Volume 1)

Editor

Atta-ur-Rahman, ***FRS***

Kings College
University of Cambridge
Cambridge
UK

CONTENTS

CHAPTERS

PREFACE

Human immunodeficiency virus (HIV) is responsible for AIDS (Acquired Immune Deficiency Syndrome), due to which the immune system of the body is badly affected and natural defense mechanisms become compromised. This opens the way for many infectious diseases to attack simultaneously. The treatment of HIV has been directed to decrease mortality and increase the number of clinically secured patients. Volume 1 of the book series *"**Frontiers in Clinical Drug Research - HIV**"* presents important recent developments in the form of cutting edge reviews written by eminent professionals.

Highly active antiretroviral therapy (HAART) uses multiple drugs that can act on special viral targets which in turn maintain the functions of the immune system. Chapter 1 by Phillips and Svard summarizes the current status in terms of development of drugs to target various stages of the disease and to refine the use of current drugs.

Viral suppression reduces the function and replication of a virus. It also decreases the amount of virus in the blood. Successful antiretroviral therapy is being used for sustained HIV viral suppression and immunological recuperation in HIV infected patients. Casseb and Arruda in Chapter 2 discuss the advances in the field of antiretroviral agents (ART) that focus on two main types of inhibitors, integrase inhibitors and entry inhibitors.

In the next chapter Brakier-Gingras *et al.* review the characteristics of the mechanism accounting for HIV-1 frameshifting. They present the different approaches investigated to develop novel anti-HIV-1 drugs interfering with the frameshift, including the high-throughput screening of libraries of chemical compounds with a bicistronic reporter, the use of antisense oligonucleotides binding to the frameshift stimulatory signal, and the selection and modification of chemical compounds that bind to the frameshift stimulatory signal.

Single Nucleotide Polymorphism (SNP) is a genetic variation in human genome that causes resistance to drugs applied for the management of HIV/AIDS. Astakhova in Chapter 4 comprehensively describes the approaches of current SNP sensing in HIV-1 cDNA and RNA. In addition, several promising technologies that are being used for the diagnosis of HIV are also highlighted in this review.

The nucleosides having unusual branched sugars are known to work as potential antiviral agents. Haraguchi *et al.* in Chapter 5 describe the new synthetic methods for the synthesis of 1' and 4'-branched-sugar nucleosides. This review also addresses the anti-viral activities, pharmacology and clinical developments (Phase I and Phase IIa) of 4'-ethynylstavudine (4'-Ed4T) that has more potent anti-HIV activity than the parent compound stavudine (d4T).

HIV-integrase is an attractive target for the development of new anti-HIV drugs and has potent antiviral activity. The advancement in effective inhibitors of HIV replication has established the prospective efficiency of antiviral treatment for the cure of AIDS. Ashton and Hann in Chapter 6 have reviewed in detail the recent developments targeting HIV integrase.

HAART is an aggressive treatment used to restrain HIV viral replication and the progression of HIV disease. Ansari *et al.* in Chapter 7 describe the potential adverse effects of HAART on kidney.

This first volume of the book series represents the results of a considerable amount of work by eminent contributors. I am grateful for their excellent contributions. I also wish to thank the excellent team of Bentham Science Publishers, especially Ms. Fariya Zulfiqar, led by Mr. Mahmood Alam, Director Bentham Science Publishers, who deserve our appreciation.

Atta-ur-Rahman, *FRS*

Kings College
University of Cambridge
Cambridge
UK

List of Contributors

Benjamin L. Miller	Department of Biochemistry and Biophysics, and Dermatology, University of Rochester, Rochester, New York, USA
Elijah Paintsil	Department of Pediatrics, School of Medicine, Yale University, New Haven, CT 06520, USA
Hiroki Kumamoto	School of Pharmacy, Showa University, Tokyo 142-8555, Japan
Hiromichi Tanaka	School of Pharmacy, Showa University, Tokyo 142-8555, Japan
Jenny Svärd	Unit of Infectious Diseases, Department of Medicine Huddinge, Karolinska Institutet, Stockholm, Sweden
Johanie Charbonneau	Department of Biochemistry, University of Montreal, Montreal, Quebec, H3T 1J4, Canada
Jorge Casseb	Laboratory of Investigation in Dermatology and Immunodeficiencies – LIM56, Department of Dermatology, School of Medicine at University of Sao Paulo, Sao Paulo, Brazil
Kazuhiro Haraguchi	Department of Pharmaceutical Sciences, Nihon Pharmaceutical University, Saitama 362-0806, Japan
Kira Astakhova	Nucleic Acid Center, Department of Physics, Chemistry and Pharmacy, Campusvej 55, 5230 Odense M, Denmark
Léa Brakier-Gingras	Department of Biochemistry, University of Montreal, Montreal, Quebec, H3T 1J4, Canada
Liã Bárbara Arruda	Institute of Tropical Medicine of Sao Paulo, University of Sao Paulo, Sao Paulo, Brazil
Mark Ashton	Department of Pharmacy, Health and Wellbeing, University of Sunderland, Sunderland, Tyne and Wear, UK
Masanori Baba	Division of Antiviral Chemotherapy, Center for Chronic Viral Diseases, Graduate School of Medical and Dental Sciences, Kagoshima University, Kagoshima 890-8544, Japan
Matthew Phillips	Department of Sexual and Reproductive Healthcare, Royal Bolton Hospital, Bolton, UK
Naheed Ansari	Division of Nephrology, Department of Medicine, Jacobi Medical Center, Albert Einstein College of Medicine, Bronx, New York 10461, USA
Parikshit T. Hameer	Division of Nephrology, Department of Medicine, Jacobi Medical Center, Albert Einstein College of Medicine, Bronx New York 10461, USA
Shingo Takeda	School of Pharmacy, Showa University, Tokyo 142-8555, Japan

Siddhartha Yedla	Division of Nephrology, Department of Medicine, Jacobi Medical Center, Albert Einstein College of Medicine, Bronx, New York 10461, USA
Takayuki Hamasaki	Division of Antiviral Chemotherapy, Center for Chronic Viral Diseases, Graduate School of Medical and Dental Sciences, Kagoshima University, Kagoshima 890-8544, Japan
Victoria Hann	Department of Pharmacy, Health and Wellbeing, University of Sunderland, Sunderland, Tyne and Wear, UK
Yasuo Urata	Oncolys BioPharma Inc., 4-1-28 Toranomon, Minato-ku, Tokyo 105-0001, Japan
Yung-Chi Cheng	Department of Pharmacology, School of Medicine, Yale University, New Haven, CT 06520, USA
Yutaka Kubota	School of Pharmacy, Showa University, Tokyo 142-8555, Japan

CHAPTER 1

Antiretroviral Drugs: Current Therapy, Recent Developments and Future Perspectives

Matthew Phillips[1,*] and Jenny Svärd[2]

[1]Department of Sexual and Reproductive Healthcare, Royal Bolton Hospital, Bolton, UK and [2]Unit of Infectious Diseases, Department of Medicine Huddinge, Karolinska Institutet, Stockholm, Sweden

Abstract: The treatment of human immunodeficiency virus (HIV) infection has been a great success story of our time; from the widespread panic in the early 1980's when the virus was identified as the cause of AIDS, to the availability of a whole plethora of drugs to treat and effectively control HIV infection, developed after millions of dollars of research funding investments. However, this treatment is not entirely problem-free. From the early days of antiretroviral (ARV) monotherapy, to the mid 1990's when triple therapy (highly active antiretroviral treatment, HAART) was discovered to be not only more effective but less toxic, there has been ongoing work to change the face of HIV treatment. This work can be broadly split into three categories, being:

1. developing drugs to target different stages of the life cycle.
2. developing novel drugs and refining the use of current drugs to reduce toxicities and side effects.
3. reducing the pill burden and the impact of daily therapy.

In part I, the life cycle of HIV and the targets of current therapy will be presented in terms of their individual actions and side effects. This section is completed by an exploration of wider issues surrounding anti-HIV therapy including distribution, cost and regular access. Part II will examine three key aspects of new drugs in development. This examination will be of new ARV agents in development, including some agents very recently licensed. The first aspect will be drugs in the pipeline which are directed against existing drug targets; potential differences between these drugs compared to current agents will be outlined. The second aspect is the most exciting, focusing on the development of novel drugs for novel targets in the HIV life cycle. The final aspect of part II will be to examine the role of these new drugs in adding to an already complex treatment arena - are these drugs for patients who have failed other therapies, or do their new actions and side effect profiles make them more useful for first line treatment? Will their expense or mode of delivery make them simply inaccessible to people living with HIV?

***Corresponding author Matthew Phillips:** Department of Sexual and Reproductive Healthcare, Royal Bolton Hospital, Bolton, UK; Tel: +4416110545; Fax: +44161 8875; Email: phillima@tcd.ie

Atta-ur-Rahman (Ed)

Part III will contain the conclusions pertaining to the preceding section, and will examine potential for the development of even newer drugs in terms of targets, efficacy, toxicities and acceptability. The two facets that will be explored are the potential for the correction of deficits in current treatment and potential new drugs.

Keywords: Adverse effects, adherence, antiretroviral drug development, HIV, HIV life cycle.

PART I: STAGES IN THE HIV LIFE CYCLE TARGETED BY CURRENT ARV DRUGS

The human immunodeficiency virus (HIV) is a retrovirus of the lentivirus family. Being a retrovirus, it requires reverse transcription to take place prior to incorporation into the host DNA. The genes coding for the proteins of HIV have been identified and are presented in Table **1** [1], and the structure of HIV in Fig. **1**.

Table 1: HIV-encoded proteins with their corresponding gene and function

Protein Type	Gene	Function
Structural	*Gag*	Encodes for capsid, matrix and nucleocapsid
	Pol	Encodes for viral enzymes
	Env	Encodes for envelope glycoproteins
Regulatory	*Tat*	Regulates HIV transcription
	Rev	Induces transition from early to late genes
Accessory	*Vpu*	Enhances virus particle release
	Vpr	Facilitates import of prointegration complex and cell growth arrest
	Vif	Maintains replication of HIV in lymphocytes and macrophages
	Nef	Down-regulates CD4 receptors and stimulates HIV infectivity

Life Cycle of HIV Replication

1. Binding, Fusion and Entry

At the initial stage, HIV comes into contact with a CD4-expressing cell (such as a helper T cell or macrophage). The main glycoprotein needed for this interaction is gp120 on the virion surface, which forms a trimer together with a transmembrane component, gp41. The presence of chemokine co-receptor (CCR5 or CXCR4), expressed on the surface of the CD4 cell, is also required in addition to the CD4 molecule. These interactions allow the virion to bind firmly in preparation for fusion with the cell membrane and release of the viral core into the CD4+ cell (Fig. **2**).

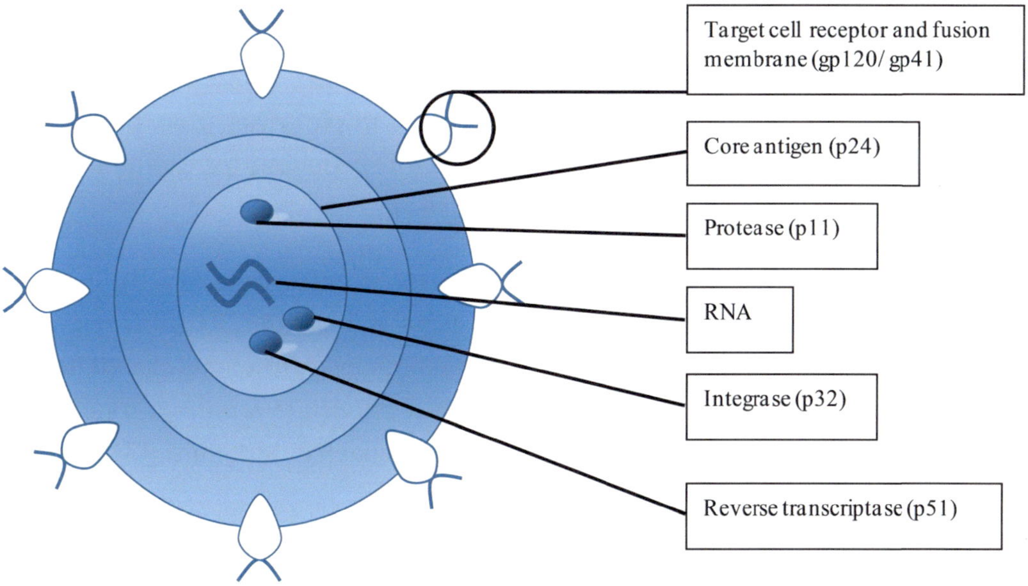

Figure 1: Schematic structure of the human immunodeficiency virus (HIV).

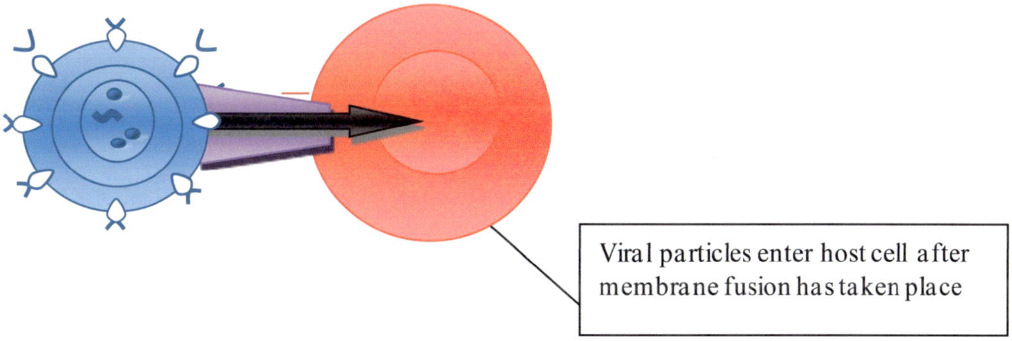

Figure 2: Viral entry.

Drugs Which Inhibit Binding, Fusion and Entry

There are currently two drug classes that act at this step: a selective CCR5 inhibitor (maraviroc) and a fusion inhibitor (enfuvirtide).

The human genetic sequence for CCR5 co-receptor expression is located on the p-arm, position 21, chromosome 3. A naturally occurring deletion mutation, denominated CCR5-Δ32, results in a non-functional receptor and confers a certain degree of protection against HIV infection [2]. CCR5 inhibitors work by binding to the CCR5 co-receptor on the CD4+ cell, thereby blocking cell entry. Specifically, maraviroc binds to the transmembrane cavity, preventing the gp120 protein binding functionally to the CD4+ cell [3]. However, maraviroc monotherapy can lead to emergence of CXCR4-tropic virus from pre-existing minor variant reservoirs [4, 5]. The relevance of this finding for triple therapy in the clinical setting remains to be clarified.

The only currently licensed entry/fusion inhibitor is enfuvirtide (T-20). It acts at the stage after gp120 has interacted with the CD4 and CCR5/CXCR4 receptor. At this stage, the transmembrane gp41 protein undergoes a structural change from a non-fusible protein to a fusion enabled protein. Enfuvirtide mimics a fragment of gp41, preventing reconfiguration to a fusion enabled structure [3], thereby preventing fusion of the virion to the CD4+ cell.

2. Reverse Transcription

After the viral proteins are released into the host cell, the RNA must undergo reverse transcription before being integrated into the host DNA. The viral reverse transcriptase (RT) performs this function (Fig. **3**).

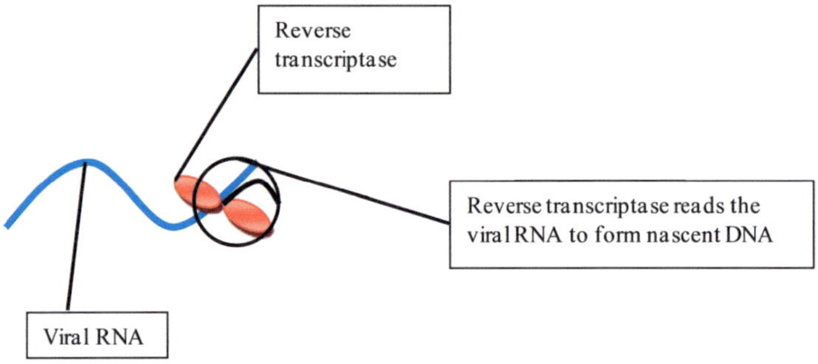

Figure 3: HIV reverse transcription.

Drugs Which Inhibit Reverse Transcription

There are two large groups of ARV drugs operational at this stage, the nucleoside/nucleotide reverse transcriptase inhibitors (NRTIs) and non-nucleoside reverse transcriptase inhibitors (NNRTIs).

NRTIs are analogues of deoxyribonucleosides/nucleotides, but lack a 3'-hydroxyl group [6]. Therefore, as they are incorporated into the nascent DNA, the DNA cannot be extended any further by ongoing transcription due to chain interruption. In order to perform this action, the NRTI must be converted to its corresponding triphosphate form by intracellular kinases. Approved NRTIs are zidovudine (AZT), didanosine (ddI), zalcitabine (ddC, no longer marketed), stavudine (d4T), lamivudine (3TC), abacavir (ABC), tenofovir disproximil fumarate (TDF) and emtricitabine (FTC).

NNRTIs function in a similar but distinct capacity. They do not require triphosphorylation by kinase activity. The function of NNRTIs is to bind to the viral reverse transcriptase at the NNRTI binding pocket, which is distinct from the active site, causing an allosteric conformational change [7]. This prevents the ongoing DNA synthesis. To date, five NNRTIs have been approved: nevirapine (NVP), delavirdine (DLV), efavirenz (EFV), etravirine (ETR) and most recently rilpivirine (RPV).

3. Integration

At this step, reverse transcription of the HIV RNA is complete, and the strands are arranged into double stranded HIV cDNA ready to be integrated into the host DNA in the cell nucleus. This step has three components, of which HIV integrase mediates the first two [8, 9]. The first component is the trimming of the 3' end of the viral cDNA in order to prepare the cDNA for the second part of integration which is strand transfer. It is at this point that the 3' ends of the cDNA are annealed to receptive 5' strands in the host DNA. The final component of the integration step is repair of the strand connection sites to create functional DNA (Fig. **4**).

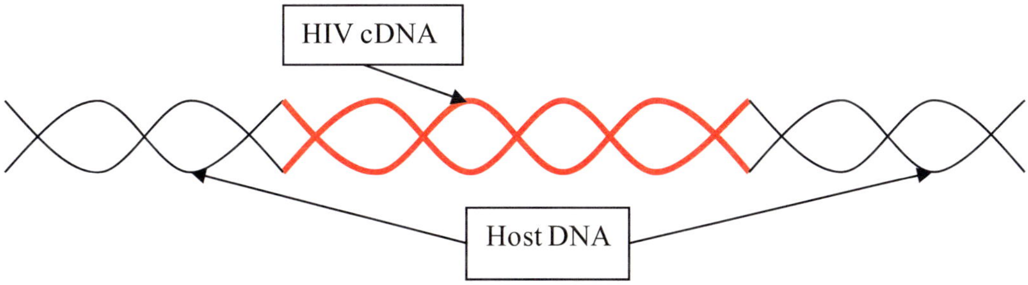

Figure 4: HIV RNA integration.

Drugs Which Inhibit Integration

Integrase inhibitor raltegravir (RAL) is now included as an optional component of first line combination ART in both US and European guidelines. Raltegravir works specifically by interfering with the strand transfer step of integration by virtue of its β-diketoacid moiety, which has specificity for the viral integrase but does not interact with human integrases [9]. Therefore, as strand transfer is prevented, the HIV genome cannot be integrated and replication cannot occur.

4. Transcription

Once the HIV DNA is fully integrated, cellular transcription can normally occur. As the HIV genome is incorporated into the host DNA, transcription will yield HIV RNA and proteins (Fig. **5**).

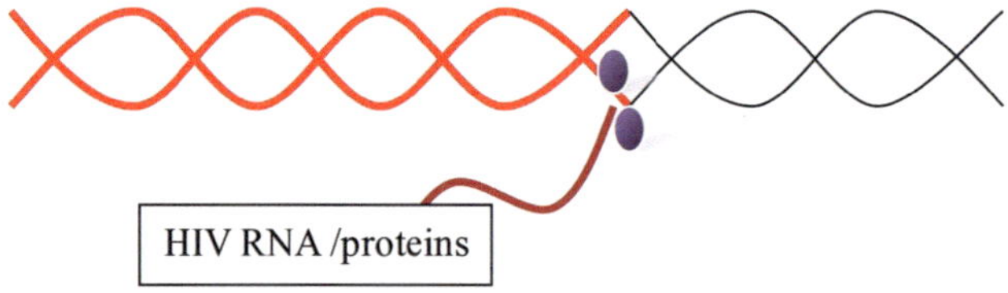

Figure 5: Transcription.

Drugs Which Inhibit Transcription

There are currently no ARV drugs which target this part of the HIV replication cycle.

5. Assembly

As the HIV polyprotein is produced, the HIV protease works by cleaving this precursor into functional products, ready for virion production (Fig. **6**).

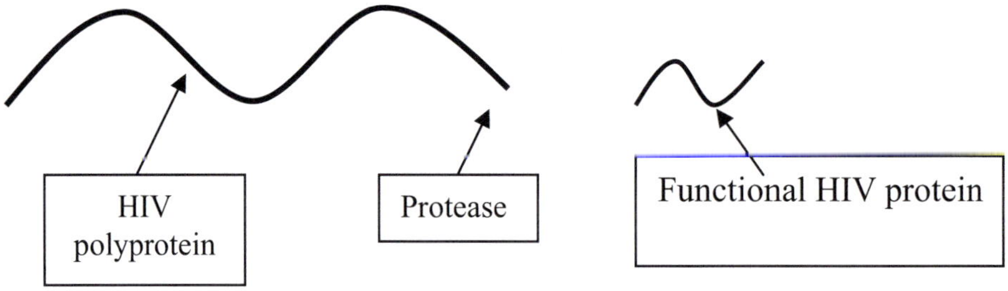

Figure 6: Assembly.

Drugs Which Inhibit Assembly/Protease Activity

HIV protease inhibitors (PIs) are the main group acting at this level. The main target of action is HIV aspartyl protease which cleaves the HIV Gag and Gag-Pol backbone [10]. As this action is inhibited, functional proteins cannot be formed and therefore virion production is halted at this stage. There are a number of PIs available: saquinavir (SQV), ritonavir (RTV), indinavir (IDV), nelfinavir (NFV), amprenavir (APV), lopinavir (LPV, only available as co-formulation with low dose ritonavir), fosamprenavir (FOS), atazanavir (ATV), tipranavir (TPV) and darunavir (DRV).

6. Budding and Maturation

Once all proteins and glycoproteins required for virion production have been cleaved, virions bud from the surface of the CD4+ cell to produce individual infective particles.

Drugs Which Inhibit Budding and Maturation

There are currently no approved drugs which act at this part of the HIV replication cycle.

At present, 25 ARV agents have been approved for use in the treatment of HIV infection. In addition, there are a number of co-formulated products available. All currently approved single drugs are summarized in Table **2**, including drug class and year of approval.

COMBINATIONS OF ANTIRETROVIRALS IN CLINICAL PRACTICE

The following combinations are as suggested by the British HIV Association (BHIVA) guidelines on the management of HIV-1. They do not cover the treatment of HIV-2. The exact treatments and their merits are outside of the scope of this chapter which aims only to comment on combinations used commonly in clinical practice. Some of the major side effects of the drug classes will be discussed. This should not be considered a guide of what to use in clinical practice, as certain drugs have very specific applications and requirements which will not be covered.

Table 2: Approved antiretroviral drugs with brand names, manufacturers and year of approval. NRTI = nucleoside/nucleotide reverse transcriptase inhibitor, NNRTI = non-nucleoside reverse transcriptase inhibitor, PI = protease inhibitor.

Generic name	Brand name	Drug class	Manufacturer	Year of Approval
Abacavir sulphate (ABC)	Ziagen	NRTI	GlaxoSmithKline	1998
Didanosine (ddI)	Videx	NRTI	Bristol Myers-Squibb	1991
Emtricitabine (FTC)	Emtriva	NRTI	Gilead	2003
Lamivudine (3TC)	Epivir	NRTI	GlaxoSmithKline	1995
Tenofovir disproximil fumarate (TDF)	Viread	NRTI	Gilead	2001
Zalcitabine (ddC)	Hivid	NRTI	Hoffman-La Roche	1992
Zidovudine (AZT)	Retrovir	NRTI	GlaxoSmithKline	1987
Delavirdine (DLV)	Rescriptor	NNRTI	Pfizer	1997
Efavirenz (EFV)	Sustiva	NNRTI	Bristol Myers-Squibb	1998
Etravirine (TMC 125)	Intelence	NNRTI	Tibotec Therapeutics	2008
Nevirapine (NVP)	Viramune	NNRTI	Boehringer Ingelheim	1991
Rilpivirine (RPV)	Edurant	NNRTI	Tibotec Therapeutics	2011
Amprenavir (APV)	Agenerase	PI	GlaxoSmithKline	
Atazanavir sulphate (ATV)	Reyataz	PI	Bristol Myers-Squibb	2003
Darunavir (DRV)	Prezista	PI	Tibotec, Inc.	2006
Fosamprenavir calcium (FPV)	Lexiva	PI	GlaxoSmithKline	2003
Indinavir (IDV)	Crixivan	PI	Merck	1996
Lopinavir/ritonavir (LPV/r)	Kaletra	PI	Abbot Laboratories	2000
Nelfinavir (NFV)	Viracept	PI	Agouron Pharmaceuticals	1997
Ritonavir (RTV)	Norvir	PI	Abbot Laboratories	1996
Saquinavir mesylate (SQV)	Invirase	PI	Hoffman-La Roche	1995
Tipranavir (TPV)	Aptivus	PI	Boehringer Ingelheim	2005
Enfuvirtide (T-20)	Fuzeon	Fusion inhibitor	Hoffman-La Roche & Trimeris	2003
Maraviroc (MVC)	Selzentry	Entry inhibitor	Pfizer	2007
Raltegravir (RAL)	Isentress	Integrase inhibitor	Merck	2007

The advantages of triple therapy over single or dual therapy is a dogma that is now well established in HIV medicine [11]. Using a single agent (such as zidovudine in the early days of ART) required very high doses of the drug [12]. This increased the risk and amplitude of side effects for the patient, and demanded a very high level of dedication from patients to be able to tolerate these side effects. Using a single agent also increases the risk of emergent drug resistance mutations as any missed dose or occurrence that results in sub-therapeutic drug levels gives the virus the opportunity to mutate. Multiple agents, usually three, reduce this chance. The agents almost always have at least two modes of action (*i.e.,* target two different stages of the HIV replicative cycle, or at the very least have different targets within a given stage). The drugs used can thus be administered in smaller doses, and at less frequent intervals. The treatment becomes more robust as the patient is able to comply with the regime more easily; furthermore a single missed dose is less likely to result in resistance development (depending on drug half-life and the genetic barrier to the individual drugs). As drugs have become more refined, different fixed dose preparations have become available which increase patient adherence as they are easy to take. The first example of a one tablet once-a-day regime was Atripla (tenofovir, emtricitabine and efavirenz), although newer combinations will be discussed in part II.

Therefore, a standard regime contains three drugs. These are commonly combined as two drugs forming a backbone (usually two NRTIs), plus a third agent from a different class of drugs (Table **3**). Some combinations of ARVs are advised against for reasons such as antagonistic effects, lack of additive benefits or increased risk of virological failure or adverse effects. These combinations are presented in Table **4**.

Side Effects

Different classes of drugs have specific side effects. Within each class, some agents have a greater propensity than others to induce these side effects. The most common of these will be discussed here.

Table 3: Recommendations for first line antiretroviral treatment (British HIV Association 2012) [13]. NRTI = nucleoside/nucleotide reverse transcriptase inhibitor, NNRTI = non-nucleoside reverse transcriptase inhibitor, PI = protease inhibitor.

<table>
<tr><th>Backbone</th><th></th><th>Third Agent</th></tr>
<tr><td rowspan="3">2 NRTIs
• tenofovir (TDF) + emtricitabine (FTC)
• abacavir (ABC) + lamivudine (3TC)
• zidovudine (AZT) + lamivudine (3TC)</td><td rowspan="3">+ any one of the agents from the right hand column</td><td>NNRTI
• efavirenz (EFV)
• nevirapine (NVP)</td></tr>
<tr><td>PI
• Any ritonavir (RTV)-boosted PI</td></tr>
<tr><td>Integrase inhibitor
• raltegravir (RAL)</td></tr>
</table>

Table 4: Drugs which should be avoided in combination [1].

Combination	**Reason**
stavudine (d4T) + zidovudine (AZT)	antagonistic effect (both thymidine analogues)
emtricitabine (FTC) + lamivudine (3TC)	no additive benefit (both cytosine analogues)
abacavir (ABC) + zidovudine (AZT) + tenofovir (TDF)	increased risk of virological failure
didanosine (ddI) + tenofovir (TDF) + efavirenz (EFV)	increased risk of virological failure
didanosine (ddI) + stavudine (d4T)	increased risk of peripheral neuropathy, lactic acidosis, acute pancreatitis

Mitochondrial Toxicity

Mitochondrial toxicity is caused by inhibition of the mitochondrial γ DNA polymerase, and is a side effect of the NRTI drug class, although not all agents cause side effects through this mechanism alone. This enzyme is responsible for DNA synthesis in mitochondria. Inhibition of this enzyme causes

- myopathy
- peripheral neuropathy
- hepatic steatosis
- lactic acidosis

The most serious side effect is lactic acidosis as this can be life threatening, and requires clinical evaluation and measurement of serum lactate. Other side effects may necessitate a switch in NRTI backbone to an agent known to have a better side effect profile (for example stavudine may give rise to side effects which improve when switched to abacavir).

Peripheral Neuropathy

This can be a painful complication of HIV treatment and is most common with NRTI use, especially didanosine and stavudine. Once peripheral neuropathy has been identified within a patient, drug switch should take place quickly as the neuropathy is not reversible. However, it may be amenable to analgesic agents.

Rash

A very common side effect is usually seen with NNRTIs, although more frequently with nevirapine than efavirenz. A rash occurring when commencing abacavir therapy should bring into consideration the abacavir hypersensitivity reaction, which is described below. The rash is usually maculopapular. Systemic reactions should alert the clinician to the possibility of reactions such as Stevens-Johnson syndrome, which occurs in about 0.5% of patients [1]. Nevirapine is normally introduced in a stepwise dosing pattern to minimize the risk of rash.

Nausea

Nausea and vomiting are very common side effects of all ARVs, especially in the first few days to weeks of taking the medication, although other reasons for nausea should be explored [14].

Abnormal Dreams

Although rarely reported with any ARV, it is commonly associated with efavirenz therapy. Abnormal dreams and accompanying sleep disturbance induced by efavirenz usually settle within 2-4 weeks; however they may persist beyond three months [15] and occasionally in long-term treatment (> 1 year) [16]. There is also research showing a higher risk of efavirenz-associated side effects in individuals homozygous for the *CYP2B6* 516T mutation [17], as it leads to decreased efavirenz metabolism and higher plasma concentrations [18].

Lipid Abnormalities

PIs are particularly associated with changes in lipid metabolism [19, 20] with some studies noting a 20% increase in total cholesterol and a 22% increase in triglycerides over 12 months [21]. There have been multiple studies comparing different PIs and different backbone combinations in terms of lipid profiles [22-24]. It is important to balance the risk of cardiovascular disease in a patient alongside their HAART regimen to decide which will be the best third agent for any given patient.

Abacavir Hypersensitivity

A strong association between abacavir hypersensitivity and the HLA-B*5701 genotype has been demonstrated. In addition, screening for this genotype has been shown to be both cost-effective [25] and successful in reducing incidence of hypersensitivity reactions [26]. These usually occur within the first two weeks of treatment and can have a variety of symptoms including:

- headache
- fever
- maculopapular or urticarial rash
- dyspnoea
- abnormal liver function tests (LFTs)
- gastrointestinal (GI) tract disturbance.

If hypersensitivity reactions occur, abacavir should be stopped and never restarted as mortality can be as high as 4% in those re-challenged with the drug.

Issues Regarding Wider Access

Although this chapter focuses on new developments in HIV medicines, it would not be appropriate to forget the differential access to drugs that patients experience. There are many reasons for this problem, and although the most commonly cited is global issues of cost and geopolitical considerations, considerable variation can occur even in resource-rich settings. There has been much research on difficulties in access. In resource-poor settings, most often African countries, reasons include high cost of care and drugs for the patient [27, 28] in addition to the physical travel, as well as a high cost for the healthcare system for engaging the services of an appropriate professional [29-31]. However, sociological barriers which may affect health-seeking behavior include being worried about stigma [28, 29, 31] when exposing their HIV status in smaller communities, as well as fears of confidentiality being breached by healthcare staff [27, 30]. A shortfall of appropriate clinical staff has also been identified as a critical factor [32].

In more developed countries, issues regarding a patient's lifestyle can decrease their abilities to access HIV medication [33]. Chaotic or party lifestyles have been found to be factors, and the inextricable link to mental health has been identified as a barrier to HIV care in general [34]. Co-existent substance abuse has also been found to reduce access to ART [35].

It is beyond the scope of this chapter to discuss the complex issues surrounding access to ARV drugs in a global health arena, but one should bear in mind that although effective treatments exist, there are many other limiting factors which may have a significant impact on a patient's chance of receiving ART. Although we have not discussed specific costs, it is sufficient to see that access barriers exist in resource poor settings due to the price of specific drugs and treatments.

In the next part of this chapter, ARV drugs in the pipeline will be discussed before finally moving on to what might change in future ARV drug development.

PART II: ANTIRETROVIRAL DRUGS IN THE PIPELINE AND RECENTLY APPROVED DRUGS

Existing Drug Targets

New NRTIs

Although zidovudine monotherapy initially gave hope to HIV-infected patients whose condition had been previously untreatable, the success did not last long as drug resistance development shortly followed. In today's modern combination ART however, NRTIs constitute the backbone. As previously discussed, the main limitations of currently available NRTIs include mitochondrial toxicity [36] and drug resistance development [37].

Amdoxovir (AMDX, (-)-beta-D-2, 6-diaminopurine dioxolane) is a water-soluble pro-drug of (-)-beta-D-dioxolane guanine (DXG) which in its triphosphorylated form is a potent and selective inhibitor of the viral reverse transcriptase (RT) [38]. Like abacavir, amdoxovir is a guanosine analogue and does not give rise to thymidine analogue mutations (TAMs). On the contrary, amdoxovir-resistance associated mutations K65R and L74V introduced into a genetic background of zidovudine resistance (D67N, K70R, T215Y, T219Q) reverses the virus to become zidovudine-sensitive [39]. On account of this suppression of TAM-mediated resistance, a phase II randomized double-blind placebo-controlled study was carried out to assess antiviral activity and tolerability of amdoxovir-zidovudine combinations in HIV-infected subjects. The outcome showed synergistic reduction in VL variability [40]. Despite these promising results, clinical trials have been discontinued due to resistance development and adverse effects [41].

A longer half-life (60h) [42] than most NRTIs makes *elvucitabine* (L-cytosine nucleoside analogue of stavudine) an interesting investigational NRTI with potential for a reduced need of strict adherence and lower risk of drug resistance development. The ACH443-015 Study Team demonstrated comparable safety and efficacy to lamivudine (3TC), in addition to no emergence of resistance mutations at 96 weeks [43]. One concern is bone marrow toxicity, however as elvucitabine is more potent than stavudine lower concentrations can be used and potentially avoid this adverse effect [44].

Apricitabine, a deoxycytidine analogue, displayed retained antiviral activity against HIV-1 isolates resistant against a range of commonly used NRTIs (zidovudine, lamivudine, abacavir) in early *in vitro* assays [45]. A subsequent clinical trial in treatment-naïve HIV-infected patients confirmed promising ARV efficacy and additionally showed good tolerability with no emergence of resistance mutations after 10 days of monotherapy [46]. Cahn *et al.* [47] also demonstrated viral suppression by apricitabine in treatment-experienced patients previously on failing lamivudine-containing regimens, where all patients maintained their M184V mutation present at baseline. As no patients developed

K65R or L74V mutations after 48 weeks of treatment [48], apricitabine can be considered a suitable replacement of lamivudine or emtricitabine. On the other hand, co-administration with other deoxycytidine analogues such as lamivudine and emtricitabine should be avoided as competition for intracellular phosphorylation by deoxycytidine kinase results in reduced antiviral activity of apricitabine [49].

GS-7340, a novel pro-drug of tenofovir, displays preferential distribution and accumulation in lymphatic tissues and PBMCs [50] and can thus achieve a more potent intracellular activity in the major sites of HIV replication. A comparison of GS-7340 *vs.* tenofovir disproximil fumarate (TDF) monotherapy (14 days in HIV-1 infected subjects) by Markowitz *et al.* [51] demonstrated 94% higher plasma c_{max} by TDF while intracellular PBMC concentrations were ~30-fold higher in the group treated with GS-7340. A subsequent dose-comparing study by the same investigators confirmed superior antiviral efficacy of 25mg and 40mg GS-7340 over 300mg TDF [52]. The potency and targeting by this new pro-drug could dramatically reduce the risk of tenofovir-associated adverse effects. Birkus *et al.* [53] investigated potential pharmacokinetic interactions with antiviral protease inhibitors *in vitro* and found none for the HIV PIs examined. However, hepatitis C virus PIs telaprevir and bocepravir both reduced the antiviral effect of GS-7340 through inhibition of cathepsin A which plays a pivotal role in the intracellular activation of the pro-drug. A phase II study assessing GS-7340 in combination with cobicistat, darunavir and emtricitabine is estimated to be completed in December 2013.

Thymidine analogue *BMS-986001* has showed good virologic response in a 10-day placebo-controlled monotherapy study in treatment-experienced subjects: viral load reductions of 0.97-1.28 $\log_{10}$ copies/ml were achieved with 100 to 600mg once-daily dosing [54]. Although structurally similar to stavudine, BMS-986001 is a weaker inhibitor of mitochondrial DNA polymerase and is therefore expected to result in lower risk of mitochondrial toxicity (supported by *in vitro* results using human primary cells) [55]. In two patients receiving BMS-986001, mixed population TAMs (K70K/R and K219K/R) were detected at day 17, nevertheless both of these patients had experienced a 10-fold decline in HIV-1 RNA. Since *in vitro* resistance profiling has demonstrated significantly reduced susceptibility by K70R mutants however [56], further *in vivo* investigations on drug resistance development are warranted. A safety, efficacy and dose-response study of BMS-986001 as part of triple therapy with efavirenz and lamivudine in an ART-naïve population is currently recruiting participants.

New NNRTIs

Efavirenz is currently the most widely used NNRTI and forms part of first line ART in US, European and WHO guidelines. However, teratogenic potential [57] and discontinuation due to central nervous system (CNS) side effects such as insomnia, dizziness and headache [58] may limit the use of this NNRTI. Nevirapine [59], delavirdine [60] and the more recently approved etravirine [61] are all associated with rash. Moreover, nevirapine increases the risk of hepatotoxicity [62]. Delavirdine is not widely available outside the US and etravirine is approved only for use in treatment-experienced patients. The first-line NNRTIs efavirenz and nevirapine both have a low genetic barrier to drug resistance development, with only a single mutation required to confer high-level drug resistance [63]. Hence, newer NNRTIs with improved resistance profiles and improved tolerability are warranted. Nevertheless, this drug class is often preferred over PIs because of higher efficacy and better tolerability [64] in addition to a lower cost [65].

By combining molecular modeling and *in vitro* virological screening, *rilpivirine* (TMC278) was developed in 2001 [66]. Like etravirine, it is a diarylpyrimidine, a so-called second-generation NNRTI. It has a longer half-life, higher potency and a fewer side-effects [67]. Importantly, CNS effects which are highly common adverse events in efavirenz-based treatment are less frequent with rilpivirine [68]. In addition, rilpivirine inhibits replication of viral isolates resistant to efavirenz and nevirapine, and displays a high genetic barrier to resistance development [69]. Clinical trials in ART-naïve subjects have showed comparable antiviral efficacy to efavirenz over 48 weeks (ECHO and THRIVE studies [70]) and over 96 weeks (TMC278-C204 Study Group [68]). However, in patients experiencing viral failure with high baseline viral load (VL >100,000 copies/ml), NNRTI resistance-associated mutations were surprisingly more common in the rilpivirine group [71]. Rilpivirine was approved for use in HIV treatment by the US Food and Drug

Administration (FDA) and European Medicines Agency (EMA) in 2011, and is now also available as a once-daily fixed-dose combination with tenofovir and emtricitabine (named Complera in the US, Eviplera in Europe).

Lersivirine (UK-453061), another novel second-generation NNRTI, achieved mean VL reductions up to 1.8 log_{10} copies/ml after eight days of monotherapy in NNRTI-naïve HIV-1 infected patients, when steady-state had been achieved. The most frequently reported treatment-emerged adverse events were headache, fatigue and nausea, although these were generally considered mild [72]. While not as potent as efavirenz in RT enzyme assays (IC_{50} lersivirine 118 nM *vs.* efavirenz 7.2 nM), lersivirine better retains activity against K103N (80% *vs.* efavirenz 7%) and Y181C (57% *vs.* efavirenz 43%) single mutants. The improved resistance profile relative to efavirenz was retained also with other NNRTI mutations present. By X-ray crystallography, the similar binding modes of lersivirine to wildtype and K103N RT were demonstrated, setting lersivirine apart from other currently used NNRTIs [73].

RDEA806, an NNRTI in phase II clinical trials, was the result of a large-scale screening using a cell-based assay to identify a compound with good potency against both wildtype and NNRTI-resistant strains (K103N, Y181C, K103N/Y181C, K103N/L100I) [74]. 9 days of monotherapy in HIV-1 positive ART-naïve individuals achieved mean VL reductions of up to 1.95 log_{10} copies/ml (400mg twice daily), while increases in CD4+ T cell counts were only significant for 800mg and 1000mg once-daily. No emergence of NNRTI resistance-associated mutations were detected in these subjects. Although generally well tolerated, the most common adverse events experienced by the study subjects were diarrhea, upper abdominal discomfort, fatigue, headache and erythema [75]. Some concerns have been raised regarding the association between a metabolite of RDEA806 and hyperuricemia, which may become a problem in HIV patients with advanced disease or underlying renal dysfunction [76].

A safety and tolerability study of *GSK2248761* (formerly known as IDX-899), a candidate NNRTI with *in vitro* activity against efavirenz-resistant strains [77], demonstrated a favorable pharmacokinetic profile in healthy volunteers. With the exception of one case of moderate vomiting, all other adverse events were mild in severity [78]. Mean VL reductions of at least 1.78 log_{10} copies/ml were noted after eight days of monotherapy in treatment-naïve HIV-1 infected patients. On analysis of the RT sequence, none of these subjects displayed recognized NNRTI mutations [79]. The FDA placed GSK2248761 on clinical hold in 2011 due to five reports of seizures in treatment-experienced patients [80], further evaluation of these events is pending.

MK-4965 was developed through a combination of methods including crystallography, structure-activity relationship analyses and molecular modeling [81]. In a HIV-1 RT biochemical assay, this novel NNRTI has displayed similar potency to efavirenz against wildtype RT, and furthermore retained efficacy against efavirenz-resistant K103N RT. Additionally, a similar IC_{50} was measured with Y181C RT which confers resistance to nevirapine and reduces susceptibility to etravirine. However, in HIV multiple-cycle replication assays in the presence of 10% fetal bovine serum (FBS), etravirine exhibited approximately two-fold higher potency than MK-4965 against virus harboring K103N or K103N/Y181C mutations. In contrast, in presence of 50% human serum where antiviral activity of all tested compounds were reduced due to high levels of protein binding, MK-4965 displayed slightly better potency towards K103N or K103N/Y181C viruses compared to etravirine [82]. The clinical development of MK-4965 was however terminated due to indications of toxicity in an animal study [83].

A screening of diphenylether compounds led to the selection of *RO-0335* as a novel candidate NNRTI with broad and potent antiviral activity against common NNRTI-resistant strains. *In vitro* selection experiments did not lead to emerging K103N mutants, and Y181C arose at relatively high concentrations only ($\geq$ 500nM). The predominant path to susceptibility loss appears to be through the V106A/F227C double mutation which is distinct from the K103N mutation pathway, although this results in a considerable loss in viral fitness [84]. A pro-drug of RO-0335, *R1206*, substantially increases bioavailability in rats, dogs and monkeys [85].

New PIs

At present, very few HIV protease inhibitors (PIs) are in the pipeline. Karpoormath *et al.* [86] recently presented a new type of peptidic HIV protease inhibitors derived from pentacycloundecane, with IC_{50} values ranging between 0.6 to 5μM against wildtype HIV-1 protease activity *in vitro*. *In silico* analysis was performed which further confirmed the ability of these compounds to fit into the active enzyme pocket.

New Integrase Inhibitors

Currently, raltegravir is the only approved integrase inhibitor on the market. In long-term studies, raltegravir has proven effective in reducing viral load in treatment-experienced patients receiving an optimized background therapy [87, 88], however raltegravir is also approved for first line use in both Europe [89] and the USA [90].

Elvitegravir is an integrase inhibitor which, like raltegravir, inhibits the strand transfer step when both ends of the viral DNA are covalently linked to the cellular genomic DNA. Shimura *et al.* [91] demonstrated *in vitro* EC_{50} values of 0.4-2.8 nM against laboratory strains. After elvitegravir drug selection, an analysis of emerged mutations was carried out which revealed substitutions mostly in the central core catalytic domain of integrase. A 10-day monotherapy [92] showed substantial antiviral activity with a viral load reduction of at least 1.48 $\log_{10}$ copies/ml with twice-daily dosing in both treatment-naïve and treatment-experienced patients. Furthermore, with ritonavir-boosting a mean reduction of 1.91 $\log_{10}$ copies/ml was achieved with only 50mg elvitegravir once-a-day. None of the patients in this study displayed evidence of integrase inhibitor resistance. In a phase III study comparing addition of elvitegravir or raltegravir in treatment-experienced patients receiving a fully active PI/r-based background regimen during 48 weeks, non-inferiority of elvitegravir was demonstrated, with similar levels of adverse events [93]. An advantage of elvitegravir is the once-daily dosing compared to twice daily with raltegravir, made possible by ritonavir boosting as elvitegravir is predominantly metabolized by CYP3A4 [94]. Raltegravir, on the other hand, is not metabolized *via* the oxidative pathway but rather mediated by UDP-glucuronosyltransferases (UGTs), mainly UGT1A1 [95]. However, due to similar patterns of resistance mutations [93], elvitegravir is not likely to be useful in patients who have developed raltegravir resistance. Nevertheless, one notable difference is that elvitegravir does not interact with the amino acid at position 143, consequently elvitegravir remains active against raltegravir-resistant Y143R integrase mutants [96].

Dolutegravir, a second generation integrase inhibitor in late stages of clinical development, is interesting for two reasons: First, it has a somewhat different resistance profile to raltegravir and elvitegravir: the main resistance-associated mutation appears to be Q148 although secondary mutations may be necessary for reduced susceptibility [97], while there are a number of primary resistance-associated mutations for raltegravir (Y143R, Q148H/K/R, N155H) and elvitegravir (T66I, E92Q, S147G, Q148H/K/R, N155H) [98]. *In vitro*, dolutegravir exhibits a slower dissociation rate from HIV-1 integrase-DNA complexes, both for wildtype and E92, Y143, Q148, and N155 variants [99]. This is probably due to structural differences between dolutegravir and the other integrase inhibitors affecting the interactions between the inhibitors and the catalytic site [100]. Secondly, it has a long half-life and does not require boosting for a once-daily formulation [101]. SPRING 1, a multi-center dose-ranging study in ART-naïve patients, showed 87% response rates for all tested doses of dolutegravir at week 48 compared to 82% for efavirenz, in combination with dual NRTIs [102]. For treatment-experienced patients with integrase inhibitor resistance mutations in the VIKING I study [103], 78% achieved viral suppression after 11 days of once-daily dosing in addition to background therapy. Since reduced susceptibility was noted against virus with Q148 plus additional mutations, the VIKING II study [97] was carried out with twice-daily dosing during 11 days, which resulted in viral suppression in 96% of the patients (despite more extensive integrase inhibitor resistance at baseline).

S/GSK1265744, developed as a back-up compound to dolutegravir, is currently being evaluated for both oral dosing and as a long-acting parenteral formulation. *In vitro* studies have indicated glucoronidation as primary route of metabolism, potentially reducing the risk of drug interactions. In healthy subjects, co-administration with etravirine (inducer of CYP3A4 and inhibitor of CYP2C9, CYP2C19 and P-glycoprotein) had no effect on S/GSK1265744 pharmacokinetics while it reduced exposure to raltegravir and dolutegravir [104]. Moreover, S/GSK1265744 has displayed *in vitro* activity against a number of raltegravir-resistant strains [105]. A phase I dose-escalation study using a nano-suspension formulation by intramuscular or subcutaneous injection achieved sustained plasma concentrations previously demonstrated to reduce viral load by >2.5 $\log_{10}$ copies/ml, indicating that once-monthly dosing may be possible [106]. A phase

IIb study is currently recruiting treatment-naïve participants, for an induction dose-ranging phase with backbone NRTIs, followed by a maintenance phase in combination with raltegravir without NRTIs [107].

A novel type of integrase inhibitors, denominated LEDGINs, has been identified through rational drug design [108]. These small molecules bind to the pocket targeted by LEDGF/p75, a strong binding partner of HIV-1 integrase in eukaryotic cells, causing inhibition through an allosteric mechanism. Compound *BI-C* [109] displayed an EC_{50} value of 4-14 nM against laboratory HIV-1 strains and retained full antiviral activity against N155S, Q148H, and E92Q variants, consistent with the non-catalytic site mechanism of action. In addition, it also displayed favorable pharmacokinetic profiles in rat and monkey. Preclinical biochemical and antiviral evaluation of LEDGINs demonstrated inhibition of both 3' processing and strand transfer with activity against a broad range of clades including strains with reduced susceptibility against strand transfer inhibitors [110]. Additionally, antiviral assays using combinations of LEDGINs with strand transfer inhibitors resulted in additive effects.

New Entry Inhibitors

Co-Receptor Antagonists

Currently, the only approved co-receptor antagonist is maraviroc, targeting CCR5 and hence in theory active only against R5-tropic virus strains. It is included in both European and US guidelines as an alternative third agent to PIs or NNRTIs.

Vicriviroc, a novel CCR5 inhibitor in late clinical trials, was previously considered for use in treatment-experienced patients as the phase II VICTOR E1 study showed significant improvement in viral suppression and immune recovery in patients with R5-tropic virus who had failed on triple ART [111]. However, due to disappointing results in phase III studies [112] where no significant difference could be demonstrated between vicriviroc and placebo in addition to an optimized background therapy, the manufacturer decided not to seek FDA approval for this drug [113].

A 10-day monotherapy trial [114] investigating the safety and activity of *AMD11070*, a novel allosteric CXCR4 antagonist [115], demonstrated a tropism shift from dual- or mixed-tropic viruses to solely R5-tropic in 3 out of 4 patients who responded to therapy. Nevertheless, the study population also contained five patients who did not respond to AMD11070 monotherapy, potentially as a result of prominent X4-tropic viral populations. The authors remarked on the similarity to results obtained with AMD3100, which also showed a lack of efficacy in clinical studies. Although not effective as a single drug, it may be possible to benefit from AMD11070 in combination with CCR5 antagonists to prohibit the selection for X4-tropic strains.

New Fusion Inhibitors

At present, enfuvirtide is the only approved fusion inhibitor [116], derived from the viral gp41. The synthetic peptide binds to the coiled-coil formation of gp41, preventing the structural transitions necessary for virus-cell fusion [117]. By virtue of its peptide structure, this type of fusion inhibitor is only available in injectable form and reserved for salvage therapy only.

Despite its high efficacy, at the time when enfuvirtide was developed the full sequence of gp41 was still not known. Hence, after the full structure of gp41 was solved [118], an improved fusion inhibitor with a higher binding activity could be designed: *sifuvirtide*. Using *in vitro* p24 antigen assays, sifuvirtide displayed an EC_{50} of 4.3 nM against a laboratory strain (HIV-1_{IIIB}) and 0.96nM against a clinical isolate [119]. For comparison, the HIV-1_{IIIB} EC_{50} of enfuvirtide was 213 nM. These results were confirmed in a separate study [120] where sifuvirtide exhibited superior *in vitro* antiviral activity to enfuvirtide in *env*-luciferase replicon model systems representing A, B and C subtypes as well as strains with enfuvirtide resistance mutations. Currently, sifuvirtide is undergoing phase II trials in China.

Monoclonal Antibodies

PRO 140 is a humanized monoclonal CCR5 antibody which acts synergistically with small molecule CCR5 inhibitors (maraviroc, vicriviroc and TAK-779, an investigational agent which was subsequently discontinued) *in vitro* [121]. In HIV-infected subjects, PRO 140 has demonstrated efficacy both as single intravenous infusions (VL reduction 1.83 log_{10} copies/ml in the 5mg/kg group) [122] and as weekly/biweekly subcutaneous infusion (VL reduction 1.65 log_{10} copies/ml in the 324mg weekly group) [123].

PRO 542 is a tetravalent CD4-immunoglobulin fusion protein which binds to the viral surface glycoprotein gp120, preventing binding to CD4+ cells and consequently viral entry. Following indications of good HIV-1 neutralizing abilities *in vitro* [124] as well as prevention of HIV-1 infection in Hu-PBL-SCID mice (a model of AIDS) [125] and human primary cells [126], a phase I single dose study gave preliminary evidence of antiviral activity of PRO 542 in HIV-infected adults [127]. A follow-on study demonstrated a significant reduction of approximately 0.5 log_{10} copies/ml up to 4 weeks after a single 25mg/kg intravenous dose of PRO 452 [128]. This effect may not be linear, as indicated by a pediatric study where a doubling in dose did not result in a proportional reduction in viremia [129]. However, no new clinical study results have been published since.

More recent clinical data are available on *ibalizumab*, a humanized monoclonal anti-CD4 antibody which causes post-gp120-binding conformational changes and prevents co-receptor interactions [130]. A 24 week phase II randomized, double-blind, controlled study in 82 treatment-experienced patients with optimized background therapy showed significantly greater viral load reductions in both treatment arms (10mg/kg weekly for 8 weeks followed by either 10mg/kg or 15mg/kg twice weekly) compared to placebo [131]. Of note is that anti-ibalizumab antibodies have been detected in some patients in a 9 week study [132] at week 3, however these later declined and became undetectable. Furthermore, there was no association between presence of anti-ibalizumab antibodies and adverse events. A case study by Fessel *et al.* [133] described a highly treatment-experienced HIV positive patient who initiated ibalizumab therapy consisting of monthly infusions, resulting in a rapid decline in VL of approximately 4.0 log_{10}. Following an unintended administration of placebo at week 32, the patient experienced a rapid rise in VL and emergence of resistance to the background regimen (etravirine and enfuvirtide). After re-instatement of ibalizumab at week 36, VL declined again to approximately 2.0 log_{10} below pre-ibalizumab levels.

Attachment Inhibitor

A novel small molecule inhibitor of gp120 attachment to CD4, *BMS-626529*, has displayed antiviral efficacy *in vitro* with EC_{50} values in the range of <10 nM against most laboratory strains tested as well as subtype A, B and C clinical isolates [134]. Although the mechanism of action is not fully elucidated, studies of a similar compound (*BMS-488043*) suggest induction of conformational changes within gp120 which prevent binding to CD4 [135].

An 8-day monotherapy study of *BMS-663068* (pro-drug of BMS-626529) in HIV-1 infected individuals resulted in VL reductions of 1.6-1.8 $\log_{10}$ copies/ml with ritonavir-boosting, and a decrease of 1.2 $\log_{10}$ copies/ml for unboosted BMS-663068 [136]. However, in BMS-626529 naïve HIV-1 patients gp120 mutations have been detected [137] which correspond to those emerged after *in vitro* drug selection pressure assays with BMS-626529 [138]. For one substitution (M434I), prevalence was as high as 15.2 % for CRF02_AG. This indicates limited usefulness of BMS-663068/BMS-626529 treatment in patients infected with certain strains, although the relevance of these mutations *in vivo* warrants further investigation.

Pharmacoenhancers ("Boosters")

The cytochrome P450 (CYP450)-inhibiting properties of ritonavir were initially considered a limitation of its use due to a high risk of drug-drug interactions. Later however, it soon became clear that this HIV PI could be used in subantiviral doses to "boost" the bioavailability and half-lives of co-administered PIs or other ARVs [139]. Nevertheless, even in low doses ritonavir is associated with adverse events [140] and is temperature sensitive, rendering co-formulation with partner drugs difficult.

Cobicistat was designed to be a specific inhibitor of CYP3A4, as opposed to ritonavir which has a broad CYP450 specificity, and without intrinsic ARV activity. Additionally, cobicistat is not an inducer of pregnane X receptor (PXR) which is the case for ritonavir [141, 142] and several other ARVs of different subclasses [143]. Therefore the risk of drug-drug interactions and other off-target effects is greatly reduced [144]. Using midazolam as a CYP3A4 substrate,

Mathias *et al.* [144] demonstrated 95% reduced clearance by a single dose of 200mg cobicistat, equivalent of the effect by 100mg ritonavir (96% reduction). The most frequently reported adverse effects in patients receiving cobicistat monotherapy were headache, drowsiness, and abnormal dreams [144].

A phase II study [145] comparing the pharmacoenhancer effects of cobicistat *versus* ritonavir in a quadruple antiretroviral combination therapy, containing atazanavir and emtricitabine/tenofovir in a fixed combination, was carried out over 48 weeks. Both arms displayed similar degrees of viral suppression and immunologic recovery. The proportion of patients experiencing treatment-emergent adverse events found in at least five percent of patients on either treatment was higher in the ritonavir-arm (48%) compared to the cobicistat arm (36%). A different comparison was performed by Cohen *et al.* [146] where a once-daily formulation of elvitegravir/cobicistat/lamivudine/tenofovir (the "Quad" pill) was found to achieve a high VL suppression and resulted in fewer CNS and psychiatric adverse effects compared to efavirenz/lamivudine/tenofovir, the most commonly used antiretroviral combination in clinical practice today.

Novel Drug Targets

Capsid Assembly Inhibitors

A number of new compounds have been described which target the viral capsid protein (CA), a component of the Gag precursor protein and a previously unexploited antiretroviral drug target. The first one, *CAP-1*, was characterized by Tang *et al.* [147]: 95% inhibition of viral infectivity was demonstrated using 100 μM in latently infected U1 cells, while cell viability and virus production measured by p24 protein remained unaffected. Electron microscopy analysis of the produced viral particles revealed a greater degree of size heterogeneity compared to untreated cells, as well as aberrant core morphologies. Other studies have highlighted the importance of core structure and stability for functional viral replication [148, 149].

CAI (capsid assembly inhibitor) was identified through phage display screening of peptides with high affinity and specificity for CA [150]. Inhibition of assembly by CAI was confirmed *in vitro*. By using X-ray crystallography to identify the critical amino acid residues for CA-CAI interaction, Zhang *et al.* [151] re-designed the peptide structure to a more stable α-helical structure to achieve improved cell penetrating abilities while retaining CA inhibition. This new peptide, denominated *NYAD-1*, was able to completely block both immature and mature virus assembly in cell-free and cell-based systems. Similarly to results obtained for CAI, electron microscopy analysis of Gag- or Gag/Pol-expressing cells treated with NYAD-1 showed altered particle morphology compared to untreated controls. NYAD-1 also displayed broad *in vitro* antiviral activity against both laboratory strains and primary isolates, with IC_{50} values in the range of approximately 4-22 μM. However, the peptidic nature of CAI and NYAD-1 limits the types of possible delivery modes and may restrict their use as ARV agents.

A new type of small molecule capsid assembly inhibitor has been described by Blair *et al.* [152], with a distinct binding site from CAP-I, CAI and NYAD-1. Two selected compounds of this class displayed antiviral activity against both laboratory strains and clinical isolates with EC_{50} values in the micromolar range. One of them, *PF-3759857*, was also active against HIV-2 (EC_{50}= 4.7 μM). Elucidation of the mechanism of action pointed towards effects on both viral coat uncoating (early stage) and viral coat assembly (late stage), by disrupting CA-CA interactions. Further progress on this promising new drug target is awaited.

Multiple Targets

Betulinic acid, naturally occurring in the bark of several plant species, has exhibited antioxidant, antibacterial, anti-inflammatory, antimalarial, anti-helmintic and anti-HIV properties [153, 154]. However, the mode of action as an ARV is not entirely clear. Zhao *et al.* [155] presented results from an *in vitro* study of ionic betulinic acid derivatives as potential inhibitors of the HIV protease: in particular a cholinium salt of betulinic acid showed equivalent inhibitory capacity to pepstatin A, combined with high water solubility (in contrast to unmodified betulinic acid which has low solubility in aqueous solutions). Apart from inhibition of HIV-1 protease activity, other mechanisms behind the antiviral activity of betulinic acid have been suggested: inhibition of HIV-1 replication and maturation, inhibition of virus-cell membrane fusion as well as inhibition of HIV-1 reverse transcription [156, 157]. *Bevirimat* ([3-O-

(3',3'-dimethylsuccinyl) betulinic acid]) has been demonstrated to specifically block cleavage of the Gag capsid precursor into mature protein [158]. Single oral doses were well tolerated and reduced viral load in ART-naïve HIV-1 infected patients [159].

Betulin and betulinic acid have also been used in a pilot study as hepatitis C virus (HCV) therapy with significant reductions in HCV viral load and alanine aminotransferase (ALT) levels. Furthermore, a decrease in subjective symptoms such as fatigue, abdominal discomfort and depression was noted [160]. The results from this small and uncontrolled study will however need further evaluation.

Role of Newly Developed Drugs in ART

Potential Use in Treatment-Naïve Patients

Many of the antiretroviral drugs in development at the moment are predominantly intended for use in heavily treatment-experienced patients with limited options. However, somc of the newer drugs are at least initially reserved for treatment-naïve HIV-infected individuals: the recently approved NNRTI rilpivirine has been associated with fewer side-effects than efavirenz [70], rilpivirine therapy resulted in higher prevalence of resistance mutations at failure [71]. The new version of the "Quad" pill incorporating two novel drugs; cobicistat and GS-7340, in addition to already approved darunavir and emtricitabine, will be evaluated in HIV patients who have not received prior treatment.

Potential Use in Treatment-Experienced Patients

Patients with extensive drug resistance require either novel drug targets or novel compounds within existing drug classes with documented efficacy against resistant strains. By virtue of the activity of apricitabine in the presence of TAMs [47], this novel NRTI currently in phase III trials will initially be licensed for use in patients with limited therapeutic options [161] – potentially to replace lamivudine or emtricitabine. Co-administration with one of these NRTIs is however not recommended as they compete for phosphorylation by the same kinase [48]. Lersivirine may prove an interesting option for patients with NNRTI resistance; however the high prevalence of patients experiencing nausea in a phase IIb study [162] is of concern. Although only currently tested in ART-naïve subjects, second generation NNRTI RDAE806 has the potential for use in treatment-experienced patients owing to a high barrier to resistance [163].

Elvitegravir showed efficacy when added to an active PI/r-based background therapy in treatment-experienced patients with confirmed resistance to two drug classes or equivalent [93]. It could improve therapy outcome in this patient group, provided there is no resistance to raltegravir present. Dolutegravir and S/GSK1265744, on the other hand, have different resistance profiles to raltegravir and retains activity against raltegravir-resistant strains *in vivo* [97] or *in vitro* [105].

As monoclonal antibodies such as PRO 140, PRO 542 and ibalizumab as well as new fusion inhibitor sifuvirtide require intravenous administration, these are more likely to be used in heavily treatment-experienced patients.

Use in Resource-Limited Settings

As previously discussed, many resource-limited settings have a restricted access to antiretroviral drugs and a growing population of treatment-experienced patients, potentially with extensive nucleoside resistance [164]. For this reason, it is important to identify new antiretroviral agents which may be suitable for this setting. A randomized controlled trial investigating the addition of raltegravir to optimized background therapy demonstrated successful viral suppression, even in patients with a phenotypic sensitivity score of 0 (effectively on raltegravir monotherapy) [87]. It is possible that newer integrase inhibitors elvitegravir and dolutegravir could be even more suitable in developing countries. In July 2011, Gilead granted rights to other pharmaceutical partners to manufacture generic versions of elvitegravir, cobicistat and also the "Quad" pill incorporating these two drugs plus tenofovir/emtricitabine [165]. This should ensure lower drug costs while maintaining high quality. However, dolutegravir may retain efficacy longer due to a higher resistance barrier [99], and additionally it does not require pharmacokinetic boosting [101].

Considering the low manufacturing cost and dose of rilpivirine combined with a long half-life, this new NNRTI offers great potential treatment of HIV-infected patients in resource-limited settings [166]. Furthermore, no evidence of teratogenicity has been found with rilpivirine, which could make it an alternative for women of childbearing potential [167]. A drawback is evidence of drug interaction potential with CYP3A4 inducers rifampicin and rifabutin, the two most commonly used drugs for treatment of tuberculosis. Co-administration studies resulted in a reduction in rilpivirine c_{max} of 69% by rifampicin [168] and of 35% by rifabutin [169].

A large part of the HIV-infected population in the developing world consists of women of child-bearing age. For women who are pregnant or attempting to conceive, ART options are limited, as efavirenz is not recommended due to evidence of fetal central nervous system abnormalities in monkeys [170]. Lersivirine on the other hand bears promise of potential use in pregnant women, as a lack of teratogenicity has been demonstrated in mice [171] and rabbits [172]. However, it may not be possible to extrapolate these results to humans and further studies are needed.

Alternative Modes of Delivery

Non-adherence is a major cause of viral rebound and drug resistance development. Therefore, long-acting ARV formulations enabling dosing with long intervals could potentially prevent treatment failure due to missed doses. An injectable nanosuspension of rilpivirine has been evaluated in healthy volunteers as a non-oral alternative where a 600mg monthly intramuscular injection achieved comparable to once-daily 25mg dosing [166, 173]. However, suitable co-administered ARVs would have to be identified in order for the patient to benefit from the long-interval administration. A strong candidate is novel integrase inhibitor S/GSK1265744 [106]. A study investigating viral suppression maintenance by S/GSK1265744/rilpivirine in treatment-naïve individuals is currently recruiting participants.

Another strategy for improving adherence is single-pill combinations, in order to simplify therapy by allowing one-pill-once-a-day dosing. Currently, three multi-class pills have been approved by the FDA, combining efavirenz/emtricitabine/tenofovir, rilpivirine/emtricitabine/tenofovir and most recently elvitegravir/cobicistat/tenofovir/emtricitabine. A potential disadvantage of fixed-dose combinations is the lack of flexibility in terms of drugs and dosage.

Since the majority of new HIV infections in sub-Saharan Africa are contracted through heterosexual intercourse [174], prophylactic microbicides represents an approach of potentially high importance for preventing transmission. Three new NNRTIs; *dapivirine* (TMC120), *UC781*, and *MIV-160*, are currently being developed as microbicides for women at risk of contracting HIV. Drug resistance selection *in vitro* by serial passages under conditions of increasing drug concentrations yielded a high degree of cross-resistance to efavirenz, nevirapine and delavirdine, although some susceptibility to etravirine and lersivirine was retained. This raises concern of cross-resistance development when using single NNRTI-based microbicides, especially since individuals in the target group may in fact have an undiagnosed HIV infection [175]. Entry inhibitor sifuvirtide, with previously demonstrated efficacy against enfuvirtide-resistant strains [120], has also been evaluated as a microbicide gel formulation. Potent antiviral activity was demonstrated *in vitro* against subtype B, C, CRF07_BC, CRF01_AE, as well as absence of cytokine induction after intravaginal administration in mice [176]. However, a thorough safety assessment will be necessary before progressing to human trials.

PART III: DISCUSSION AND FUTURE PERSPECTIVES

Part III contains the conclusions pertaining to the preceding discussion, and examines potential for the development of even newer drugs in terms of targets, efficacy, toxicity and acceptability.

The two facets that will be explored are the potential for the correction of deficits in current treatment and potential new drugs, based on possible mechanisms of action from a molecular perspective.

Categorization of ARV Drugs in the Pipeline

As has been shown, much of current research is based on the refinement of existing ARV drug classes and side effects, as well as improving drug resistance profiles. There is some research exploring new drug targets, although relatively limited.

The advances shown in the previous discussion can be broadly categorized as shown in Fig. **7**. Each of these categories will be explored separately, before finally discussing which components should be prioritized in the future.

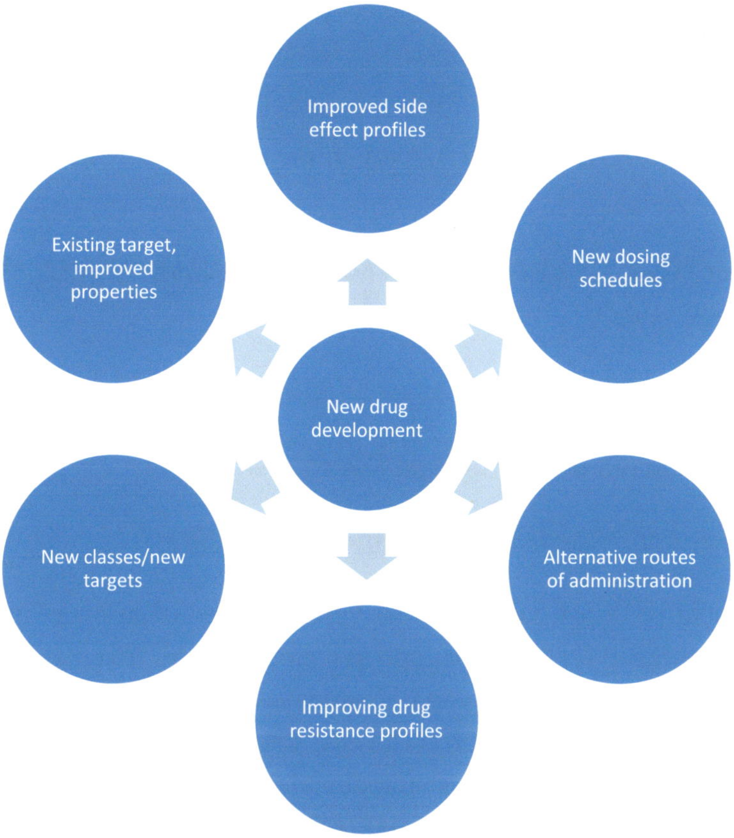

Figure 7: Themes of current antiretroviral drug development.

Improved Side Effect Profiles

Rilpivirine (NNRTI): Fewer CNS Side Effects

Side effects of certain drugs or drug classes are major contributors to non-adherence to ARV medication, and therefore resistance development. Furthermore, for patients who manage to adhere even in the face of adverse effects, this may contribute to a decrease in quality of life and cause significant co-morbidity. The formulation of an NNRTI with fewer CNS side effects is particularly useful for patients, as this type of toxicity is quoted as one of the most common reasons for patients to discontinue of switch from an efavirenz containing regimen [177, 178]. More importantly, rilpivirine is now available in a co-formulation alongside emtricitabine and tenofovir, and so can be used as a once-daily preparation.

Improving Drug Resistance Profiles

Amdoxovir (NRTI): does not induce TAMs

Apricitabine (NRTI): retained activity in the presence of NRTI resistant virus

Rilpivirine (NNRTI): higher genetic barrier than other NNRTIs (but not at high viral loads?)

Lersivirine (NNRTI): activity against K103N

MK-4965 (NNRTI): activity against K103N and Y181C

Elvitegravir (integrase inhibitor): active against Y143

The development of drugs with new resistance profiles is an ongoing endeavour of utmost importance to provide options for heavily treatment-experienced patients. In order to produce new ARV drugs which are active against mutant viral strains with resistance to current drugs, one or both of the following two criteria needs to be fulfilled: the new compounds need to either induce a different mutation pattern than established drugs of the same class, owing to novel structures and different interaction patterns with viral proteins. Examples of this are amdoxovir and abacavir which do not induce TAMs. The other alternative is a high genetic barrier, meaning that several accumulated mutations are required to achieve resistance. Preferably, these mutations should represent a high fitness cost. Rilpivirine has displayed a higher genetic barrier than current NNRTIs, however this may not be true at very high viral loads.

Increasingly, with changes in preparations and less toxic drugs, adherence is becoming easier for many patients. However, special groups to consider at risk of non-adherence and mutations are those with chaotic life structure, and mobile populations [179, 180]. Those with a chaotic life, whether due to employment type, drug use, or other clinical diagnoses, are at much higher risk of not adhering to their regime. This can be addressed and supported somewhat in the clinic, but is not always successful. For this group of people, it is important to constantly address the question of what to do in the presence of mutations and multi-class resistance - if technology and strategies remain static, then at some point this population will suffer. Mobile populations present a similar challenge. Many populations in developed and developing countries are mobile due to housing and food insecurity and adherence to ARVs becomes a severe challenge for this population [180, 181]. This problem is magnified by globally displaced populations, for whom problems of entitlement and citizenship may compound the ability to access ARVs. A lack of access to a secure supply of HAART might lead to subtherapeutic drug levels and resistance development. For this group, ongoing work in seeking to facilitate access to treatment in order to overcome resistance mutations emerging is imperative.

Existing Drug Targets - Improved Properties

BMS-986001 (NRTI): potentially reduced mitochondrial toxicity

GS-7340 (NRTI): tenofovir pro-drug

Sifuvirtide (fusion inhibitor): improved binding

As the vast majority of ART medications are oral, improved bioavailability and distribution is an important, although slightly neglected area of research. The GS-7340 compound, which is a pro-drug of tenofovir, displays two characteristics which make it attractive: it shows a preferential distribution to lymphoid tissues and PBMCs - targeting the sites of highest proliferation and infection of HIV. In addition, GS-7340 achieves higher plasma levels than tenofovir at lower doses, which has biological plausibility for decreasing the risk of tenofovir associated side effects, although this has not yet been tested or confirmed. Sifuvirtide shows improved binding at its target fusion site compared to enfuvirtide, and correspondingly improved antiviral activity *in vitro*. Results from phase II clinical trials will show whether this makes sifuvirtide more effective in patients. Although the structure of BMS-986001 resembles that of stavudine, *in vitro* results indicate weaker inhibition of mitochondrial DNA polymerase, presumably translating into a reduced risk of mitochondrial toxicity (associated with stavudine use) in patients.

New Dosing Schedules

Elvucitabine (NRTI): long half-life

Rilpivirine (NNRTI): co-formulated with backbone

Elvitegravir (integrase inhibitor): once daily administration with ritonavir boosting

Dolutegravir (integrase inhibitor): once daily administration

PRO 140 (monoclonal antibody): weekly/biweekly infusions

S/GSK1265744 (integrase inhibitor): once-monthly intramuscular/subcutaneous injections

A key part of designing an ARV regime is the timing and frequency of dose, as well as the number of tablets to be taken. It is well recognized that adherence can be affected negatively if the regime and schedule are not compatible with the patient's lifestyle. Ongoing work in this area is aimed a reducing the number of doses and tablets to be taken each day. Until recently, the formulation of Atripla (tenofovir + emtricitabine + efavirenz) in one tablet, once daily preparation was the pinnacle achievement in dosing. However, more recently a new preparation named Eviplera (tenofovir + emtricitabine + rilpivirine, Complera in the US) has become available, and the "Quad" pill is in development (tenofovir + emtricitabine + elvitegravir + cobicistat). Other drugs with twice daily administration, such as integrase inhibitors, are having the boundaries pushed in term of drugs which can be administered once daily. Yet more excitingly, drugs are being developed which can be given twice or once weekly, or even once monthly. A major drawback at the moment is that some are delivered intravenously, which will have an obvious impact on the patient's life and different demands on the healthcare services. Delivery through intramuscular or subcutaneous injections may offer new opportunities for increased dosing intervals.

Alternative Routes of Administration

S/GSK1265744 (integrase inhibitor): nano-suspension (intramuscular/ subcutaneous injection)

PRO 140 (monoclonal antibody): intravenous infusion

PRO 542 (monoclonal antibody): intravenous infusion

Ibalizumab (monoclonal antibody): intravenous infusion

Currently, only zidovudine is available in an intravenous format, and enfuvirtide is available for subcutaneous injection. This is extremely limiting for patient care settings such as the intensive care unit where it may not be appropriate to administer drugs *via* the oral route. The development of further intravenous agents presents novel options for managing such patients. Another new and promising avenue in HIV care is represented by long-acting ARVs delivered by other non-oral routes with potential for once-monthly dosing, such as S/GSK1265744.

New Classes/New Targets

LEDGINs (integrase inhibitors): new binding target

AMD11070 (co-receptor inhibitor): CXCR4 inhibition

PRO 140 (monoclonal antibody): anti-CCR5 antibody

PRO 542 (monoclonal antibody): CD4-fusion immunoglobulin, targets gp120

Ibalizumab (monoclonal antibody): anti-CD4 antibody

BMS-626529 (attachment inhibitor): probable induction of gp120 changes

Cobicistat (pharmacoenhancer): CYP3A4 inhibitor

CAP-1 (capsid assembly inhibitor): target capsid assembly protein

NYAD-1 (capsid assembly inhibitor): target capsid assembly protein

PF- 3759857 (capsid assembly inhibitor): target capsid assembly and uncoating

Bevirimat (maturation inhibitor): blocks cleavage of Gag capsid precursor

New classes and targets represent the bulk of drugs in development at the moment. The LEDGINs are an interesting new type of integrase inhibitors - they bind at a different site to current drugs of the same class, and therefore may well be of value in the future for those who fail integrase inhibitor therapy with existing drugs. The development of drugs which target the CXCR4 co-receptor may also play an important role, especially in conjunction with CCR5 inhibitors. It is plausible that CXCR4 and CCR5 inhibitors could work synergistically. Although indicated *in vitro* [182], this has not been tested in patients.

Monoclonal antibody development shows a lot of promise for treatment, but the intravenous mode of delivery comes with restrictions. Of course, they remain of great use in salvage therapy and for those who cannot take medications orally- however otherwise they are limited. Their route of administration makes it very unlikely they will ever become first line drugs, however it might be envisaged that if a preparation that can be made with an extremely long half-life which lends itself to once a month, or even less frequent dosing, it could be a more attractive drug for first line ART.

Entirely novel targets which have been covered are those of capsid assembly inhibitors, and a single combined protease and maturation inhibitor, bevirimat. These new targets are opening up entirely new avenues of potential for development. These two new classes represent previously untargeted parts of the HIV life cycle, and may therefore change the way HAART regimes are constructed. At this point however, capsid assembly inhibitors are not yet evaluated in patients and clinical trials are necessary to assess safety, efficacy and potential toxicity. Although single dose studies of bevirimat have demonstrated tolerability and antiviral effect in HIV patients [159], further pharmacokinetic evaluation is warranted.

All in all, the exploration of novel targets presents us with a potential therapeutic leap. And as our understanding of HIV at the cellular level increases, it may become possible to rationalise exactly which stage of the life cycle should be targeted in a given patient with a particular strain of HIV.

Where Next?

Using the six themes we have used to explore the drugs that are currently in development, we can comment on where future focuses of HIV drug discovery might lie (Fig. **8**).

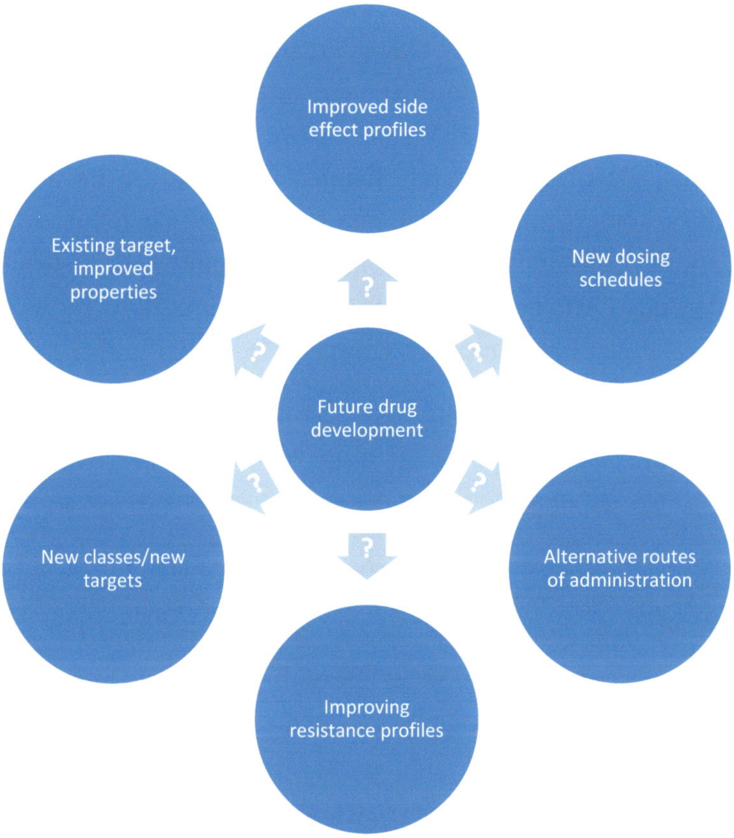

Figure 8: Future potential directions in antiretroviral drug development.

Improved Side Effect Profiles

The management of side effects of medications is a burgeoning issue within HAART. Effective HAART means that a 20 year old asymptomatic HIV+ patient can expect to live until they are 66 [183] - this brings with it a plethora of potential problems in managing cardiovascular, CNS, bone and renal disease, as well as the issue of glucose intolerance which is under scrutiny at the moment [184]. Previously, the prospect of ageing with HIV was low enough not to have to consider these diseases which normally accumulate with age, or occur due to senescence. Now, when the reverse is true, system-specific impact of drugs is one of the prime factors for considering the constitution of a HAART regime.

The ongoing search for drugs with fewer and more tolerable side effects is an important driver of new advances in ARVs. Ideal drugs would achieve excellent viral suppression with minimal early side effects and preferably no middle to long term effects. Drugs such as efavirenz have excellent evidence for powerful, durable suppression of HIV [64, 185-187]. However, the CNS side effects, such as strange dreams, sleeplessness, and changes in mood are mostly short lived [188], however in some groups of patients can last much longer and be much more severe [16]. Tenofovir is an excellent NRTI, again with a strong record of durability [189] - however, its use may be limited in the future as we understand more about the renal and bone side effects associated with tenofovir [190-192].

Therefore, pharmacotherapy in the future might use two complementary strategies. Hopefully, there will be ongoing development of drugs with less toxicity, such as the motivation that lead to the discovery of rilpivirine as an alternative to efavirenz. The second route, although not strictly drug discovery, is of reliable predictive markers of toxicity. Similar to the undisputed association between HLA-B*5701 polymorphism and abacavir hypersensitivity, it might be that leading the edge in tailor made medicine will look at other genetic markers to determine if individuals will be tolerant of bone or renal effects of tenofovir, for instance.

Improving Resistance Profiles

Research focusing on the development of drugs within an existing class with improved, higher genetic barriers to resistance is an integral component of HIV drug discovery. As discussed previously, although adherence to HAART might be changing with new formulations, and access to HAART might be widening, there will always be subgroups of patients who will need drugs active against a range of viral strains with various degrees of drug resistance. The biggest challenge is to find drugs in any class which do not become inactive through a single mutation in the virus, therefore making them more robust to any changes in drug taking.

Ideally, mutations induced by the drug should be detrimental to the virus itself. Probably the best known example of this is the mutation induced by lamivudine and emtricitabine (M184V). This particular mutation confers resistance to these NRTIs. However, a virus harbouring this mutation is also less able to reproduce, producing a 'less fit' virus. Drugs of this type are particularly useful in salvage regimes. Hence, the impact by the mutations induced on viral fitness is as important as the number of mutations required for drug resistance, both contributing to the genetic barrier.

Existing Drug Targets - Improved Properties

Work continues through using rationalization techniques to produce drugs which work more effectively at lower doses. For example, the tenofovir pro-drug GS-7340, is not only required in a lower dose so may avoid toxicities that are tenofovir dose-related, but also accumulates in target lymphoid tissues and PBMCs more effectively than tenofovir does. So, even though essentially this might be considered the same drug, careful attention to design and delivery have enabled the development of this new preparation. Similarly, sifuvirtide has been seen on an *in vitro* basis to bind more effectively to its target than enfuvirtide. Preparations can, and should undergo regular revisiting as knowledge and technology are advanced, as the form and frequency of delivery can often have a profound effect on a patient's life. For instance, if a drug must always be consumed at least two hours after a meal because of the interaction with food and or gastric acid, then the patient must adhere to eating at very specific times every day for the duration of that drug. Rational design and the addition of extra features, such as improvements from an instant release preparation to a extended release preparation (nevirapine [193]) can have excellent quality of life impacts on individual people by reducing regimes from two or three times daily to once daily. In addition, changes to the molecular structure of certain preparations may enable them to be more stable and less dependent on people's eating habits.

Naturally following this, it is the aim to design molecules with the ability to enter all body compartments. Although blood plasma levels may become adequate, penetration into sites such as the CNS and the genital tract may occur to a much lesser degree. The development of universally penetrating drugs is an important aim for future research. There is a relatively high prevalence of neurocognitive impairment in those infected with HIV [194], and as that population ages, it will be important to minimize any suspicion of ongoing HIV replication within the CNS. Although there are drugs with a certain degree of CNS penetration at present, ongoing work in this area is needed in order to increase understanding of the mechanism of neurocognitive impairment due to HIV.

New Dosing Schedules

Dosing schedules are intensely important to individuals undergoing anti-HIV treatment. They are required to adhere strictly to regimes to prevent the chance of emergent mutations and ensure full virological control. There is therefore an obvious difference between asking patients to take their medication three times a day, as compared to once a day. Most recently, Atripla and Eviplera/Complera triple drug fixed dose combinations (FDCs) have been approved, with the promise of the Quad pill on the horizon. FDCs offer the fantastic opportunity for patients to schedule their drug taking to once a day, thereby increase compatibility with their respective lifestyles. However, FDCs have three obvious disadvantages. The first disadvantage is that doses cannot be adjusted as the preparations are fixed; it might be necessary to switch to the individual components if there is a need to dose adjust, such as in renal failure. The second disadvantage is that if the single pill is forgotten, then the patient has no exposure to anti-HIV drugs at all. This will have varying consequences depending on the individual pharmacokinetics of the constituent drugs. The final disadvantage, which may change in the next few years, is that of cost. The new formulations are all under patents and therefore prices are set by the pharmaceutical companies, whereas constituent drug costs may well be less, especially on expanded access programmes. Certainly, for the time being, FDCs are less accessible to resource limited settings. However, there may be a chance to achieve even more intelligent dosing schedules. If drugs with a very long half-life were developed, it might be feasible to change to once weekly or even once monthly schedules. This is only really feasible if the drug can be delivered in a slow release preparation, which seems unlikely with an orally administered drug. However, there are examples of long acting drugs such as depot medroxy progesterone (Depo provera), a progestogenic hormone administered intramuscularly every three months as a contraceptive. It may not yet be feasible, but it can be visualized that such an injection could enable excellent adherence and decrease the chance of virological failure in a patient undergoing HAART, as well as reduce their daily pill burden. Developments in drug delivery and schedules should continue exploring the possibility of "less than once daily" medications.

Alternative Routes of Administration

As mentioned above, it is conceivable that long lasting drugs would be very useful to patients. We have considered intramuscular (IM) administration above, while main route at the moment is oral dosing. However, enfuvirtide exists as a subcutaneous preparation, zidovudine is available as both oral and intravenous (IV) and as discussed above there are a few different intravenous monoclonal antibodies undergoing clinical trials. However, intravenous drugs are only useful to patients in one of three settings. The first setting is when the patient cannot take medications orally and there is an obvious need for parenteral therapy. The second circumstance is the need for a rapid rise in plasma drug levels - a situation mostly seen during labour, when women can be given zidovudine intravenously to induce rapidly high levels of the drug IV. The final scenario where IV drugs are useful is when they enable less than daily dosing. It can be easily envisaged that some patients might find a once monthly infusion more acceptable than oral medications every day.

Another method for drug delivery, again used in hormone therapy, is by coating an inert substance which is then implanted subcutaneously (for example etonogestrel implant contraceptives). The drug is released so slowly that the implant lasts for months to years. Although not currently available, the formulation of ARV drugs which could be coated and then implanted would be a massive advance in HAART. These would improve ease of use, ensure a steady supply of reliable HAART for those in less stable home or national circumstances, and would maximize patient convenience in terms of obtaining further supplies of HAART.

New Classes/New Targets

As described above, there has been some research within the area of ARV drug discovery focusing on the identification of new targets and new classes. Most notably, monoclonal antibody technology has enabled a range of novel drugs to be developed with new modes of action. In relation to the life cycle of HIV, CXCR4 inhibitors are being developed to act at the fusion step and inhibit virus-cell binding at the beginning of the life cycle, while bevirimat is under investigation for its ability to block maturation and protease activity at the later stages. The development of a maturation inhibitor was an obvious strategy, as there are currently no drugs in clinical use which act at this stage. However, in addition to this rational new target, LEDGINs are being investigated for their usefulness in ART. Although essentially integrase inhibitors, LEDGINs target a new site previously unexploited in the strand transfer pathway, and therefore may not be subject to failure from the same mutations that affect other integrase inhibitors.

Future developments will be based on rational drug design. Better understanding of the exact processes underlying the HIV life cycle will facilitate the identification of target-specific compounds. An ideal new class would be an entry inhibitor which does not rely on a single receptor blockade, which can therefore prevent entry to any CD4+ cell, in addition to a maturation inhibitor that prevents production of new virions.

CONCLUSION

This chapter has explored the life cycle of HIV, mechanisms of action of established ARV drugs, recent development in the pipeline and possibilities for the future. Whilst we have focused on the pure science of HIV drug development, we must always bear in mind that inequality of access to drugs remains an important issue. This is not just a developed world *versus* developing world issue - people with chaotic lifestyles and substance addictions may also be unable to access treatment in resource-rich settings. Individuals with certain mental illness may not be able to access, or adhere, to treatment. Certainly those in economically and/or politically unstable regions may not be able to adhere due to lack of supply of the medicine, or inability to reach the contact point where medicines can be obtained. The most worthy advance in HIV treatment will be equality of secured access to ARVs for all.

In the meantime, as scientists it is important to push the barriers for greater advances: fewer pills, reduced risk of toxicity and dosing at longer intervals, to give better virological and immunological control. In this chapter we have seen that all of these objectives may well be possible, although not necessarily within the same drug, and not necessarily within the next few years. However, it is of paramount importance even with improvements being made within the field of ARV agents, to persevere in the endeavor to continue the development of newer drugs in the face of adverse events and drug resistance development. HIV patients are now ageing to a point that no-one thought possible 20 years ago. We must rise to the challenge of the changing needs of this population which cannot yet be predicted, by constantly increasing our understanding and challenging the usefulness of the drugs at our disposal, and in order to provide ourselves with an armory of different options for future use.

ACKNOWLEDGEMENTS

Declared none.

CONFLICTS OF INTEREST

Dr. Jenny Svärd: None to declare.

DISCLOSURE

Dr. Matthew Phillips: Has received lecturing fees and sponsorship from ViiV healthcare, Janssen Cilag, Gilead and Abbott. No sponsorship has been worth more than $1000 US.

REFERENCES

[1] Pattman R, Snow M, Handy P, Sankar KN, Elawad B, Eds. Oxford Handbook of Genitourinary Medicine, HIV and AIDS (Oxford Handbooks Series) Oxford: Oxford University Press 2005.

[2] Samson M, Libert F, Doranz BJ, *et al.* Resistance to HIV-1 infection in caucasian individuals bearing mutant alleles of the CCR-5 chemokine receptor gene. Nature 1996; 382(6593): 722-5.

[3] Briz V, Poveda E, Soriano V. HIV entry inhibitors: mechanisms of action and resistance pathways. J Antimicrob Chemother 2006; 57(4): 619-27.

[4] Archer J, Braverman MS, Taillon BE, *et al.* Detection of low-frequency pretherapy chemokine (CXC motif) receptor 4 (CXCR4)-using HIV-1 with ultra-deep pyrosequencing. AIDS 2009; 23(10): 1209-18.

[5] Westby M, Lewis M, Whitcomb J, *et al.* Emergence of CXCR4-using human immunodeficiency virus type 1 (HIV-1) variants in a minority of HIV-1-infected patients following treatment with the CCR5 antagonist maraviroc is from a pretreatment CXCR4-using virus reservoir. J Virol 2006; 80(10): 4909-20.

[6] Michailidis E, Marchand B, Kodama EN, *et al.* Mechanism of inhibition of HIV-1 reverse transcriptase by 4'-Ethynyl-2-fluoro-2'-deoxyadenosine triphosphate, a translocation-defective reverse transcriptase inhibitor. J Biol Chem 2009; 284(51): 35681-91.

[7] Sluis-Cremer N, Tachedjian G. Mechanisms of inhibition of HIV replication by non-nucleoside reverse transcriptase inhibitors. Virus Res 2008; 134(1-2): 147-56.

[8] Pommier Y, Johnson AA, Marchand C. Integrase inhibitors to treat HIV/AIDS. Nat Rev Drug Discov 2005; 4(3): 236-48.

[9] Temesgen Z, Siraj DS. Raltegravir: first in class HIV integrase inhibitor. Ther Clin Risk Manag 2008; 4(2): 493-500.

[10] Monini P, Sgadari C, Barillari G, Ensoli B. HIV protease inhibitors: antiretroviral agents with anti-inflammatory, anti-angiogenic and anti-tumour activity. J Antimicrob Chemother 2003; 51(2): 207-11.

[11] Jordan R, Gold L, Cummins C, Hyde C. Systematic review and meta-analysis of evidence for increasing numbers of drugs in antiretroviral combination therapy. BMJ 2002; 324(7340): 757.

[12] Fischl MA, Richman DD, Grieco MH, *et al.* The efficacy of azidothymidine (AZT) in the treatment of patients with AIDS and AIDS-related complex. A double-blind, placebo-controlled trial. N Engl J Med 1987; 317(4): 185-91.

[13] British HIV Association: Guidelines for the treatment of HIV-1 positive adults with antiretroviral therapy 2012. Accessed: 24 June 2012. Available from: http://www.bhiva.org/TreatmentofHIV1_2012.aspx.

[14] Chubineh S, McGowan J. Nausea and vomiting in HIV: a symptom review. Int J STD AIDS 2008; 19(11): 723-8.

[15] Lochet P, Peyriere H, Lotthe A, *et al.* Long-term assessment of neuropsychiatric adverse reactions associated with efavirenz. HIV Med 2003; 4(1): 62-6.

[16] Gutierrez F, Navarro A, Padilla S, *et al.* Prediction of neuropsychiatric adverse events associated with long-term efavirenz therapy, using plasma drug level monitoring. Clin Infect Dis 2005; 41(11): 1648-53.

[17] Haas DW, Ribaudo HJ, Kim RB, *et al.* Pharmacogenetics of efavirenz and central nervous system side effects: an Adult AIDS Clinical Trials Group study. AIDS 2004 ; 18(18): 2391-400.

[18] Rotger M, Tegude H, Colombo S, *et al.* Predictive value of known and novel alleles of CYP2B6 for efavirenz plasma concentrations in HIV-infected individuals. Clin Pharmacol Ther 2007; 81(4): 557-66.

[19] Malvestutto CD, Aberg JA. Coronary heart disease in people infected with HIV. Cleve Clin J Med 2010; 77(8): 547-56.

[20] SoRelle R. Vascular and lipid syndromes in selected HIV-infected patients. Circulation 1998; 98(9): 829-30.

[21] Levy AR, McCandless L, Harrigan PR, *et al.* Changes in lipids over twelve months after initiating protease inhibitor therapy among persons treated for HIV/AIDS. Lipids Health Dis 2005; 4: 4.

[22] Carey D, Amin J, Boyd M, Petoumenos K, Emery S. Lipid profiles in HIV-infected adults receiving atazanavir and atazanavir/ritonavir: systematic review and meta-analysis of randomized controlled trials. J Antimicrob Chemother 2010; 65(9): 1878-88.

[23] Gyalrong-Steur M, Bogner JR, Seybold U. Changes in lipid profiles after switching to a protease inhibitor-containing cART--unfavourable effect of fosamprenavir in obese patients. Eur J Med Res 2011; 16(2): 85-92.

[24] Hill A, Sawyer W, Gazzard B. Effects of first-line use of nucleoside analogues, efavirenz, and ritonavir-boosted protease inhibitors on lipid levels. HIV Clin Trials 2009; 10(1): 1-12.

[25] Hughes DA, Vilar FJ, Ward CC, *et al.* Cost-effectiveness analysis of HLA B*5701 genotyping in preventing abacavir hypersensitivity. Pharmacogenetics 2004; 14(6): 335-42.

[26] Rauch A, Nolan D, Martin A, *et al.* Prospective genetic screening decreases the incidence of abacavir hypersensitivity reactions in the Western Australian HIV cohort study. Clin Infect Dis 2006; 43(1): 99-102.

[27] Boyer S, Marcellin F, Ongolo-Zogo P, *et al.* Financial barriers to HIV treatment in Yaounde, Cameroon: first results of a national cross-sectional survey. Bull World Health Organ 2009; 87(4): 279-87.

[28] Kunihira NR, Nuwaha F, Mayanja R, Peterson S. Barriers to use of antiretroviral drugs in Rakai district of Uganda. Afr Health Sci 2010; 10(2): 120-9.

[29] Boender TS, Sigaloff KC, Kayiwa J, *et al.* Barriers to Initiation of Pediatric HIV Treatment in Uganda: A Mixed-Method Study. AIDS Res Treat 2012; 2012: 817506.

[30] Duff P, Kipp W, Wild TC, Rubaale T, Okech-Ojony J. Barriers to accessing highly active antiretroviral therapy by HIV-positive women attending an antenatal clinic in a regional hospital in western Uganda. J Int AIDS Soc 2010; 13: 37.

[31] Fox MP, Mazimba A, Seidenberg P, *et al.* Barriers to initiation of antiretroviral treatment in rural and urban areas of Zambia: a cross-sectional study of cost, stigma, and perceptions about ART. J Int AIDS Soc 2010; 13: 8.

[32] Hirschhorn LR, Oguda L, Fullem A, Dreesch N, Wilson P. Estimating health workforce needs for antiretroviral therapy in resource-limited settings. Hum Resour Health 2006; 4: 1.

[33] Wood E, Montaner JS, Bangsberg DR, *et al.* Expanding access to HIV antiretroviral therapy among marginalized populations in the developed world. AIDS 2003; 17(17): 2419-27.

[34] Freeman M, Patel V, Collins PY, Bertolote J. Integrating mental health in global initiatives for HIV/AIDS. Br J Psychiatry 2005; 187: 1-3.

[35] Strathdee SA, Palepu A, Cornelisse PG, *et al.* Barriers to use of free antiretroviral therapy in injection drug users. JAMA 1998; 280(6): 547-9.

[36] Lewis W, Day BJ, Copeland WC. Mitochondrial toxicity of NRTI antiviral drugs: an integrated cellular perspective. Nat Rev Drug Discov 2003; 2(10): 812-22.

[37] Wainberg MA, Sawyer JP, Montaner JS, *et al.* Challenges for the clinical development of new nucleoside reverse transcriptase inhibitors for HIV infection. Antivir Ther 2005; 10(1): 13-28.

[38] Furman PA, Jeffrey J, Kiefer LL, *et al.* Mechanism of action of 1-beta-D-2,6-diaminopurine dioxolane, a prodrug of the human immunodeficiency virus type 1 inhibitor 1-beta-D-dioxolane guanosine. Antimicrob Agents Chemother 2001; 45(1): 158-65.

[39] Bazmi HZ, Hammond JL, Cavalcanti SC, *et al.* In vitro selection of mutations in the human immunodeficiency virus type 1 reverse transcriptase that decrease susceptibility to (-)-beta-D-dioxolane-guanosine and suppress resistance to 3'-azido-3'-deoxythymidine. Antimicrob Agents Chemother 2000; 44(7): 1783-8.

[40] Murphy RL, Kivel NM, Zala C, *et al.* Antiviral activity and tolerability of amdoxovir with zidovudine in a randomized double-blind placebo-controlled study in HIV-1-infected individuals. Antivir Ther 2010; 15(2): 185-92.

[41] Ghosh RK, Ghosh SM, Chawla S. Recent advances in antiretroviral drugs. Expert Opin Pharmacother 2011; 12(1): 31-46.

[42] Colucci P, Pottage JC, Robison H, Turgeon J, Ducharme MP. Effect of a single dose of ritonavir on the pharmacokinetic behavior of elvucitabine, a nucleoside reverse transcriptase inhibitor, administered in healthy volunteers. Antimicrob Agents Chemother 2009; 53(2): 646-50.

[43] Elvucitabine data released at CROI. AIDS Patient Care STDS 2010; 24(3): 198.

[44] Dutschman GE, Grill SP, Gullen EA, *et al.* Novel 4'-substituted stavudine analog with improved anti-human immunodeficiency virus activity and decreased cytotoxicity. Antimicrob Agents Chemother 2004; 48(5): 1640-6.

[45] Gu Z, Allard B, de Muys JM, *et al.* In vitro antiretroviral activity and in vitro toxicity profile of SPD754, a new deoxycytidine nucleoside reverse transcriptase inhibitor for treatment of human immunodeficiency virus infection. Antimicrob Agents Chemother 2006; 50(2): 625-31.

[46] Cahn P, Cassetti I, Wood R, *et al.* Efficacy and tolerability of 10-day monotherapy with apricitabine in antiretroviral-naive, HIV-infected patients. AIDS 2006; 20(9): 1261-8.

[47] Cahn P, Altclas J, Martins M, *et al.* Antiviral activity of apricitabine in treatment-experienced HIV-1-infected patients with M184V who are failing combination therapy. HIV Med 2011; 12(6): 334-42.

[48] Cahn P, Wainberg MA. Resistance profile of the new nucleoside reverse transcriptase inhibitor apricitabine. J Antimicrob Chemother 2010; 65(2): 213-7.

[49] Bethell R, De MJ, Lippens J, *et al.* In vitro interactions between apricitabine and other deoxycytidine analogues. Antimicrob Agents Chemother 2007; 51(8): 2948-53.

[50] Lee WA, He GX, Eisenberg E, *et al.* Selective intracellular activation of a novel prodrug of the human immunodeficiency virus reverse transcriptase inhibitor tenofovir leads to preferential distribution and accumulation in lymphatic tissue. Antimicrob Agents Chemother 2005; 49(5): 1898-906.

[51] Markowitz M, Zolopa A, Ruane P, *et al.* GS-7340 demonstrates greater declines in HIV-1 RNA than TDF during 14 days of monotherapy in HIV-1-infected subjects (Abstract 152LB). 18th Conference on Retroviruses and Opportunistic Infections; 2011 Feb 27-Mar 2; Boston, MA, USA.

[52] Ruane P, DeJesus E, Berger D, *et al.* GS-7340 25 mg and 40 mg Demonstrate Superior Efficacy to Tenofovir 300 mg in a 10-day Monotherapy Study of HIV-1+ Patients (Abstract 103). 19th Conference on Retroviruses and Opportunistic Infections; 2012 Mar 5-8; Seattle, WA, USA.

[53] Birkus G, Bam R, Frey C, *et al.* Intracellular Activation Pathways for GS-7340 and the Effect of Antiviral Protease Inhibitors (Abstract 577). 19th Conference on Retroviruses and Opportunistic Infections; 2012 Mar 5-8; Seattle, USA.

[54] Hwang C, Zhu L, Chan H, *et al.* Antiviral activity, exposure-response, and resistance analyses of monotherapy with the novel HIV NRTI BMS-986001 in ART-experienced subjects (Abstract O_06). 13th International Workshop on Clinical Pharmacology of HIV Therapy; 2012 Apr 16-18; Barcelona, Spain.

[55] Wang F, Flint O. The HIV NRTI BMS-986001 does not degrade mitochondrial DNA in long term primary cultures of cells isolated from human kidney, muscle and subcutaneous fat (Abstract TUPE042). XIX International AIDS Conference; 2012 Jul 22-27; Washington D.C., USA.

[56] Li Z, Terry B, Olds W, *et al.* The in vitro cross-resistance profile of the NRTI BMS-986001 against known NRTI resistance mutations (Abstract no. 2). International Workshop on HIV & Hepatitis Virus Drug Resistance; 2012 Jun 5-9; Sitges, Spain.

[57] Chersich MF, Urban MF, Venter FW, *et al.* Efavirenz use during pregnancy and for women of child-bearing potential. AIDS Res Ther 2006; 3: 11.

[58] van LM, Bannister WP, Mocroft A, *et al.* Absence of a relation between efavirenz plasma concentrations and toxicity-driven efavirenz discontinuations in the EuroSIDA study. AntivirTher 2009; 14(1): 75-83.

[59] Sabin CA, Fisher M, Churchill D, *et al.* Long-term follow-up of antiretroviral-naive HIV-positive patients treated with nevirapine. J Acquir Immune Defic Syndr 2001; 26(5): 462-5.

[60] Kuritzkes DR, Bassett RL, Johnson VA, *et al.* Continued lamivudine *versus* delavirdine in combination with indinavir and zidovudine or stavudine in lamivudine-experienced patients: results of Adult AIDS Clinical Trials Group protocol 370. AIDS 2000; 14(11): 1553-61.

[61] Girard PM, Campbell T, Grinsztejn B, *et al.* Pooled week 96 results of the phase III DUET-1 and DUET-2 trials of etravirine: further analysis of adverse events and laboratory abnormalities of special interest. HIV Med 2012.

[62] McKoy JM, Bennett CL, Scheetz MH, *et al.* Hepatotoxicity associated with long- *versus* short-course HIV-prophylactic nevirapine use: a systematic review and meta-analysis from the Research on Adverse Drug events And Reports (RADAR) project. Drug Saf 2009; 32(2): 147-58.

[63] Ghosn J, Chaix ML, Delaugerre C. HIV-1 resistance to first- and second-generation non-nucleoside reverse transcriptase inhibitors. AIDS Rev 2009; 11(3): 165-73.

[64] Staszewski S, Morales-Ramirez J, Tashima KT, *et al.* Efavirenz plus zidovudine and lamivudine, efavirenz plus indinavir, and indinavir plus zidovudine and lamivudine in the treatment of HIV-1 infection in adults. Study 006 Team. N Engl J Med 1999; 341(25): 1865-73.

[65] Plosker GL, Perry CM, Goa KL. Efavirenz: a pharmacoeconomic review of its use in HIV infection. Pharmacoeconomics 2001; 19(4): 421-36.

[66] Janssen PA, Lewi PJ, Arnold E, *et al.* In search of a novel anti-HIV drug: multidisciplinary coordination in the discovery of 4-[[4-[[4-[(1E)-2-cyanoethenyl]-2,6-dimethylphenyl]amino]-2-pyrimidinyl]amino]benzonitrile (R278474, rilpivirine). J Med Chem 2005; 48(6): 1901-9.

[67] Fernandez-Montero JV, Vispo E, Anta L, de MC, Soriano V. Rilpivirine: a next-generation non-nucleoside analogue for the treatment of HIV infection. ExpertOpinPharmacother 2012; 13(7): 1007-14.

[68] Pozniak AL, Morales-Ramirez J, Katabira E, *et al.* Efficacy and safety of TMC278 in antiretroviral-naive HIV-1 patients: week 96 results of a phase IIb randomized trial. AIDS 2010; 24(1): 55-65.

[69] Azijn H, Tirry I, Vingerhoets J, *et al.* TMC278, a next-generation nonnucleoside reverse transcriptase inhibitor (NNRTI), active against wild-type and NNRTI-resistant HIV-1. Antimicrob Agents Chemother 2010; 54(2): 718-27.

[70] Cohen CJ, Molina JM, Cahn P, *et al.* Efficacy and safety of rilpivirine (TMC278) *versus* efavirenz at 48 weeks in treatment-naive HIV-1-infected patients: pooled results from the phase 3 double-blind randomized ECHO and THRIVE Trials. J Acquir Immune Defic Syndr 2012; 60(1): 33-42.

[71] Rimsky L, Vingerhoets J, Van EV, *et al.* Genotypic and phenotypic characterization of HIV-1 isolates obtained from patients on rilpivirine therapy experiencing virologic failure in the phase 3 ECHO and THRIVE studies: 48-week analysis. J Acquir Immune Defic Syndr 2012; 59(1): 39-46.

[72] Fatkenheuer G, Staszewski S, Plettenburg A, *et al.* Activity, pharmacokinetics and safety of lersivirine (UK-453,061), a next-generation nonnucleoside reverse transcriptase inhibitor, during 7-day monotherapy in HIV-1-infected patients. AIDS 2009; 23(16): 2115-22.

[73] Corbau R, Mori J, Phillips C, *et al.* Lersivirine, a nonnucleoside reverse transcriptase inhibitor with activity against drug-resistant human immunodeficiency virus type 1. Antimicrob Agents Chemother 2010; 54(10): 4451-63.

[74] Romero DL, Morge RA, Biles C, *et al.* Discovery, synthesis, and bioactivity of bis(heteroaryl)piperazines. 1. A novel class of non-nucleoside HIV-1 reverse transcriptase inhibitors. J Med Chem 1994; 37(7): 999-1014.

[75] Moyle G, Boffito M, Stoehr A, *et al.* Phase 2a randomized controlled trial of short-term activity, safety, and pharmacokinetics of a novel nonnucleoside reverse transcriptase inhibitor, RDEA806, in HIV-1-positive, antiretroviral-naive subjects. Antimicrob Agents Chemother 2010; 54(8): 3170-8.
[76] Yeh L, Shen Z, Kerr B, *et al.* RDEA594: a potent URAT1 inhibitor without affecting other important renal transporters, OAT1 and OAT3 (Abstract THU0452). Annual European Conference on Rheumatology; 2009 June 10-13; Copenhagen, Denmark.
[77] Richman D, Jakubik J, Chapron C, *et al.* Genotypic Resistance and Phenotypic Cross-resistance Profile in vitro for a Novel NNRTI: IDX899 (Abstract 729). 15th Conference on Retroviruses and Opportunistic Infections; 2008 Feb 3-6; Boston, MA, USA.
[78] Zhou XJ, Pietropaolo K, Damphousse D, *et al.* Single-dose escalation and multiple-dose safety, tolerability, and pharmacokinetics of IDX899, a candidate human immunodeficiency virus type 1 nonnucleoside reverse transcriptase inhibitor, in healthy subjects. Antimicrob Agents Chemother 2009; 53(5): 1739-46.
[79] Zala C, St CM, Dudas K, *et al.* Safety and efficacy of GSK2248761, a next-generation nonnucleoside reverse transcriptase inhibitor, in treatment-naive HIV-1-infected subjects. Antimicrob Agents Chemother 2012; 56(5): 2570-5.
[80] Idenix P. The FDA places GSK2248761 ('761, formerly IDX899) on clinical hold (9 Feb 2011). Accessed: 24 June 2012. Available from: http://phx.corporate-ir.net/phoenix.zhtml?c=131556&p=irol-newsArticle&ID=1527182&highlight=.
[81] Tucker TJ, Sisko JT, Tynebor RM, *et al.* Discovery of 3-{5-[(6-amino-1H-pyrazolo[3,4-b]pyridine-3-yl)methoxy]-2-chlorophenoxy}-5-chloro benzonitrile (MK-4965): a potent, orally bioavailable HIV-1 non-nucleoside reverse transcriptase inhibitor with improved potency against key mutant viruses. J Med Chem 2008; 51(20): 6503-11.
[82] Lai MT, Munshi V, Touch S, *et al.* Antiviral activity of MK-4965, a novel nonnucleoside reverse transcriptase inhibitor. Antimicrob Agents Chemother 2009; 53(6): 2424-31.
[83] Lai MT, Lu M, Felock PJ, *et al.* Distinct mutation pathways of non-subtype B HIV-1 during in vitro resistance selection with nonnucleoside reverse transcriptase inhibitors. Antimicrob Agents Chemother 2010; 54(11): 4812-24.
[84] Javanbakht H, Ptak RG, Chow E, *et al.* In vitro resistance development for RO-0335, a novel diphenylether nonnucleoside reverse transcriptase inhibitor. Antiviral Res 2010; 86(2): 212-9.
[85] Klumpp K, Dunn J, Heilek G, *et al.* R1206, a representative of a new class of potent diphenylether non-nucleoside reverse transcriptase inhibitors broadly active against NNRTI resistant HIV-1 variants and achieving high systemic exposures and benign safety profiles in animal species (Oral presentation) 16th Intl HIV Drug Resistance Workshop; 2007 June 12-16; Barbados.
[86] Karpoormath R, Sayed Y, Govender P, *et al.* Pentacycloundecane derived hydroxy acid peptides: a new class of irreversible non-scissile ether bridged type isoster as potential HIV-1 wild type C-SA protease inhibitors. Bioorg Chem 2012; 40(1): 19-29.
[87] Grinsztejn B, Nguyen BY, Katlama C, *et al.* Safety and efficacy of the HIV-1 integrase inhibitor raltegravir (MK-0518) in treatment-experienced patients with multidrug-resistant virus: a phase II randomised controlled trial. Lancet 2007; 369(9569): 1261-9.
[88] Steigbigel RT, Cooper DA, Kumar PN, *et al.* Raltegravir with optimized background therapy for resistant HIV-1 infection. N Engl J Med 2008; 359(4): 339-54.
[89] Clumeck N, Pozniak A, Raffi F. European AIDS Clinical Society (EACS) guidelines for the clinical management and treatment of HIV-infected adults. HIV Med 2008; 9(2): 65-71.

[90] Thompson MA, Aberg JA, Cahn P, *et al.* Antiretroviral treatment of adult HIV infection: 2010 recommendations of the International AIDS Society-USA panel. JAMA 2010; 304(3): 321-33.

[91] Shimura K, Kodama E, Sakagami Y, *et al.* Broad antiretroviral activity and resistance profile of the novel human immunodeficiency virus integrase inhibitor elvitegravir (JTK-303/GS-9137). J Virol 2008; 82(2): 764-74.

[92] DeJesus E, Berger D, Markowitz M, *et al.* Antiviral activity, pharmacokinetics, and dose response of the HIV-1 integrase inhibitor GS-9137 (JTK-303) in treatment-naive and treatment-experienced patients. J Acquir Immune Defic Syndr 2006; 43(1): 1-5.

[93] Molina JM, Lamarca A, Andrade-Villanueva J, *et al.* Efficacy and safety of once daily elvitegravir *versus* twice daily raltegravir in treatment-experienced patients with HIV-1 receiving a ritonavir-boosted protease inhibitor: randomised, double-blind, phase 3, non-inferiority study. Lancet Infect Dis 2012; 12(1): 27-35.

[94] Klibanov OM. Elvitegravir, an oral HIV integrase inhibitor, for the potential treatment of HIV infection. Curr Opin Investig Drugs 2009; 10(2): 190-200.

[95] Kassahun K, McIntosh I, Cui D, *et al.* Metabolism and disposition in humans of raltegravir (MK-0518), an anti-AIDS drug targeting the human immunodeficiency virus 1 integrase enzyme. Drug Metab Dispos 2007; 35(9): 1657-63.

[96] Metifiot M, Vandegraaff N, Maddali K, *et al.* Elvitegravir overcomes resistance to raltegravir induced by integrase mutation Y143. AIDS 2011; 25(9): 1175-8.

[97] Eron J, Kumar P, Lazzarin A, *et al.* DTG in Subjects with HIV Exhibiting RAL Resistance: Functional Monotherapy Results of VIKING Study Cohort II (Abstract 151LB). 18th Conference on Retroviruses and Opportunistic Infections; 2011 Feb 27-Mar 2; Boston, MA, USA.

[98] Ceccherini-Silberstein F, Malet I, D'Arrigo R, *et al.* Characterization and structural analysis of HIV-1 integrase conservation. AIDS Rev 2009; 11(1): 17-29.

[99] Hightower KE, Wang R, Deanda F, *et al.* Dolutegravir (S/GSK1349572) exhibits significantly slower dissociation than raltegravir and elvitegravir from wild-type and integrase inhibitor-resistant HIV-1 integrase-DNA complexes. Antimicrob Agents Chemother 2011; 55(10): 4552-9.

[100] DeAnda F, Hattori K, Yoshinaga T, Kawasuji T, Underwood MR. Structural Models of HIV-1 Integrase and DNA in Complex with S/GSK1349572, Raltegravir and Elvitegravir: Structure-based Rationale for INI Resistance Profiles (Abstract 59). International HIV and Hepatitis Drug Resistance Workshop; 2010 Jun 8-12; Dubrovnik, Croatia.

[101] Min S, Song I, Borland J, *et al.* Pharmacokinetics and safety of S/GSK1349572, a next-generation HIV integrase inhibitor, in healthy volunteers. Antimicrob Agents Chemother 2010; 54(1): 254-8.

[102] van LJ, Maggiolo F, Arribas JR, *et al.* Once daily dolutegravir (S/GSK1349572) in combination therapy in antiretroviral-naive adults with HIV: planned interim 48 week results from SPRING-1, a dose-ranging, randomised, phase 2b trial. Lancet Infect Dis 2012; 12(2): 111-8.

[103] Eron J, Durant J, Poizot-Martin I, *et al.* Activity of a next generation integrase inhibitor (INI), S/GSK1349572, in subjects with HIV exhibiting raltegravir resistance: initial results of VIKING study (ING112961) (Abstract MOAB0105). XVIII International AIDS Conference; 2010 July 18-23; Vienna, Austria.

[104] Ford S, Chen S, Gould E, *et al.* Etravirine Has No Effect on the Pharmacokinetics of S/GSK1265744, a Novel HIV Integrase Inhibitor (Abstract P_15). 13th International Workshop on Clinical Pharmacology of HIV Therapy; 2012 Apr 16-18; Barcelona, Spain.

[105] Underwood MR, St CM, Johns BA, *et al.* S/GSK1265744: a next generation integrase inhibitor (INI) with activity against raltegravir-resistant clinical isolates (Abstract MOAA0103). XVIII International AIDS Conference; 2010 Jul 18-23; Vienna, Austria.

[106] Spreen W, Ford S, Chen S, *et al.* Pharmacokinetics, safety and tolerability of the HIV integrase inhibitor S/GSK1265744 long acting parenteral nanosuspension following single dose administration to healthy adults (Abstract TUPE040). XIX International AIDS Conference 2012 Jul 22-27; Washington D.C., USA.

[107] ClinicalTrials.gov. Dose Ranging Study of GSK1265744 Plus Nucleoside Reverse Transcriptase Inhibitors for Induction of Human Immunodeficiency Virus-1 (HIV-1) Virologic Suppression Followed by Virologic Suppression Maintenance by GSK1265744 Plus Rilpivirine. Accessed: 22 Oct 2012. Available from: http://clinicaltrials.gov/ct2/show/NCT01641809.

[108] Christ F, Voet AMA, Nicolet S, *et al.* First-in-class Inhibitors of LEDGF/p75-integrase Interaction and HIV Replication (Abstract 49). 17th Conference on Retroviruses and Opportunistic Infections; 2010 Feb 16-19; San Fransisco, USA.

[109] Fenwick C, Bethell R, Bonneau P, *et al.* Identification of BI-C, a Novel HIV-1 Non-catalytic Site Integrase Inhibitor (Abstract 523). 18th Conference on Retroviruses and Opportunistic Infections 2011 Feb 27-Mar 2; Boston, MA, USA.

[110] Christ F, Pickford C, Shaw S, *et al.* Preclinical Evaluation of HIV Replication Inhibitors that Target the HIV Integrase-LEDGF/p75 Interaction (Abstract 98). 19th Conference on Retroviruses and Opportunistic Infections; 2012 Mar 5-8; Seattle, USA.

[111] Suleiman J, Zingman BS, Diaz RS, *et al.* Vicriviroc in combination therapy with an optimized regimen for treatment-experienced subjects: 48-week results of the VICTOR-E1 phase 2 trial. J Infect Dis 2010; 201(4): 590-9.

[112] Gathe J, Diaz R, Fatkenheuer G, *et al.* Phase 3 Trials of Vicriviroc in Treatment-experienced Subjects Demonstrate Safety but Not Significantly Superior Efficacy over Potent Background Regimens Alone (Abstract 54LB). 17th Conference on Retroviruses and Opportunistic Infections; 2010 Feb 16-19; San Fransisco, CA, USA.

[113] Alcorn K. Merck will not seek vicriviroc licenses in treatment-experienced (21 Jan 2010). Accessed: 24 June 2012. Available from: http://www.aidsmap.com/Merck-will-not-seek-vicriviroc-licenses-in-treatment-experienced/page/1437505/.

[114] Moyle G, DeJesus E, Boffito M, *et al.* Proof of activity with AMD11070, an orally bioavailable inhibitor of CXCR4-tropic HIV type 1. Clin Infect Dis 2009; 48(6): 798-805.

[115] Mosi RM, Anastassova V, Cox J, *et al.* The molecular pharmacology of AMD11070: an orally bioavailable CXCR4 HIV entry inhibitor. Biochem Pharmacol 2012; 83(4): 472-9.

[116] Fletcher CV. Enfuvirtide, a new drug for HIV infection. Lancet 2003; 361(9369): 1577-8.

[117] Chen CH, Matthews TJ, McDanal CB, Bolognesi DP, Greenberg ML. A molecular clasp in the human immunodeficiency virus (HIV) type 1 TM protein determines the anti-HIV activity of gp41 derivatives: implication for viral fusion. J Virol 1995; 69(6): 3771-7.

[118] Chan DC, Fass D, Berger JM, Kim PS. Core structure of gp41 from the HIV envelope glycoprotein. Cell 1997; 89(2): 263-73.

[119] Wang RR, Yang LM, Wang YH, *et al.* Sifuvirtide, a potent HIV fusion inhibitor peptide. Biochem Biophys Res Commun 2009; 382(3): 540-4.

[120] He Y, Xiao Y, Song H, *et al.* Design and evaluation of sifuvirtide, a novel HIV-1 fusion inhibitor. J Biol Chem 2008; 283(17): 11126-34.

[121] Murga JD, Franti M, Pevear DC, Maddon PJ, Olson WC. Potent antiviral synergy between monoclonal antibody and small-molecule CCR5 inhibitors of human immunodeficiency virus type 1. Antimicrob Agents Chemother 2006; 50(10): 3289-96.

[122] Jacobson JM, Saag MS, Thompson MA, *et al.* Antiviral activity of single-dose PRO 140, a CCR5 monoclonal antibody, in HIV-infected adults. J Infect Dis 2008; 198(9): 1345-52.

[123] Jacobson JM, Thompson MA, Lalezari JP, *et al.* Anti-HIV-1 activity of weekly or biweekly treatment with subcutaneous PRO 140, a CCR5 monoclonal antibody. J Infect Dis 2010; 201(10): 1481-7.

[124] Allaway GP, Ryder AM, Beaudry GA, Maddon PJ. Synergistic inhibition of HIV-1 envelope-mediated cell fusion by CD4-based molecules in combination with antibodies to gp120 or gp41. AIDS Res Hum Retroviruses 1993; 9(7): 581-7.

[125] Gauduin MC, Allaway GP, Olson WC, *et al.* CD4-immunoglobulin G2 protects Hu-PBL-SCID mice against challenge by primary human immunodeficiency virus type 1 isolates. J Virol 1998; 72(4): 3475-8.

[126] Ketas TJ, Frank I, Klasse PJ, *et al.* Human immunodeficiency virus type 1 attachment, coreceptor, and fusion inhibitors are active against both direct and trans infection of primary cells. J Virol 2003; 77(4): 2762-7.

[127] Jacobson JM, Lowy I, Fletcher CV, *et al.* Single-dose safety, pharmacology, and antiviral activity of the human immunodeficiency virus (HIV) type 1 entry inhibitor PRO 542 in HIV-infected adults. J Infect Dis 2000; 182(1): 326-9.

[128] Jacobson JM, Israel RJ, Lowy I, *et al.* Treatment of advanced human immunodeficiency virus type 1 disease with the viral entry inhibitor PRO 542. Antimicrob Agents Chemother 2004; 48(2): 423-9.

[129] Fletcher CV, DeVille JG, Samson PM, *et al.* Nonlinear pharmacokinetics of high-dose recombinant fusion protein CD4-IgG2 (PRO 542) observed in HIV-1-infected children. J Allergy Clin Immunol 2007; 119(3): 747-50.

[130] Moore JP, Sattentau QJ, Klasse PJ, Burkly LC. A monoclonal antibody to CD4 domain 2 blocks soluble CD4-induced conformational changes in the envelope glycoproteins of human immunodeficiency virus type 1 (HIV-1) and HIV-1 infection of CD4+ cells. J Virol 1992; 66(8): 4784-93.

[131] Norris D, Morales J, Gathe J, *et al.* Phase 2 efficacy and safety of the novel entry inhibitor, TNX-355, in combination with optimized background regimen (OBR) (Abstract TUPE0058). XVI International AIDS Conference; 2006 Aug 13-18; Toronto, Canada.

[132] Jacobson JM, Kuritzkes DR, Godofsky E, *et al.* Safety, pharmacokinetics, and antiretroviral activity of multiple doses of ibalizumab (formerly TNX-355), an anti-CD4 monoclonal antibody, in human immunodeficiency virus type 1-infected adults. Antimicrob Agents Chemother 2009; 53(2): 450-7.

[133] Fessel WJ, Anderson B, Follansbee SE, *et al.* The efficacy of an anti-CD4 monoclonal antibody for HIV-1 treatment. Antiviral Res 2011; 92(3): 484-7.

[134] Nowicka-Sans B, Gong YF, McAuliffe B, *et al.* In vitro antiviral characteristics of HIV-1 attachment inhibitor BMS-626529, the active component of the prodrug BMS-663068. Antimicrob Agents Chemother 2012.

[135] Ho HT, Fan L, Nowicka-Sans B, *et al.* Envelope conformational changes induced by human immunodeficiency virus type 1 attachment inhibitors prevent CD4 binding and downstream entry events. J Virol 2006; 80(8): 4017-25.

[136] Nettles R, Schurmann D, Zhu L, *et al.* Pharmacodynamics, Safety, and Pharmacokinetics of BMS-663068: A Potentially First-in-class Oral HIV Attachment Inhibitor (Abstract 49). 18th Conference on Retroviruses and Opportunistic Infections; 2011 Feb 27-Mar 2; Boston, MA, USA.

[137] Charpentier C, Larrouy L, Visseaux B, *et al.* Prevalence of subtype-related polymorphisms associated with in vitro resistance to attachment inhibitor BMS-626529 in HIV-1 'non-B'-infected patients. J Antimicrob Chemother 2012; 67(6): 1459-61.

[138] Nowicka-Sans B, Gong YF, H T, *et al.* Antiviral activity of a new small molecule HIV-1 attachment inhibitor, BMS-626529, the parent of BMS-663068 (Abstract 518). 18th Conference on Retroviruses and Opportunistic Infections; 2011 Feb 27-Mar 2; Boston, MA, USA.

[139] Moyle GJ, Back D. Principles and practice of HIV-protease inhibitor pharmacoenhancement. HIV Med 2001; 2(2): 105-13.

[140] Malan N, Krantz E, David N, *et al.* Efficacy and Safety of Atazanavir-based Therapy in Antiretroviral Naive HIV-1 Infected Subjects, Both with and without Ritonavir: 48-week Results from AI424-089 (Abstract 107LB). 13th Conference on Retroviruses and Opportunistic Infections; 2006 Feb 5-8; Denver, CO, USA.

[141] Dussault I, Lin M, Hollister K, *et al.* Peptide mimetic HIV protease inhibitors are ligands for the orphan receptor SXR. J Biol Chem 2001; 276(36): 33309-12.

[142] Gupta A, Mugundu GM, Desai PB, Thummel KE, Unadkat JD. Intestinal human colon adenocarcinoma cell line LS180 is an excellent model to study pregnane X receptor, but not constitutive androstane receptor, mediated CYP3A4 and multidrug resistance transporter 1 induction: studies with anti-human immunodeficiency virus protease inhibitors. Drug Metab Dispos 2008; 36(6): 1172-80.

[143] Svard J, Spiers JP, Mulcahy F, Hennessy M. Nuclear receptor-mediated induction of CYP450 by antiretrovirals: functional consequences of NR1I2 (PXR) polymorphisms and differential prevalence in whites and sub-Saharan Africans. J Acquir Immune Defic Syndr 2010; 55(5): 536-49.

[144] Mathias AA, German P, Murray BP, *et al.* Pharmacokinetics and pharmacodynamics of GS-9350: a novel pharmacokinetic enhancer without anti-HIV activity. Clin Pharmacol Ther 2010; 87(3): 322-9.

[145] Elion R, Cohen C, Gathe J, *et al.* Phase 2 study of cobicistat *versus* ritonavir each with once-daily atazanavir and fixed-dose emtricitabine/tenofovir df in the initial treatment of HIV infection. AIDS 2011; 25(15): 1881-6.

[146] Cohen C, Elion R, Ruane P, *et al.* Randomized, phase 2 evaluation of two single-tablet regimens elvitegravir/cobicistat/emtricitabine/tenofovir disoproxil fumarate *versus* efavirenz/emtricitabine/tenofovir disoproxil fumarate for the initial treatment of HIV infection. AIDS 2011; 25(6): F7-12.

[147] Tang C, Loeliger E, Kinde I, *et al.* Antiviral inhibition of the HIV-1 capsid protein. J Mol Biol 2003; 327(5): 1013-20.

[148] Forshey BM, von SU, Sundquist WI, Aiken C. Formation of a human immunodeficiency virus type 1 core of optimal stability is crucial for viral replication. J Virol 2002; 76(11): 5667-77.

[149] Reicin AS, Ohagen A, Yin L, Hoglund S, Goff SP. The role of Gag in human immunodeficiency virus type 1 virion morphogenesis and early steps of the viral life cycle. J Virol 1996; 70(12): 8645-52.

[150] Sticht J, Humbert M, Findlow S, *et al.* A peptide inhibitor of HIV-1 assembly in vitro. Nat Struct Mol Biol 2005; 12(8): 671-7.

[151] Zhang H, Zhao Q, Bhattacharya S, *et al.* A cell-penetrating helical peptide as a potential HIV-1 inhibitor. J Mol Biol 2008; 378(3): 565-80.

[152] Blair WS, Pickford C, Irving SL, *et al.* HIV capsid is a tractable target for small molecule therapeutic intervention. PLoS Pathog 2010; 6(12): e1001220.

[153] Aiken C, Chen CH. Betulinic acid derivatives as HIV-1 antivirals. Trends Mol Med 2005; 11(1): 31-6.

[154] Yogeeswari P, Sriram D. Betulinic acid and its derivatives: a review on their biological properties. Curr Med Chem 2005; 12(6): 657-66.

[155] Zhao H, Holmes SS, Baker GA, *et al.* Ionic derivatives of betulinic acid as novel HIV-1 protease inhibitors. J Enzyme Inhib Med Chem 2011.

[156] Kanamoto T, Kashiwada Y, Kanbara K, *et al.* Anti-human immunodeficiency virus activity of YK-FH312 (a betulinic acid derivative), a novel compound blocking viral maturation. Antimicrob Agents Chemother 2001; 45(4): 1225-30.

[157] Kashiwada Y, Hashimoto F, Cosentino LM, *et al.* Betulinic acid and dihydrobetulinic acid derivatives as potent anti-HIV agents. J Med Chem 1996; 39(5): 1016-7.

[158] Li F, Goila-Gaur R, Salzwedel K, *et al.* PA-457: a potent HIV inhibitor that disrupts core condensation by targeting a late step in Gag processing. Proc Natl Acad Sci USA 2003; 100(23): 13555-60.

[159] Smith PF, Ogundele A, Forrest A, *et al.* Phase I and II study of the safety, virologic effect, and pharmacokinetics/pharmacodynamics of single-dose 3-o-(3',3'-dimethylsuccinyl)betulinic acid (bevirimat) against human immunodeficiency virus infection. Antimicrob Agents Chemother 2007; 51(10): 3574-81.

[160] Shikov AN, Djachuk GI, Sergeev DV, *et al.* Birch bark extract as therapy for chronic hepatitis C--a pilot study. Phytomedicine 2011; 18(10): 807-10.

[161] Avexa L. ASX Release: Avexa and FDA agree path forward for ATC (28 Mar 2011). Accessed: 22 Oct 2012. Available from: http://www.avexa.com.au/freestyler/files/961373.pdf.

[162] Vernazza P, Wang C, Pozniak A, *et al.* Efficacy and safety of lersivirine (UK-453,061) *vs.* efavirenz in antiretroviral treatment-naïve HIV-1-infected patients: week 48 primary analysis results from an ongoing, multicentre, randomised, double-blind, phase IIb trial (study A5271015) (Abstract TUAB0101). 6th IAS Conference on HIV Pathogenesis, Treatment and Prevention; 2011 Jul 17-20; Rome, Italy.

[163] Xu W, Groschel B, Straney R, *et al.* Resistance to RDEA806 requires multiple mutations which have limited cross-resistance to other NNRTIs (Abstract H-1222). 48th Interscience Conference on Antimicrobial Agents and Chemotherapy; 2008 Oct 25-28; Washington, D.C., USA.

[164] Taiwo B, Murphy RL, Katlama C. Novel antiretroviral combinations in treatment-experienced patients with HIV infection: rationale and results. Drugs 2010; 70(13): 1629-42.

[165] Gilead Website: Pipeline Products, July 2011. Accessed: 24 June 2012. Available from: http://www.gilead.com/pipeline_products.

[166] Ford N, Lee J, Andrieux-Meyer I, Calmy A. Safety, efficacy, and pharmacokinetics of rilpivirine: systematic review with an emphasis on resource-limited settings. HIV AIDS (Auckl) 2011; 3: 35-44.

[167] Desmidt M, Willems B, Dom P, *et al.* Absence of a teratogenic potential from a novel next-generation NNRTI, TMC278 (Abstract PE7.1/4). 12th European AIDS Conference 2009 11-14 Nov; Cologne, Germany.

[168] van Heeswijk R, Hoetelmans R, Kestens D, *et al.* The effects of CYP3A4 modulation on the pharmacokinetics of TMC278, an investigational non-nucleoside reverse transcriptase inhibitor (NNRTI) (Abstract 74). 7th International Workshop of Clinical Pharmacology; 2006 Apr 20-22; Lisbon, Portugal.

[169] Crauwels H, Van Heeswijk R, Kestens D, *et al.* The pharmacokinetic (PK) interaction between rifabutin and TMC278, an investigational non-nucleoside reverse transcriptase inhibitor (NNRTI)

(Abstract TUPE0080). XVIIth International AIDS Conference; 2008 Aug 3-8; Mexico City, Mexico.

[170] Nightingale SL. From the Food and Drug Administration. JAMA 1998; 280(17): 1472.

[171] Cappon GD, Bowman CJ, Campion SN, *et al.* Developmental Toxicity Study of Lersivirine in Mice. Birth Defects Res B Dev Reprod Toxicol 2012.

[172] Campion SN, Bowman CJ, Cappon GD, *et al.* Developmental Toxicity of Lersivirine in Rabbits when Administered throughout Organogenesis and when Limited to Sensitive Windows of Axial Skeletal Development. Birth Defects Res B Dev Reprod Toxicol 2012.

[173] Verloes R, van't Klooster G, Baert L, *et al.* TMC278 long acting - a parenteral nanosuspension formulation that provides sustained clinically relevant plasma concentrations in HIV-negative volunteers (Abstract TUPE0042). AIDS 2008 - XVII International AIDS Conference; 2008 3-8 Aug; Mexico City, Mexico.

[174] UNAIDS Report on the Global AIDS Epidemic 2010. Accessed: 24 June 2012. Available from: http://unaids.org/globalreport/Global_report.htm.

[175] Selhorst P, Vazquez AC, Terrazas-Aranda K, *et al.* Human immunodeficiency virus type 1 resistance or cross-resistance to nonnucleoside reverse transcriptase inhibitors currently under development as microbicides. Antimicrob Agents Chemother 2011; 55(4): 1403-13.

[176] Li L, Ben Y, Yuan S, *et al.* Efficacy, Stability, and Biosafety of Sifuvirtide Gel as a Microbicide Candidate against HIV-1. PLoS One 2012; 7(5): e37381.

[177] Spire B, Carrieri P, Garzot MA, L'Henaff M, Obadia Y. Factors associated with efavirenz discontinuation in a large community-based sample of patients. AIDS Care 2004 Jul; 16(5): 558-64.

[178] van Luin M, Bannister WP, Mocroft A, *et al.* Absence of a relation between efavirenz plasma concentrations and toxicity-driven efavirenz discontinuations in the EuroSIDA study. Antivir Ther 2009; 14(1): 75-83.

[179] Leserman J, Ironson G, O'Cleirigh C, Fordiani JM, Balbin E. Stressful life events and adherence in HIV. AIDS Patient Care STDS 2008; 22(5): 403-11.

[180] Taylor BS, Garduno LS, Reyes EV, *et al.* HIV care for geographically mobile populations. Mt Sinai J Med 2011; 78(3): 342-51.

[181] Weiser SD, Frongillo EA, Ragland K, *et al.* Food insecurity is associated with incomplete HIV RNA suppression among homeless and marginally housed HIV-infected individuals in San Francisco. J Gen Intern Med 2009; 24(1): 14-20.

[182] Nakata H, Steinberg SM, Koh Y, *et al.* Potent synergistic anti-human immunodeficiency virus (HIV) effects using combinations of the CCR5 inhibitor aplaviroc with other anti-HIV drugs. Antimicrobial agents and chemotherapy 2008; 52(6): 2111-9.

[183] May M, Gompels M, Delpech V, *et al.* Impact of late diagnosis and treatment on life expectancy in people with HIV-1: UK Collaborative HIV Cohort (UK CHIC) Study. BMJ 2011; 343: d6016.

[184] Florescu D, Kotler DP. Insulin resistance, glucose intolerance and diabetes mellitus in HIV-infected patients. Antivir Ther 2007; 12(2): 149-62.

[185] Arribas JR, Pulido F, Miro JM, *et al.* High effectiveness of efavirenz-based highly active antiretroviral therapy in HIV-1-infected patients with fewer than 100 CD4 cells/microl and opportunistic diseases: the EfaVIP Study (Efavirenz in Very Immunosuppressed Patients). AIDS 2002; 16(11): 1554-6.

[186] Bartlett JA, DeMasi R, Quinn J, Moxham C, Rousseau F. Overview of the effectiveness of triple combination therapy in antiretroviral-naive HIV-1 infected adults. AIDS 2001; 15(11): 1369-77.

[187] Tashima K, Staszewski S, Nelson M, *et al.* Durable viral suppression on EFV-based HAART: 168 week follow-up (Abstract TuPeB4547). 15th International AIDS Conference; 2004 11-16 July; Bangkok, Thailand.
[188] Clifford DB, Evans S, Yang Y, *et al.* Impact of efavirenz on neuropsychological performance and symptoms in HIV-infected individuals. Ann Intern Med 2005; 143(10): 714-21.
[189] Gallant JE, Deresinski S. Tenofovir disoproxil fumarate. Clin Infect Dis 2003; 37(7): 944-50.
[190] Carr A, Hoy J. Low bone mineral density with tenofovir: does statistically significant mean clinically significant? Clin Infect Dis 2010; 51(8): 973-5.
[191] Scherzer R, Estrella M, Li Y, *et al.* Association of tenofovir exposure with kidney disease risk in HIV infection. AIDS 2012; 26(7): 867-75.
[192] Stellbrink HJ, Orkin C, Arribas JR, *et al.* Comparison of changes in bone density and turnover with abacavir-lamivudine *versus* tenofovir-emtricitabine in HIV-infected adults: 48-week results from the ASSERT study. Clin Infect Dis 2010; 51(8): 963-72.
[193] Buscher A, Hartman C, Kallen MA, Giordano TP. Impact of antiretroviral dosing frequency and pill burden on adherence among newly diagnosed, antiretroviral-naive HIV patients. Int J STD AIDS 2012; 23(5): 351-5.
[194] Lindl KA, Marks DR, Kolson DL, Jordan-Sciutto KL. HIV-associated neurocognitive disorder: pathogenesis and therapeutic opportunities. J Neuroimmune Pharmacol 2010; 5(3): 294-309.

CHAPTER 2

New Developments for Anti-HIV Treatment

Liã Bárbara Arruda[1] and Jorge Casseb[2,*]

[1]Institute of Tropical Medicine of Sao Paulo, University of Sao Paulo, Sao Paulo, Brazil and [2]Laboratory of Investigation in Dermatology and Immunodeficiencies – LIM56, Department of Dermatology School of Medicine at University of Sao Paulo, Sao Paulo, Brazil

Abstract: Viral suppression is necessary to control the evolution of drug resistance, reduce the chronic immune activation, which is associated with morbidity and mortality in HIV-infected patients, reducing viral transmission, including transmission of drug resistance. In general, the proportion of viremic patients who achieved suppression increases with the number of pharmacokinetically active antiretroviral therapy regimen in. Guidelines to antiretroviral treatment today recommend the use of at least three antiretroviral agents (ART) selected from different drug classes, which may include inhibitors of reverse transcriptase nucleoside (NRTI), reverse transcriptase inhibitors Non-nucleoside inhibitors (NNRTIs) inhibitors protease (PI's), entry inhibitors and integrase inhibitors. There is regarding when to start therapy, what drugs should be used, how to manage the risk of toxicity and how to improve adherence to treatment. The impact of co-morbidities conditions in the selection of drugs and the risk of emergence of resistant viruses must also be considered as deciding factors. Thus, this review covers the last advances in ART, specifically focusing integrase inhibitors and entry inhibitors.

Keywords: Entry inhibitors, HIV-1, HAART, integrase inhibitors.

INTRODUCTION

At the time of the first description of the Acquired Immunodeficiency Syndrome (AIDS) and its causal agent Human Immunodeficiency Virus (HIV), options for antiviral therapy were limited and no antiretrovirals had been identified yet [1]. The first ideas for anti-HIV drugs aimed to inhibit viral enzymes, thus the development of reverse transcriptase (RT) inhibitors started with the discovery of the antiretroviral activity of the nucleoside analog zidovudine (AZT) and soon the

***Corresponding author Jorge Casseb:** Institute of Tropical Medicine of Sao Paulo - University of Sao Paulo, Brazil; Tel: 551130617193; Fax: 551130817190; Email: jcasseb10@gmail.com development of others nucleoside analogs [1, 2]. The experience with these drugs in monotherapy showed that the inhibition of HIV replication by treatment was achievable and the resistant viruses were selected in a very short time [1, 3]. In the middle of 90's, the antiretroviral therapy was improved by the development of the nonnucleoside RT inhibitors (NNRTI). Several members of both drug classes are used today in antiretroviral combination therapy [1].

In 1995, the first protease inhibitor (PI) was approved for clinical use and the combination therapy of two nucleoside analogs with a PI or an NNRTI was found to be superior to achieve viral suppression [1, 4, 5]. The highly active antiretroviral therapy (HARRT) era began reaching the immune reconstitution, but limited by a high pill burden and side effects [1, 6, 7]. Currently, PIs are coadministered with low-dose as a pharmaceutical booster, which leads to a expressive reduction of viral resistance [1]. Therefore, the HAART has resulted in a dramatic decrease for the morbidity and mortality of HIV-1 infection [8]. However, the drug resistance may emerge with treatment failure, mainly caused by low adherence by the patient to the treatment. Thus, the regimens should be not only effective against HIV, but also minimize adverse events and maximize adherence to sustain the infection under control [8, 9].

New targets have been explored aiming the development of anti-HIV drugs with different mechanism of action. In 2007, maraviroc (MVC) was the first chemokine receptor 5 (CCR5) antagonist approved for clinical use. MCV interacts with the host coreceptor and blocks the binding of the viral gp120. However, this drug is only effective against CCR5-tropic (R5) viruses and a tropism test is mandatory before and along the CCR5 antagonist administration [1, 10]. The most recent new anti-HIV drug class is the first integrase (IN) inhibitor, raltegravir (RAL), approved in 2008 and dolutegravir (DTG) in 2013. This drug is a strand transfer inhibitor class which binds to the IN close to the DDE motif in the active site blocking the enzyme activity, which prevents the proviral DNA insertion into the host genome [1, 11, 12].

CCR5 ANTAGONIST

HIV envelope proteins recognize and bind to CD4 surface receptor, anchoring the virus to the surface of the host cell, and enabling additional interactions with a coreceptor protein [13-15]. The main coreceptors used by HIV-1 are chemokine receptors CCR5 and CXCR4 [13]. The use of CCR5 or CXCR4 coreceptors is determined by the amino acid sequence of HIV-1 of the viral surface protein gp120, especially of the third variable region (V3 loop) [13, 16]. R5 viruses are predominant in the early phase of infection, whereas CXCR4-tropic (X4) viruses usually become detectable only at later stages which is associated with accelerated loss of CD4 cells and faster progression to AIDS [17-18]. After the appearance of X4 viruses, the R5 and X4 populations most often coexist in the host and also appear strains able to use both CCR5 and CXCR4 coreceptors which characterizes the dual tropic (D) R5X4 viruses [13, 17].

Approximately 1% of Caucasians are homozygous for a nonfunctional CCR5 receptor, caused by a deletion of 32 base pairs in the CCR5 gene (CCR5-Δ32 mutation). These individuals are healthy and partially resistant to HIV-1 infection. Based on this fact, blocking the CCR5 receptor could significantly decrease HIV replication without interfering in the immune cell activity [1, 19].

As CCR5 antagonists only interact with the CCR5 molecule, they are only effective against R5 viruses; therefore, a tropism test is mandatory before CCR5 antagonist administration [1, 10, 13]. Currently, the tropism determination can be performed by a phenotypic tropism test (PTT) or a genotypic tropism test (GTT) [20, 21]. PPT are considered the gold-standard test for tropism determination, but its high cost and restricted logistic are important limitations for its wide application, mainly in developing countries [20, 22]. Recently, the European Guidelines have been encouraging the application GTT using bioinformatics systems for coreceptor usage prediction [21]. This strategy consists in the bulk sequencing of the V3-loop sequence followed by the prediction using the geno2pheno[coreceptor] tool [1, 23].

The efficacy of Maraviroc (Selzentry®, Celsentri ®, ViiV Healthcare) against R5 virus has been tested in three trials [1, 24]. The MOTIVATE (MCV optimized therapy in viremic antiretroviral treatment-experienced patients) 1 and 2 studies were designed to assess the efficacy and safety of MVC given once or twice daily when added to optimized background therapy in patients with R5 virus who had experienced failure in the HAART administration [24-26]. The findings from

MOTIVATE 1 and 2 studies showed that MVC was associated with significantly better virologic suppression rates in patients prior antiretroviral (ART) experience who harbor R5 and non-R5 viruses [24]. The MERIT (MVC *versus* efavirenz in treatment naïve patients) study evaluated MVC as firs-line treatment, showing that MVC was noninferior to efavirenz in suppressing replication of HIV infection and it achieved virologic suppression rates only slightly less than efavirenz [24, 27]. Usually, the treatment failure is associated with viral tropism switch and in very few cases it has been described as consequence of specific mutations in the V3 loop that lead to resistance [24, 28].

Two other compounds of CCR5 antagonist class had reached clinical studies but have been withdrawn. Aplaviroc (GlaxoSmithKline) showed *in vitro* activity against HIV; however phase II studies were terminated prematurely because of severe hepatotoxicity which led to discontinuation of clinical development of aplaviroc (APL) [1, 24]. Vicriviroc completed the testing in phase I-III clinical studies of HIV-infected individuals but subsequently was withdrawn from further clinical development because the primary efficacy endpoints have not been met [1, 24].

Contrary the CCR5 coreceptor, the blocking of the CXCR4 leads to a serious immune commitment as the chemokine SDF1 can only interact with CXCR4. The CXCR4 antagonist AMD3100 showed very promising results *in vitro*, but produced such severe side effects that the clinical studies has to be aborted; however, other drugs from this series are currently being tested [1, 29].

INTEGRASE INHIBITORS

After the fusion, the process of reverse transcriptase begins. The double-strand cDNA is transported into the nucleus within the preintegration complex (PIC), which comprises a number of viral and cell proteins. After it is transported into the nucleus, a DNA copy is integrated into the genome of the host cell due to the catalytic activity of the viral IN. The integration of viral DNA is an essential step required to complete the life cycle of HIV [1, 11].

The integration process comprises two main steps: the first step, referred to as 3'-end processing, occurs in the cytoplasm within the PIC. The terminal GT dinucleotides are removed from each 3'-end to produce new 3'-hydroxyl ends (CA-3'-OH). After the PIC is transported through the nuclear pore, the second step begins to join the viral DNA to the host DNA. The joining reaction, termed strand transfer, includes a cleavage of the target DNA and ligation of the CA-3'-OH viral DNA ends to the 5'-O-phosphate ends of the target DNA. The integration reaction is completed by the repair of the single-stranded gaps between the viral and target DNA, probably accomplished by host cell DNA repair enzymes [30-34].

HIV-1 IN is a protein consisting of 288 amino acid (aa) residues and comprises three domains: the N-terminal domain (aa 1-50), including an HH-CC zinc-binding motive; the catalytic core domain (aa 51–212), containing the active centre (DDE motif: D46, D116 and E152); and the C-terminal domain (aa 213–288) which allows the binding to the cellular DNA [1, 11, 35]. For the integration to be possible, IN demands the presence of ions of cofactor metal ions (Mg^{2+} or Mn^{2+}), which are coordinated with two residues from the catalytic triad (D64 and D116) [11, 36].

Inhibitors of integrase that have now been developed are strand transfer inhibitors (INSTIs) that block the insertion position on the host DNA. These drugs bind to the IN close to the DDE motif in the active site and competitively block the IN activity. The proviral DNA cannot be inserted into the host genome and is circularized by cellular repair enzymes, stopping the viral replication irreversibly [1, 34, 37].

Raltegravir (RAL, Isentress®, Merck) has demonstrated potent and durable activity against HIV-1, while maintaining a favorable safety profile. Results from clinical trials indicate that is safe and highly effective in the treatment of both antiretroviral-naive and antiretroviral-experienced patients [1, 9]. RAL with optimized background therapy (OBT) provides an alternative regimen for patients with limited remaining treatment options and may be a viable treatment option for patients with contraindication or intolerance to other ART [9, 38]. Resistance to RAL has been associated with amino acid substitutions at three key positions in the IN protein: Y143R/C, Q148H/ R/K or H155H, alone, or accompanied by other mutations such as T66I, L74M, E92Q, T97A, E138K+G140S/A GY143H, V151I and G163R [1, 38-40].

Elvitegravir (EVG, GS-9137, Gilead), also an INSTI, is undergoing a phase III clinical trial. EVG has demonstrated good efficacy and safety, with minimal side effects. It presents the advantage of an oral once-daily dosage, however the drug requires boosting and this leads to a number of drug-drug interactions and necessary dose adjustment when dosing with certain drugs [1, 41]. Resistance to EVG is associated with the mutations T66I/A/K, E92Q, E138K, Q146P, S147G, Q148R/H/K and N155H [42], which are close to the resistance mutations selected by RAL; therefore, cross-resistance for both drugs is expected [1, 43].

Dolutegravir (S/GSK1349572) is an investigational INSTI with activity against most isolates resistant to RAL or EVG [44]. Pharmacokinetic studies in people have shown a long plasma half-life without the need for booster and showed the potential for a higher barrier to resistance compared with RAL and EVG [45]. The 96-week outcomes from the SPRING-1 trial, a randomized, partially blinded, dose-finding study of dolutegravir *versus* efavirenz, showed dolutegravir was effective when given once daily without booster and was well tolerated at all assessed doses and no resistance was detected, and has recently been approved by FDA [44-46].

FUTURE AND ADVANCES

Advances in the development of new antiretroviral drugs, the combination of therapeutic regimens and the development of coformulations that reduced the number of tablets to be administered have led to high rates of therapeutic success. These changes lead to a significant improvement in rates of HIV suppression and response count of T CD4+ cells to baseline therapy. Thus, it seems reasonable to think that a better control of HIV infection worldwide will be achieve soon, specially using single tablet containing the full anti-HIV regimen.

ACKNOWLEDGEMENTS

Declared none.

CONFLICT OF INTEREST

The authors confirm that this chapter contents have no conflict of interest.

REFERENCES

[1] Sierra-Aragon S, Walter H. Targets for inhibition of HIV replication: entry, enzyme action, release and maturation. Intervirology 2012; 55(2): 84-97.

[2] Schuurman R, Nijhuis M, van Leeuwen R, *et al.* Rapid changes in human immunodeficiency virus type 1 RNA load and appearance of drug-resistant virus populations in persons treated with lamivudine (3TC). J Infect Dis 1995; 171(6): 1411-9.

[3] Staszewski S. Zidovudine and lamivudine: results of phase III studies. J Acquir Immune Defic Syndr Hum Retrovirol 1995; 10 Suppl 1: S57.

[4] Larder BA. Viral resistance and the selection of antiretroviral combinations. J Acquir Immune Defic Syndr Hum Retrovirol 1995; 10 Suppl 1: S28-33.

[5] Vella S. Rationale and experience with reverse transcriptase inhibitors and protease inhibitors. J Acquir Immune Defic Syndr Hum Retrovirol 1995; 10 Suppl 1: S58-61.

[6] Cohen J. AIDS therapy. Failure isn't what it used to be.but neither is success. Science 1998; 279(5354): 1133-4.

[7] Carr A, Samaras K, Burton S, Law M, Freund J, Chisholm DJ, *et al.* A syndrome of peripheral lipodystrophy, hyperlipidaemia and insulin resistance in patients receiving HIV protease inhibitors. AIDS 1998; 12(7): F51-8.

[8] Alencar CS, Nishiya AS, Ferreira S, Giret MT, Diaz RS, Sabino EC. Evaluation of primary resistance to HIV entry inhibitors among brazilian patients failing reverse transcriptase/protease inhibitors treatment reveal high prevalence of maraviroc resistance-related mutations. AIDS Res Hum Retroviruses 2010; 26(12): 1267-71.

[9] Rokas KE, Bookstaver PB, Shamroe CL, Sutton SS, Millisor VE, Bryant JE, *et al.* Role of raltegravir in HIV-1 management. Ann Pharmacother 2012; 46(4): 578-89.

[10] Alkhatib G, Berger EA. HIV coreceptors: from discovery and designation to new paradigms and promise. Eur J Med Res 2007; 12(9): 375-84.

[11] Korolev SP, Agapkina YY, Gottikh MB. Clinical Use of Inhibitors of HIV-1 Integration: Problems and Prospects. Acta Naturae 2011; 3(3): 12-28.

[12] Hazuda DJ, Felock P, Witmer M, Wolfe A, Stillmock K, Grobler JA, *et al.* Inhibitors of strand transfer that prevent integration and inhibit HIV-1 replication in cells. Science 2000; 287(5453): 646-50.

[13] Este JA, Telenti A. HIV entry inhibitors. Lancet 2007; 370(9581): 81-8.

[14] Eckert DM, Kim PS. Mechanisms of viral membrane fusion and its inhibition. Annu Rev Biochem 2001; 70: 777-810.

[15] Pierson TC, Doms RW. HIV-1 entry and its inhibition. Curr Top Microbiol Immunol 2003; 281: 1-27.

[16] Connor RI, Sheridan KE, Ceradini D, Choe S, Landau NR. Change in coreceptor use correlates with disease progression in HIV-1--infected individuals. J Exp Med 1997; 185(4): 621-8.

[17] Mild M, Esbjornsson J, Fenyo EM, Medstrand P. Frequent intrapatient recombination between human immunodeficiency virus type 1 R5 and X4 envelopes: implications for coreceptor switch. J Virol 2007; 81(7): 3369-76.

[18] Scarlatti G, Tresoldi E, Bjorndal A, Fredriksson R, Colognesi C, Deng HK, *et al. In vivo* evolution of HIV-1 co-receptor usage and sensitivity to chemokine-mediated suppression. Nat Med 1997; 3(11): 1259-65.

[19] Liu R, Paxton WA, Choe S, Ceradini D, Martin SR, Horuk R, *et al.* Homozygous defect in HIV-1 coreceptor accounts for resistance of some multiply-exposed individuals to HIV-1 infection. Cell 1996; 86(3): 367-77.

[20] Harrigan PR, Geretti AM. Genotypic tropism testing: evidence-based or leap of faith? AIDS 2011; 25(2): 257-64.

[21] Vandekerckhove LP, Wensing AM, Kaiser R, Brun-Vezinet F, Clotet B, De Luca A, *et al.* European guidelines on the clinical management of HIV-1 tropism testing. Lancet Infect Dis 2011; 11(5): 394-407.

[22] McGovern RA, Harrigan PR, Swenson LC. Genotypic inference of HIV-1 tropism using population-based sequencing of V3. J Vis Exp 2010: 46: 2531.

[23] Lengauer T, Sander O, Sierra S, Thielen A, Kaiser R. Bioinformatics prediction of HIV coreceptor usage. Nat Biotechnol 2007; 25(12): 1407-10.

[24] Wilkin TJ, Gulick RM. CCR5 antagonism in HIV infection: current concepts and future opportunities. Annu Rev Med 2012; 63: 81-93.

[25] Gulick RM, Lalezari J, Goodrich J, Clumeck N, DeJesus E, Horban A, *et al.* Maraviroc for previously treated patients with R5 HIV-1 infection. N Engl J Med 2008; 359(14): 1429-41.

[26] Fatkenheuer G, Nelson M, Lazzarin A, Konourina I, Hoepelman AI, Lampiris H, *et al.* Subgroup analyses of maraviroc in previously treated R5 HIV-1 infection. N Engl J Med 2008; 359(14): 1442-55.

[27] Cooper DA, Heera J, Goodrich J, Tawadrous M, Saag M, Dejesus E, *et al.* Maraviroc *versus* efavirenz, both in combination with zidovudine-lamivudine, for the treatment of antiretroviral-naive subjects with CCR5-tropic HIV-1 infection. J Infect Dis 2010; 201(6): 803-13.

[28] Saracino A, Monno L, Brindicci G, Trillo G, Altamura M, Punzi G, *et al.* Are the proposed env mutations actually associated with resistance to maraviroc? J Acquir Immune Defic Syndr 2010; 53(4): 550-2.

[29] Jones R, Nelson M. The role of receptors in the HIV-1 entry process. Eur J Med Res 2007; 12(9): 391-6.

[30] Fikkert V, Van Maele B, Vercammen J, Hantson A, Van Remoortel B, Michiels M, *et al.* Development of resistance against diketo derivatives of human immunodeficiency virus type 1 by progressive accumulation of integrase mutations. J Virol 2003; 77(21): 11459-70.

[31] Miller MD, Wang B, Bushman FD. Human immunodeficiency virus type 1 preintegration complexes containing discontinuous plus strands are competent to integrate *in vitro*. J Virol 1995; 69(6): 3938-44.

[32] Yoder KE, Bushman FD. Repair of gaps in retroviral DNA integration intermediates. J Virol 2000; 74(23): 11191-200.

[33] Chow SA, Vincent KA, Ellison V, Brown PO. Reversal of integration and DNA splicing mediated by integrase of human immunodeficiency virus. Science 1992; 255(5045): 723-6.

[34] Savarino A. In-Silico docking of HIV-1 integrase inhibitors reveals a novel drug type acting on an enzyme/DNA reaction intermediate. Retrovirology 2007; 4: 21.

[35] Van Maele B, Debyser Z. HIV-1 integration: an interplay between HIV-1 integrase, cellular and viral proteins. AIDS Rev 2005; 7(1): 26-43.

[36] Delelis O, Carayon K, Saib A, Deprez E, Mouscadet JF. Integrase and integration: biochemical activities of HIV-1 integrase. Retrovirology 2008; 5: 114.

[37] Katlama C, Murphy R. Emerging role of integrase inhibitors in the management of treatment-experienced patients with HIV infection. Ther Clin Risk Manag 2009; 5(2): 331-40.

[38] Correll T, Klibanov OM. Integrase inhibitors: a new treatment option for patients with human immunodeficiency virus infection. Pharmacotherapy 2008; 28(1): 90-101.

[39] Loizidou EZ, Kousiappa I, Zeinalipour-Yazdi CD, Van de Vijver DA, Kostrikis LG. Implications of HIV-1 M group polymorphisms on integrase inhibitor efficacy and resistance: genetic and structural *in silico* analyses. Biochemistry 2009; 48(1): 4-6.

[40] Malet I, Delelis O, Valantin MA, Montes B, Soulie C, Wirden M, *et al.* Mutations associated with failure of raltegravir treatment affect integrase sensitivity to the inhibitor *in vitro*. Antimicrob Agents Chemother 2008; 52(4): 1351-8.

[41] Lee JS, Calmy A, Andrieux-Meyer I, Ford N. Review of the safety, efficacy, and pharmacokinetics of elvitegravir with an emphasis on resource-limited settings. HIV AIDS (Auckl) 2012; 4: 5-15.

[42] Shimura K, Kodama E, Sakagami Y, Matsuzaki Y, Watanabe W, Yamataka K, *et al.* Broad antiretroviral activity and resistance profile of the novel human immunodeficiency virus integrase inhibitor elvitegravir (JTK-303/GS-9137). J Virol 2008; 82(2): 764-74.

[43] Goethals O, Clayton R, Van Ginderen M, Vereycken I, Wagemans E, Geluykens P, *et al.* Resistance mutations in human immunodeficiency virus type 1 integrase selected with elvitegravir confer reduced susceptibility to a wide range of integrase inhibitors. J Virol 2008; 82(21): 10366-74.

[44] Olender S, Wilkin TJ, Taylor BS, Hammer SM. Advances in antiretroviral therapy. Top Antivir Med 2012; 20(2): 61-86.

[45] van Lunzen J, Maggiolo F, Arribas JR, Rakhmanova A, Yeni P, Young B, *et al.* Once daily dolutegravir (S/GSK1349572) in combination therapy in antiretroviral-naive adults with HIV: planned interim 48 week results from SPRING-1, a dose-ranging, randomised, phase 2b trial. Lancet Infect Dis 2012; 12(2): 111-8.

[46] Stellbrink HJ, Reynes J, Lazzarin A, Voronin E, Pulido F, Felizarta F, Almond S, St Clair M, Flack N, Min S; SPRING-1 Team. Dolutegravir in antiretroviral-naive adults with HIV-1: 96-week results from a randomized dose-ranging study. AIDS 2013; 27(11): 1771-8.

CHAPTER 3

Drugs Targeting the -1 Ribosomal Frameshifting that Generates the Enzymes of the Human Immunodeficiency Virus

Léa Brakier-Gingras[1,*], Johanie Charbonneau[1] and Benjamin L. Miller[2]

[1]Department of Biochemistry, University of Montreal, Montreal, Quebec, H3T 1J4, Canada and [2]Department of Biochemistry and Biophysics, and Dermatology, University of Rochester, Rochester, New York, USA

Abstract: Translation of the full-length messenger RNA of human immunodeficiency virus of type 1 (HIV-1) uses a programmed -1 ribosomal frameshift to generate the polyprotein Gag-Pol, the precursor of the viral enzymes. This recoding event occurs at a slippery sequence followed by an irregular hairpin, the frameshift stimulatory signal, which controls the efficiency of frameshifting. In this chapter, we review the characteristics of the mechanism accounting for HIV-1 frameshifting and we examine the different approaches investigated to develop novel anti-HIV-1 drugs interfering with the frameshift, including the high-throughput screening of libraries of chemical compounds with a bicistronic reporter whose second cistron is expressed *via* HIV-1 frameshift, the use of antisense oligonucleotides binding to the frameshift stimulatory signal, and the selection and modification of chemical compounds that bind to the frameshift stimulatory signal. This latter approach is the most promising and we present results based on the modification of a compound selected by screening of a resin-bound dynamic combinatorial library. This lead compound specifically bound to HIV-1 frameshift stimulatory signal, increased HIV-1 frameshift efficiency and decreased HIV-1 infectivity.

Keywords: Antiretroviral drugs, combinatorial library, HIV-1, programmed -1 ribosomal frameshift.

INTRODUCTION

The human immunodeficiency virus of type 1 (HIV-1), the causative agent of acquired immunodeficiency syndrome (AIDS), has been the subject of intensive studies during the last two decades. Treatments with a variety of drugs, the targets of which are most frequently the viral enzymes (protease, reverse transcriptase

***Corresponding author Léa Brakier-Gingras:** Department of Biochemistry, University of Montreal, Montreal, Quebec, Canada; Tel: 514-343-6316; Fax: 514-343-2210; E-mail: lea.brakier.gingras@umontreal.ca and, more recently, integrase) are used successfully to counteract viral replication [reviewed in 1-3]. However, the emergence of *in vivo* resistance to these drugs makes it urgent to develop novel types of antiretroviral drugs [reviewed in 4]. A special recoding event, a programmed -1 ribosomal frameshift that occurs during translation of the full-length messenger RNA (mRNA) of HIV-1, is responsible for the synthesis of the precursor of the viral enzymes, Gag-Pol. Clearly, targeting this event should open the way to the development of novel interesting anti-HIV-1 drugs. In this review, we first examine briefly the current prevailing models to account for HIV-1 ribosomal frameshift. We next discuss the various approaches that have been developed to interfere with this event, and, finally, we present a successful approach, describing a novel lead compound that interferes with HIV-1 frameshift and replication.

THE PROGRAMMED -1 RIBOSOMAL FRAMESHIFT IN HIV-1

Conventional translation of the full-length HIV-1 mRNA generates Gag, the precursor of the virus structural proteins, and, *via* a programmed -1 ribosomal frameshift (-1 PRF), Gag-Pol, the precursor of the viral enzymes. Conventional translation consists of the consecutive reading of codon triplets [5, reviewed in 6] but a PRF appears to result from an alternative reading, either a doublet (-1 frameshift), as is the case for HIV-1, or a quadruplet (+1 frameshift). A PRF is not incidental, but requires specific cis elements on the mRNA and occurs to a much greater extent than accidental frameshifts. This phenomenon is found in several viruses and also in some cellular genes [for general reviews on -1 PRF, see 7-9].

The -1 PRF in HIV-1 was discovered by Jacks *et al.* [10]. More than twenty years later, the mechanism accounting for this event is not completely elucidated in spite of great progress that parallels our increased understanding of the function of the ribosome and the mechanisms of translation. In short, HIV-1 -1 PRF occurs at a slippery site, a heptanucleotide sequence, U-UUU-UUA (where the dashes separate the 0 frame codons). This site is followed by a bulged hairpin, the frameshift stimulatory signal (FSS), which is required for the frameshift to take place and controls its efficiency (Fig. **1**). In other viruses, the FSS is frequently a pseudoknot, a structure where the loop of a hairpin base–pairs to a complementary stretch of nucleotides elsewhere in the RNA chain. The use of single-molecule techniques [11] has shown that the frameshift efficiency correlates with the unwinding forces required of the ribosome to disrupt the FSS. These results were applied to a pseudoknot FSS but can likely be extrapolated to hairpin FSS. In HIV-1 full-length mRNA, it is the upper part of the FSS that acts as the effective signal, the lower part being easily unwound. Several models have been proposed to account for HIV-1 -1 PRF [reviewed in 12]. Presently, the favourite models relate the frameshift event to the resistance to unwinding of the upper part of the FSS by the ribosome helicase [13]. One model, proposed by Weiss *et al.* [14], suggests that, during translocation, the tension exerted on the mRNA, due to the resistance to unwinding of the FSS, results in a break of the codon-anticodon interactions between the mRNA and the deacylated and peptidyl transfer RNAs (tRNAs), followed by a shift of these tRNAs so they occupy, respectively, the standard E and P sites, and by the re-pairing of these tRNAs to the mRNA in the -1 frame. A second model, proposed by Léger *et al.* [15], suggests that an incomplete translocation, due to the resistance to unwinding of the FSS, occurs in the cycle of elongation prior to the occupancy of the decoding site by the slippery sequence. Because of this incomplete translocation, the deacylated and peptidyl tRNAs occupy intermediate sites and the incoming aminoacyl-tRNA must also occupy an intermediate entry (A/T) site. In this model, the frameshift occurs after the arrival of the incoming tRNA and before its accommodation in the A site and peptidyl transfer. This model takes into account the fact that the codon preceding the slippery sequence influences the shift. The major difference between these two models is that the break of the codon-anticodon interactions and the shift of the tRNAs occur during translocation in the model of Weiss *et al.* while, in the model of Léger *et al.* codon-anticodon interactions are maintained during translocation and the shift occurs after this step, upon the incoming of the new aminoacyl-tRNA (see Fig. **2** for these two models). In both models, it is likely that the shift of the tRNAs is sequential rather than simultaneous. Cryo-electron microscopy studies [16] support the relationship between an interference with translocation and the -1 PRF. Finally, a third model proposed that, when the slippery sequence occupies the P and A site, the frameshift can occur before peptidyl transfer and during aminoacyl-tRNA accommodation from the A/T to the A site. This accommodation would be accompanied by a 9 Å movement of the incoming tRNA anticodon. This movement, which drags the mRNA, causes a tension in this mRNA, because of the resistance to unwinding of the FSS. This tension is relieved by a break of codon-anticodon interactions between the mRNA and the peptidyl-tRNA and the incoming aminoacyl-tRNA, followed by a shift of the mRNA in the 3' direction and by the re-pairing of the tRNAs in the -1 frame [17]. As recently discussed by Liao *et al.* [18] and Dinman [9], it is very likely that different pathways are simultaneously used and, therefore, the different models could coexist. However, the 9 Å movement of the tRNA anticodon of the incoming tRNA was not confirmed [19], which does not support the third model. It must be noted that only a fraction (5-10%) of the elongating ribosomes make a frameshift, the majority of them succeeding in unwinding the FSS without a shift of the tRNAs. In addition, Sørensen and colleagues [20] showed that the interaction of the ribosome with a FSS can lead to a permanent stalling of the ribosome. This stalling could apply to frameshifted as well as non-frameshifted ribosomes, and therefore could influence the overall translation of the mRNA while altering the frameshift efficiency. Obviously, more high-resolution as well as time-resolved techniques will be required to fully understand the mechanism of HIV-1 frameshift.

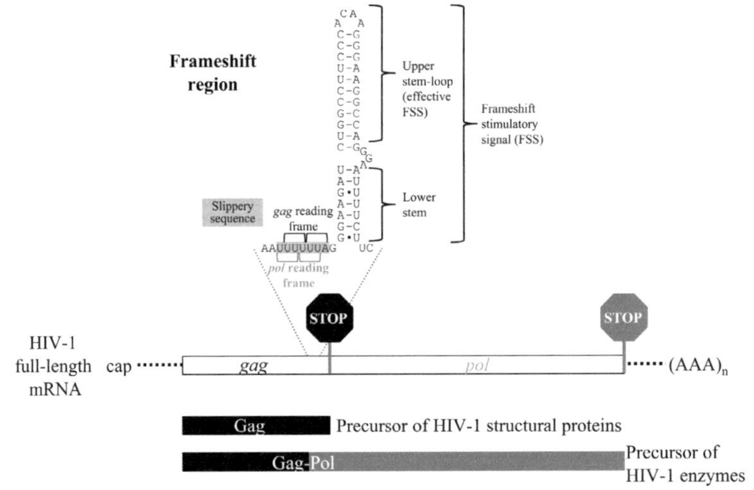

Figure 1: Schematic view of HIV-1 full-length mRNA presenting the frameshift region encompassing the slippery sequence, where the frameshift occurs, and the frameshift stimulatory signal (FSS). The Gag and Gag-Pol precursors, which are produced by translation of this mRNA, are also shown. Conventional translation of HIV-1 full-length mRNA generates Gag, the precursor of HIV-1 structural proteins whereas a programmed -1 ribosomal frameshift (-1 PRF) generates Gag-Pol, the precursor of HIV-1 enzymes.

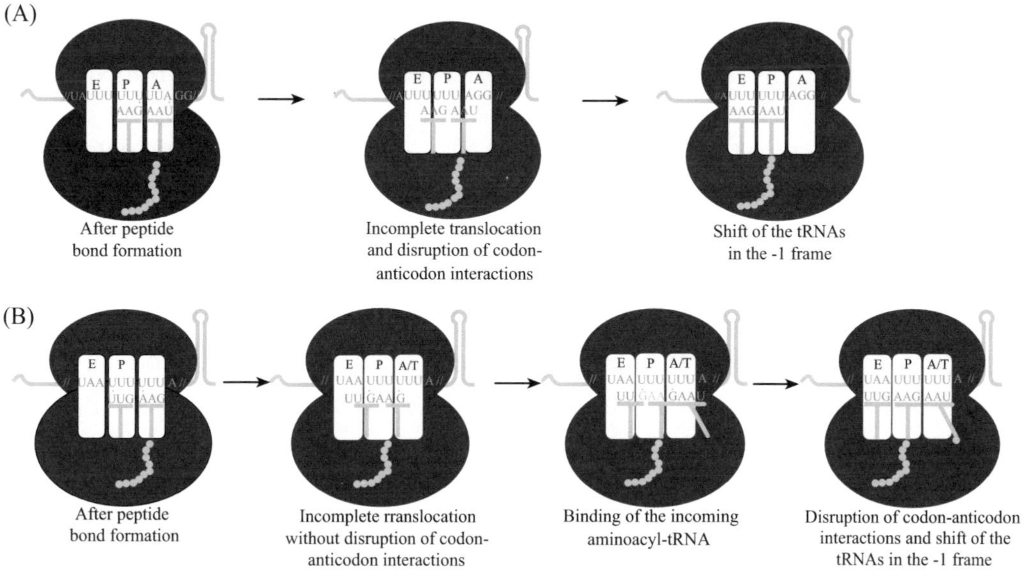

Figure 2: Models for the programmed -1 frameshift. (A) Model proposed by Weiss *et al.* [14]. The frameshift occurs during translocation of the tRNAs after peptide bond formation. During this step, the resistance of the FSS to unwinding results in an incomplete translocation of the mRNA (2 nt instead of 3 nt), accompanied by a break of the interactions between the codons of the mRNA and the anticodons of the tRNAs. The tRNAs then shift in the -1 frame and occupy their standard binding sites, and their anticodons can re-pair to the codons of the mRNA. (B) Model proposed by Léger *et al.* [15]. The resistance of FSS to unwinding also results in an incomplete translocation after peptide bond formation, not breaking the codon-anticodon interactions, with the consequence that the tRNAs occupy intermediate binding sites. The incoming aminoacyl-tRNA then binds to the mRNA but has also to occupy an intermediate entry site. The tendency of the tRNAs to occupy their standard sites drives them to shift the reading frame by breaking the codon-anticodon interactions and re-pairing in the -1 frame. Sites A/T, A, P and E are, respectively, the entry site for the aminoacyl-tRNA, the aminoacyl-tRNA binding site, the peptidyl-tRNA binding site and the deacylated tRNA exit site, corresponding to the sites successively occupied by a tRNA binding to the ribosome. Note that the incomplete translocation in (B) takes place in the cycle of elongation that precedes the cycle described in (A). As discussed in the text, the two models could coexist. In both models, whether the re-pairing also involves the E-site tRNA is still unknown. This re-pairing in the E site would allow the formation of three base-pairs in the model described in (A) but only one in the model described in (B). However, base-pairing in the E site is not stringently controlled.

Although the frameshift occurs during the elongation of translation, it has been shown that it is influenced by the rate of initiation. Indeed, every ribosome must unwind the FSS to continue its translation. Depending on the rate of initiation, the distance between successive ribosomes is sufficient or not to allow the FSS to refold [21, 22]. It is also possible that the highly structured RNA region [23] that the ribosomes must translate before reaching the frameshift region influences the movement of the ribosomes and the probability that they encounter a folded FSS.

Silencing RNA screens have been used to identify host factors affecting HIV-1 replication [24-26]. It should be possible to apply this silencing approach to find out which host factors specifically modulate HIV-1 frameshift. So far, two factors that are related to the translation machinery and identified as interfering with HIV-1 replication by Brass *et al.* [24] were found to increase HIV-1 frameshift about two-fold. These factors are the release factor eRF1 [27] and an RNA dimethylase that dimethylates two adjacent conserved adenines in the last helix of 18S rRNA[1]. In the case of eRF1, the effect on frameshift can be ascribed to a decrease in the recycling of the ribosomes [28], which slows down the initiation of translation and increases the distance between the elongating ribosomes and the probability that they encounter a folded FSS. As to the lack of dimethylation of the two adenines, it could affect the conformation of the ribosomes at the E site, facilitating the shift of the deacylated tRNA and the subsequent shift of the other tRNAs. However, the silencing of the dimethylase that increases HIV-1 frameshift was found to stimulate HIV-1 replication in contrast to the observations of Brass *et al.* [24]. The consequences of the decrease in eRF1 expression on HIV-1 replication were not verified by Kobayashi *et al.* [27]. It is interesting to observe that sparsomycin, a drug that binds to the ribosome, was also found to increase HIV-1 frameshift about two-fold and to stimulate HIV-1 replication [29]. Also, a number of signal transduction pathways can influence -1 PRF [30], which should be identified with the silencing approach. In addition, assays were performed, using a yeast three-hybrid screen, to identify cellular factors that could bind an FSS (a pseudoknot in those assays) and thus influence frameshifting, but they were unsuccessful[2]. In a recent study, however, Green *et al.* [31], using as a bait the pseudoknot allowing the synthesis of Gag-Pol in the Moloney murine retrovirus *via* the readthrough of a stop codon, identified a ribosomal protein of the large subunit, L4, which increased the readthrough. They next found that L4 seems to increase the propensity for recoding to occur in the presence of different recoding signals, among which the FSS of HIV-1. Protein

[1] unpublished results from Dulude, D. and Brakier-Gingras, L.
[2] unpublished results from Dinman, J.D. and from Brierley, I.

L4 is located inside the ribosome, lining the exit tunnel for the growing polypeptide [32] and its effect on the recoding appears to depend on an extraribosomal function.

It is easy to understand that decreasing the frameshift efficiency of HIV-1 decreases the number of complete infectious virions. But what happens when the frameshift efficiency increases? Shehu-Xilaga *et al.* [33] succeeded in artificially increasing the Gag-Pol/Gag ratio four-fold by transfecting 293T cells with HIV-1 proviral DNA and an HIV-1 Gag-Pol expression vector. Under these conditions, the viral replication was inhibited. Interestingly, it was shown that the ratio of Gag-Pol to Gag within the virions produced in these conditions was not altered. However, the dimeric genomic RNA packaged within the virions was less stable. One possible explanation is that the extra Gag-Pol present in the cytoplasm sequesters a cellular factor and prevents it from stabilizing the dimeric genomic RNA within the virions.

Finally, it is important to know that -1 PRFs are also found in cellular genes. One example is the product of the paternally expressed gene, PEG10 [34, 35], a gene derived from a retrotransposon, which plays a role in embryonic development, normal cell homeostasis and cancer [36]. Other examples are the antigene Ma3, which is associated with paraneoplastic disorders [37], and the tumor suppressor adenomatous polyposis coli (APC), a regulator of intestinal cell stem proliferation [38]. More recently, the application of the powerful ribosome profiling strategy [39] revealed that there is more alternative decoding than previously expected in human genes [40]. Also, interesting bioinformatics programs have been developed to predict frameshift signals in eukaryotes [41-43]. Altogether, these observations stress that any drug exerting a general effect on -1 PRF should be avoided.

IN SEARCH OF A DRUG INTERFERING WITH HIV-1 RIBOSOMAL FRAMESHIFT

A first assay with a monocistronic reporter heralded the start of studies aiming at targeting HIV-1 frameshift [44]. It led to the selection of one compound, a benzene derivative named RG250, which was shown later to bind not only the FSS of HIV-1 but also a number of RNA targets, including the ribosome [45].

RG250 increased the frameshift efficiency about two-fold, but, although it was found to interfere with HIV-1 replication, it now appears that this effect results from the toxicity of the drug [46]. This first assay was followed by the development and use of bicistronic reporters where the two cistrons are separated by the HIV-1 frameshift region and the expression of the second cistron is depending upon the frameshift [47-50]. A number of compounds were thus selected by high-throughput screening of a library of arginine-rich peptides or small chemical compounds, which decreased or increased frameshift efficiency about two-fold [51, (Brakier-Gingras and colleagues, unpublished)[3]]. However, with that type of reporter, the target was always found to be the ribosome, and the selected compounds did not show any specificity for HIV-1 frameshift. These results lead us to conclude that this approach is not viable, since it selects drugs that not only could affect frameshifting in cellular genes but could also interfere with the function of the ribosome, a key-component of cellular life. Surprisingly, it had been noted that drugs acting on the ribosome and increasing the frameshift about two-fold did not inhibit HIV-1 replication and even stimulated it [29][3]. Also, the group of Brierley investigated to which extent frameshift efficiency of Rous sarcoma virus (RSV) could be altered without compromising the virus replication. They found that point mutations decreasing the frameshift efficiency three-fold are inhibitory while a three-fold increase in the frameshift efficiency is well-tolerated [52].

Another approach consisted of using an antisense oligonucleotide, complementary to a sequence of the FSS. This was applied to the FSS of the coronavirus responsible for severe acute respiratory syndrome (SARS) [53]. This FSS is a pseudoknot structure and the binding of an antisense peptide-nucleic acid molecule, which stabilizes this pseudoknot, probably stalls the ribosome, interfering with the synthesis of both frameshifted and non-frameshifted products. No success with this approach was reported for HIV-1, except for the crosslinking of an oligonucleotide to HIV-1 FSS, which blocked translation of HIV-1 mRNA. Unfortunately, this procedure cannot be used for clinical applications [54]. Furthermore, a potential problem with antisense drugs is that they can induce dramatic immune modulation by binding to Toll-like receptors [55].

---

[3] unpublished results from Dulude, D. and Brakier-Gingras, L.

TARGETING THE FSS OF HIV-1

A much more promising approach than the use of bicistronic reporters reported above is to discover drugs that selectively bind to HIV-1 FSS and thereby interfere with the frameshift. This approach has been used independently by the groups of Butcher and Miller. The group of Butcher showed that guanidoneomycin B could bind to HIV-1 FSS although with a low specificity [56]. This initial study provides useful hints on the characteristics that small molecules should have to interact specifically with HIV-1 FSS. Butcher and colleagues next carried out a high-throughput screen of 34,500 small molecules to find molecules that bind to HIV-1 FSS and from that screen identified doxorubicin as a "hit". This compound binds to HIV-1 FSS with a low micromolar affinity (K_d=2.8 μM), increases the lower helix stability and binds to the bulge. However, doxorubicin lacks specificity and binds to other targets, among which double-stranded DNA to which it binds with an affinity of 4 nM [57]. This compound causes a small decrease in frameshift efficiency but this may result from the binding of doxorubicin to the ribosome.

In order to select drugs binding to HIV-1 effective FSS, the Miller group screened an 11,325 member resin-bound dynamic combinatorial library, the design of which was based on a core structure inspired by nucleic acid binding, bisintercalating natural products [58]. They selected a disulfide-containing peptide (**1**, in Fig. **3**), which was stabilized by replacing the disulfide with an olefin bioisostere (**2**, in Fig. **3**) [59]. The affinity of the disulfide-containing peptide and its stabilized derivative for the HIV-1 FSS upper stem-loop was in the high nanomolar to low micromolar range. Neither the disulfide compound nor the olefin derivative showed any affinity for "off-target" RNAs (yeast tRNAs and total yeast RNA); and titrations with the disulfide into variants of the HIV-1 FSS indicated that binding was more sensitive to changes in the loop region than in the stem. The product was not toxic to human fibroblasts at concentrations up to 1 mM. Analysis of a series of structure-activity relationships suggested that the core peptide was critical for sequence selectivity, while pendant heterocycles were essential for ligand affinity.

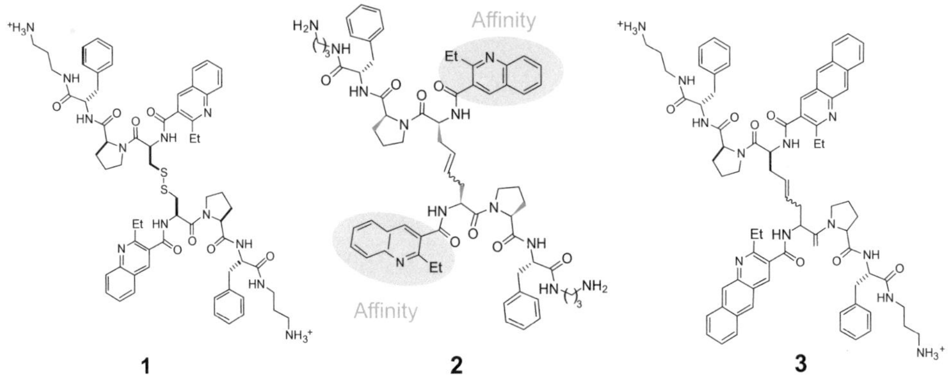

1 **2** **3**

Figure 3: Compounds targeting HIV-1 FSS developed by Miller and colleagues. (1) "hit" compound identified *via* a Resin-Bound Dynamic Combinatorial Chemistry strategy. (2) Olefin bioisostere of (1); as both *E* and *Z* olefin isomers had similar affinity for the HIV-1 FSS, this stereochemistry is left undefined. A series of analogs of (1) and (2) indicated that affinity for the FSS required the presence of the quinoline moieties, while sequence selectivity derived from the peptide core. This led to the synthesis and testing of (3), a compound with high affinity for HIV-1 FSS, and an ability to interfere with viral infectivity in a pseudotyped HIV-1 assay.

Building on these results, Miller and colleagues extended the pi-surface area of their lead compound to obtain a new structure (**3**, in Fig. **3**) with an approximately 3.7-fold higher affinity (K_D = 89 nM for the HIV-1 FSS upper stem-loop)[4]. This molecule was also found to have high selectivity for binding the HIV-1 FSS over the FSS from human T-cell leukemia virus type 2 (HTLV-2). The compound was found to increase frameshifting about two-fold in a bicistronic reporter system containing the HIV-1 FSS and transfected in 293T cells, but it had no effect on an analogous reporter system containing the HTLV-2 FSS. Compound-dependent decreases in total Fluc and Rluc production were observed for both the -1 and 0-frame systems. This is to be expected as binding of the compound to the FSS in each case could hinder the ability of ribosomes to read through this sequence. Most importantly, this compound also produced a concentration-dependent decrease in viral infectivity in a single-round pseudotyped HIV-1 assay. This decrease was obtained at concentrations, well below the point at which toxic effects were observed in standard colorimetric assays for cell viability with tetrazolium dye (MTT), indicating the observed decrease is not due to general toxicity. While the activity of the compound in this assay will need to be

[4] Ofori, L., Bennett, R.P., Smith, H.C., Miller, B.L. submitted for publication.

enhanced *via* further analog synthesis, these results nevertheless provide useful validation of the strategy of targeting the FSS. A conundrum is that drugs previously shown to increase the frameshift about two-fold when binding to the ribosome did not interfere with HIV-1 replication, as mentioned above, and a threshold of a four-fold increase appeared to be required to interfere with HIV-1 replication (see Shehu-Xhilaga *et al.* 2001). In contrast, the compound developed by the Miller group has the property to interfere with HIV-1 replication while increasing HIV-1 frameshift two-fold. This interference could result from the decreased translation of the full-length viral mRNA in the presence of the compound. Another possibility, although purely speculative, is that the compound bound to the FSS could be incorporated into the virions, and, subsequently, could interfere with viral infectivity. Further work is required to elucidate the mechanism of action of this compound. Also, it was observed that while the compounds shown in Fig. **3** are larger than typical protein-directed small molecule drugs, they still readily penetrate cells. Except in rare cases, it is likely that most RNA-targeted therapeutic candidates will be similarly large, given the surface area that must be addressed in order to attain specificity.

Of note, all the studies which aimed at finding drugs interfering with HIV-1 frameshift were done with HIV-1 group M subtype B, the group that prevails in North America and Europe. The structure of HIV-1 FSS is conserved among HIV-1 group M subtypes but there are minor differences in its sequence [60], which suggests that different compounds will need to be developed against the different subtypes.

RESISTANCE TO DRUGS TARGETING HIV-1 FRAMESHIFT STIMULATORY SIGNAL

It is likely that, as for all other drugs against HIV-1, the virus will evolve by mutating, so as to escape the effect of drugs targeting the FSS. Potential drugs interfering with HIV-1 frameshift will have to be used in combination with other drugs. It is important to notice that several mutations conferring resistance to protease were found in the HIV-1 frameshift region [61-65]. These mutations did not cause any significant increase in HIV-1 frameshift efficiency, ruling out a previous suggestion that increasing the production of protease could counteract the effect of mutations decreasing the activity of the protease at cleavage sites [66]. Also, mutations in the upper stem, the effective FSS, were generally rare. However, it cannot be excluded that mutations could occur in the upper stem and simultaneously confer resistance to protease inhibitors and to drugs binding HIV-1 FSS and altering the -1 PRF. Therefore, caution must be exerted in the choice of drugs associated with the drugs acting on HIV-1 frameshift.

CONCLUSION

Targeting the event responsible for the synthesis of HIV-1 enzymes offers the advantage of simultaneously acting on the production of protease, reverse transcriptase and integrase and thus appears as a very powerful approach to interfere with the virus propagation. This approach had remained elusive so far and all the drugs selected as interfering with the frameshift event had been found to target the ribosome. But recently, an appropriate strategy that was designed to select drugs specifically binding to HIV-1 FSS has led to successful results, with the obtention of a lead compound that was able to interfere with HIV-1 replication. It can be predicted that this approach will provide a novel interesting class of anti-HIV drugs.

ACKNOWLEDGEMENTS

L. Brakier-Gingras thanks the Canadian Institutes of Health Research (CIHR) for support of this work (grant HOP86604) and B. L. Miller thanks the National Institutes of Health / NIGMS for support of this work (grant R01GM100788).

CONFLICT OF INTEREST

The authors confirm that this chapter contents have no conflict of interest.

REFERENCES

[1] Flexner C. HIV drug development: the next 25 years. Nat Rev Drug Discov 2007; 6(12): 959-66.

[2] Sagar M. Clinical implications of new findings in HIV basic research. HIV Ther 2009; 3(4): 351-60.

[3] Desai M, Iyer G, Dikshit RK. Antiretroviral drugs: critical issues and recent advances. Indian J Pharmacol 2012; 44(3): 288-98.

[4] Johnson VA, Brun-Vezinet F, Clotet B, *et al.* Update of the drug resistance mutations in HIV-1: December 2009. Top HIV Med 2009; 17(5): 138-45.

[5] Moore PB, Steitz TA. The roles of RNA in the synthesis of protein. Cold Spring Harb Perspect Biol 2011; 3(11): a003780.

[6] Schmeing TM, Ramakrishnan V. What recent ribosome structures have revealed about the mechanism of translation. Nature 2009; 461(7268): 1234-42.

[7] Giedroc DP, Cornish PV. Frameshifting RNA pseudoknots: structure and mechanism. Virus Res 2009; 139(2): 193-208.

[8] Brierley I, Gilbert RJC, Pennell S. Pseudoknot-dependent programmed -1 ribosomal frameshifting: structures, mechanisms and models. In: Atkins JF, Gesteland RF, editors. Recoding: Expansion of Decoding Rules Enriches Gene Expression. New York, NY; Springer; 2010; pp. 149-74.

[9] Dinman JD. Control of gene expression by translational recoding. Adv Protein Chem Struct Biol 2012; 86: 129-49.

[10] Jacks T, Power MD, Masiarz FR, Luciw PA, Barr PJ, Varmus HE. Characterization of ribosomal frameshifting in HIV-1 gag-pol expression. Nature 1988; 331(6153): 280-3.

[11] Chang KC. Revealing -1 programmed ribosomal frameshifting mechanisms by single-molecule techniques and computational methods. Comput Math Methods Med 2012; 2012; article ID: 569870.

[12] Brakier-Gingras L, Dulude D. Programmed -1 ribosomal frameshift in the human immunodeficiency virus of type 1. In: Atkins JF, Gesteland, RF editors. Recoding: Expansion of Decoding Rules Enriches Gene Expression. New York, NY: Springer; 2010. pp.175-92..

[13] Qu X, Wen JD, Lancaster L, Noller HF, Bustamante C, Tinoco I, Jr. The ribosome uses two active mechanisms to unwind messenger RNA during translation. Nature 2011; 475(7354): 118-21.

[14] Weiss RB, Dunn DM, Shuh M, Atkins JF, Gesteland RF. E. coli ribosomes re-phase on retroviral frameshift signals at rates ranging from 2 to 50 percent. New Biol 1989; 1(2): 159-69.

[15] Léger M, Dulude D, Steinberg SV, Brakier-Gingras L. The three transfer RNAs occupying the A, P and E sites on the ribosome are involved in viral programmed -1 ribosomal frameshift. Nucleic Acids Res 2007; 35(16): 5581-92.

[16] Namy O, Moran SJ, Stuart DI, Gilbert RJ, Brierley I. A mechanical explanation of RNA pseudoknot function in programmed ribosomal frameshifting. Nature 2006; 441(7090): 244-7.

[17] Plant EP, Jacobs KL, Harger JW, *et al.* The 9-A solution: how mRNA pseudoknots promote efficient programmed -1 ribosomal frameshifting. RNA 2003; 9(2): 168-74.

[18] Liao PY, Choi YS, Dinman JD, Lee KH. The many paths to frameshifting: kinetic modelling and analysis of the effects of different elongation steps on programmed -1 ribosomal frameshifting. Nucleic Acids Res 2011; 39(1): 300-12.

[19] Schmeing TM, Voorhees RM, Kelley AC, Ramakrishnan V. How mutations in tRNA distant from the anticodon affect the fidelity of decoding. Nat Struct Mol Biol 2011; 18(4): 432-6.

[20] Tholstrup J, Oddershede LB, Sorensen MA. mRNA pseudoknot structures can act as ribosomal roadblocks. Nucleic Acids Res 2012; 40(1): 303-13.

[21] Gendron K, Charbonneau J, Dulude D, Heveker N, Ferbeyre G, Brakier-Gingras L. The presence of the TAR RNA structure alters the programmed -1 ribosomal frameshift efficiency of the human immunodeficiency virus type 1 (HIV-1) by modifying the rate of translation initiation. Nucleic Acids Res 2008; 36(1): 30-40.

[22] Charbonneau J, Gendron K, Ferbeyre G, Brakier-Gingras L. The 5' UTR of HIV-1 full-length mRNA and the Tat viral protein modulate the programmed -1 ribosomal frameshift that generates HIV-1 enzymes. RNA 2012; 18(3): 519-29.

[23] Watts JM, Dang KK, Gorelick RJ, *et al.* Architecture and secondary structure of an entire HIV-1 RNA genome. Nature 2009; 460(7256): 711-6.

[24] Brass AL, Dykxhoorn DM, Benita Y, *et al.* Identification of host proteins required for HIV infection through a functional genomic screen. Science 2008; 319(5865): 921-6.

[25] Bushman FD, Malani N, Fernandes J, *et al.* Host cell factors in HIV replication: meta-analysis of genome-wide studies. PLoS Pathog 2009; 5(5): e1000437.

[26] Goff SP. Host factors exploited by retroviruses. Nat Rev Microbiol 2007; 5(4): 253-63.

[27] Kobayashi Y, Zhuang J, Peltz S, Dougherty J. Identification of a cellular factor that modulates HIV-1 programmed ribosomal frameshifting. J Biol Chem 2010; 285(26): 19776-84.

[28] Shoemaker CJ, Green R. Kinetic analysis reveals the ordered coupling of translation termination and ribosome recycling in yeast. Proc Natl Acad Sci U S A. 2011; 108(51): E1392-8.

[29] Miyauchi K, Komano J, Myint L, *et al.* Rapid propagation of low-fitness drug-resistant mutants of human immunodeficiency virus type 1 by a streptococcal metabolite sparsomycin. Antivir Chem Chemother 2006; 17(4): 167-74.

[30] Turkel S, Kaplan G, Farabaugh PJ. Glucose signalling pathway controls the programmed ribosomal frameshift efficiency in retroviral-like element Ty3 in Saccharomyces cerevisiae. Yeast 2011; 28(11): 799-808.

[31] Green L, Houck-Loomis B, Yueh A, Goff SP. Large ribosomal protein 4 increases efficiency of viral recoding sequences. J Virol 2012; 86(17): 8949-58.

[32] Ben-Shem A, Garreau de Loubresse N, Melnikov S, Jenner L, Yusupova G, Yusupov M. The structure of the eukaryotic ribosome at 3.0 A resolution. Science 2011; 334(6062): 1524-9.

[33] Shehu-Xhilaga M, Crowe SM, Mak J. Maintenance of the Gag/Gag-Pol ratio is important for human immunodeficiency virus type 1 RNA dimerization and viral infectivity. J Virol 2001; 75(4): 1834-41.

[34] Shigemoto K, Brennan J, Walls E, *et al.* Identification and characterisation of a developmentally regulated mammalian gene that utilises -1 programmed ribosomal frameshifting. Nucleic Acids Res 2001; 29(19): 4079-88.

[35] Manktelow E, Shigemoto K, Brierley I. Characterization of the frameshift signal of Edr, a mammalian example of programmed -1 ribosomal frameshifting. Nucleic Acids Res 2005; 33(5): 1553-63.

[36] Lux H, Flammann H, Hafner M, Lux A. Genetic and molecular analyses of PEG10 reveal new aspects of genomic organization, transcription and translation. PLoS One 2010; 5(1): e8686.

[37] Wills NM, Moore B, Hammer A, Gesteland RF, Atkins JF. A functional -1 ribosomal frameshift signal in the human paraneoplastic Ma3 gene. J Biol Chem 2006; 281(11): 7082-8.

[38] Baranov PV, Wills NM, Barriscale KA, *et al.* Programmed ribosomal frameshifting in the expression of the regulator of intestinal stem cell proliferation, adenomatous polyposis coli (APC). RNA Biol 2011; 8(4): 637-47.

[39] Ingolia NT, Ghaemmaghami S, Newman JR, Weissman JS. Genome-wide analysis *in vivo* of translation with nucleotide resolution using ribosome profiling. Science 2009; 324(5924): 218-23.

[40] Michel AM, Roy Choudhury K, Firth AE, Ingolia NT, Atkins JF, Baranov PV. Observation of dually decoded regions of the human genome using ribosome profiling data. Genome Res 2012: 2219-29.

[41] Baranov PV, Gurvich OL, Fayet O, *et al.* RECODE: a database of frameshifting, bypassing and codon redefinition utilized for gene expression. Nucleic Acids Res 2001; 29(1): 264-7.

[42] Belew AT, Hepler NL, Jacobs JL, Dinman JD. PRFdb: a database of computationally predicted eukaryotic programmed -1 ribosomal frameshift signals. BMC genomics 2008; 9: 339.

[43] Moon S, Byun Y, Han K. FSDB: a frameshift signal database. Comput Biol Chem 2007; 31(4): 298-302.
[44] Hung M, Patel P, Davis S, Green SR. Importance of ribosomal frameshifting for human immunodeficiency virus type 1 particle assembly and replication. J Virol 1998; 72(6): 4819-24.
[45] Marcheschi RJ, Tonelli M, Kumar A, Butcher SE. Structure of the HIV-1 Frameshift Site RNA Bound to a Small Molecule Inhibitor of Viral Replication. ACS Chem Biol 2011; 6(8): 857-64.
[46] Brierley I, Dos Ramos FJ. Programmed ribosomal frameshifting in HIV-1 and the SARS-CoV. Virus Res 2006; 119(1): 29-42.
[47] Grentzmann G, Ingram JA, Kelly PJ, Gesteland RF, Atkins JF. A dual-luciferase reporter system for studying recoding signals. RNA 1998; 4(4): 479-86.
[48] Harger JW, Dinman JD. An *in vivo* dual-luciferase assay system for studying translational recoding in the yeast Saccharomyces cerevisiae. RNA 2003; 9(8): 1019-24.
[49] Dulude D, Berchiche YA, Gendron K, Brakier-Gingras L, Heveker N. Decreasing the frameshift efficiency translates into an equivalent reduction of the replication of the human immunodeficiency virus type 1. Virology 2006; 345(1): 127-36.
[50] Rakauskaite R, Liao PY, Rhodin MH, Lee K, Dinman JD. A rapid, inexpensive yeast-based dual-fluorescence assay of programmed--1 ribosomal frameshifting for high-throughput screening. Nucleic Acids Res 2011; 39(14): e97.
[51] Dulude D, Theberge-Julien G, Brakier-Gingras L, Heveker N. Selection of peptides interfering with a ribosomal frameshift in the human immunodeficiency virus type 1. RNA 2008; 14(5): 981-91.
[52] Nikolic EI, King LM, Vidakovic M, Irigoyen N, Brierley I. Modulation of ribosomal frameshifting frequency and its effect on the replication of rous sarcoma virus. J Virol 2012; 86(21): 11581-94.
[53] Ahn DG, Lee W, Choi JK, *et al.* Interference of ribosomal frameshifting by antisense peptide nucleic acids suppresses SARS coronavirus replication. Antiviral Res 2011; 91(1): 1-10.
[54] Aupeix-Scheidler K, Chabas S, Bidou L, Rousset JP, Leng M, Toulme JJ. Inhibition of *in vitro* and *ex vivo* translation by a transplatin-modified oligo(2'-O-methylribonucleotide) directed against the HIV-1 gag-pol frameshift signal. Nucleic Acids Res 2000; 28(2): 438-45.
[55] Agrawal S, Kandimalla ER. Role of Toll-like receptors in antisense and siRNA [corrected]. Nat Biotechnol 2004; 22(12): 1533-7.
[56] Staple DW, Venditti V, Niccolai N, Elson-Schwab L, Tor Y, Butcher SE. Guanidinoneomycin B recognition of an HIV-1 RNA helix. Chembiochem 2008; 9(1): 93-102.
[57] Marcheschi RJ, Mouzakis KD, Butcher SE. Selection and characterization of small molecules that bind the HIV-1 frameshift site RNA. ACS Chem Biol 2009; 4(10): 844-54.
[58] McNaughton BR, Gareiss PC, Miller BL. Identification of a selective small-molecule ligand for HIV-1 frameshift-inducing stem-loop RNA from an 11,325 member resin bound dynamic combinatorial library. J Am Chem Soc 2007; 129(37): 11306-7.
[59] Palde PB, Ofori LO, Gareiss PC, Lerea J, Miller BL. Strategies for recognition of stem-loop RNA structures by synthetic ligands: application to the HIV-1 frameshift stimulatory sequence. J Med Chem 2010; 53(16): 6018-27.
[60] Baril M, Dulude D, Gendron K, Lemay G, Brakier-Gingras L. Efficiency of a programmed -1 ribosomal frameshift in the different subtypes of the human immunodeficiency virus type 1 group M. RNA 2003; 9(10): 1246-53.
[61] Girnary R, King L, Robinson L, Elston R, Brierley I. Structure-function analysis of the ribosomal frameshifting signal of two human immunodeficiency virus type 1 isolates with increased resistance to viral protease inhibitors. J Gen Virol 2007; 88(Pt 1): 226-35.

[62] Knops E, Brakier-Gingras L, Schulter E, Pfister H, Kaiser R, Verheyen J. Mutational patterns in the frameshift-regulating site of HIV-1 selected by protease inhibitors. Med Microbiol Immunol 2011: 213-8.

[63] Larrouy L, Chazallon C, Landman R, *et al.* Gag mutations can impact virological response to dual-boosted protease inhibitor combinations in antiretroviral-naive HIV-infected patients. Antimicrob Agents Chemother 2010; 54(7): 2910-9.

[64] Knops E, Brakier-Gingras L, Schulter E, Pfister H, Kaiser R, Verheyen J. Mutational patterns in the frameshift-regulating site of HIV-1 selected by protease inhibitors. Med Microbiol Immunol 2012; 201(2): 213-8.

[65] Nijhuis M, van Maarseveen NM, Lastere S, *et al.* A novel substrate-based HIV-1 protease inhibitor drug resistance mechanism. PLoS Med 2007; 4(1): e36.

[66] Doyon L, Payant C, Brakier-Gingras L, Lamarre D. Novel Gag-Pol frameshift site in human immunodeficiency virus type 1 variants resistant to protease inhibitors. J Virol 1998; 72(7): 6146-50.

CHAPTER 4

Sensing of SNP in HIV-1 Genome Using Fluorescent Oligonucleotide Probes

Kira Astakhova*

Nucleic Acid Center, Department of Physics, Chemistry and Pharmacy, Campusvej 55, 5230 Odense M, Denmark

Abstract: Single nucleotide polymorphisms (SNPs) are gaining increasing attention in modern diagnostics and research, serving as markers on genetic predispositions, clinically evident disorders and diverse drug responses. Genome of human immunodeficiency virus (HIV-1) contains multiple SNPs due to mistakes of reverse transcriptase converting RNA genome of HIV-1 into cDNA. Some of these SNPs cause resistance to drugs applied for the treatment of HIV/AIDS. Generally, current assays for SNP diagnostics, including HIV-1, can be divided into two broad categories: 1) sophisticated, high-throughput laboratory machines, and 2) easy-to-use, portable devices. Present sophisticated SNP diagnostics of HIV-1 primarily use enzymatic reactions in different formats including sequencing, polymerase-chain reaction (PCR) and microarrays. In doing this, the enzymes help to address the required sensitivity and specificity of the detection. On the other hand, an ideal portable method for the detection of SNP would work by allowing a simple mixing of a cDNA or RNA target with a probe and obtaining a single right away without applying an enzyme or state-of-the-art equipment. Remarkable progress has been achieved in recent years within both categories of methods. To date, most enzymatic and enzyme-free diagnostic strategies apply fluorescently labeled oligonucleotides - rationally designed probes or primers containing a dye(s) of choice in the desired position(s) of a nucleotide chain. In this chapter, current SNP sensing approaches in HIV-1 cDNA and RNA are described with a main focus on recently developed fluorescent oligonucleotide probes. The chapter includes up-to-date review of sophisticated and portable biosensors for HIV diagnostics, and several exciting emerging technologies are highlighted.

Keywords: Diagnostics, enzyme-free assays, fluorescence, genotyping, HIV-1, imaging, nanoparticles, oligonucleotide probe, PCR, SNP.

INTRODUCTION

During the past decades, the human immunodeficiency virus type-1 (HIV-1) has

***Corresponding author Kira Astakhova:** Nucleic Acid Center, Department of Physics, Chemistry and Pharmacy, Campusvej 55, 5230 Odense M, Denmark; Tel: +45-6550-25-23; E-mail: ias@sdu.dk

Atta-ur-Rahman (Ed)

been the object of intensive studies [1-24]. Imaging and diagnostics of both HIV-1 RNA and cDNA are of high scientific and clinical importance, and include studies of the viral life-cycle and development of nucleic acid-based HIV clinical tests. The antiretroviral HIV/AIDS treatment reduces both the mortality and morbidity of an HIV-1 infection. However, this therapy often fails due to drug-resistant HIV-1 variants containing single point mutations (*i.e.,* single-nucleotide polymorphisms, or SNPs) in HIV-1 genome. Multiple SNPs are widely spread in the HIV-1 RNA genome due to a high number of errors during reverse transcription of retroviral RNA.

Fluorescence-based technologies offer new opportunities for detection, quantification and characterization of viral nucleic acids. Optical imaging and clinical diagnostics of both HIV-1 DNA and RNA targets can be performed using advanced fluorescent oligonucleotide probes. To date, various methods have been developed for the detection of SNPs; most of them require pre-amplification of genomic DNA/RNA (*e.g.,* by PCR), followed by SNP genotyping (*i.e.,* by an allele-specific reaction). The latter may be combined with homogeneous or solid-phase detection *e.g.,* fluorescence intensity, fluorescence polarization or mass spectrometry. Each of these methods has its own strengths and weaknesses and there is still no universal approach of choice. In the present chapter, these assays are reviewed as parts of two major categories: 1) those applied in sophisticated, high-throughput laboratory machines, and 2) techniques suitable for easy-to-use, portable devices.

Generally, a suitable method for SNP sensing must be accurate, adaptable for both homogeneous and solid-phase reaction formats and provide a robust and easily interpretable signal. So far, due to heterogeneity of viral nucleic acids, the development of effective oligonucleotide probes for their targeting requires significant optimization of the probes to each particular target. By decreasing hybridization efficiency of fluorescent oligonucleotide probes and affecting their binding-induced fluorescence signaling, such sequence variations are a big challenge when targeting HIV-1 RNA and its corresponding cDNA fragment. To create an effective sensing method fulfilling all aforementioned requirements, oligonucleotide probes providing a high affinity and intense signaling of binding a target are required. These properties have recently been reported for fluorescent derivatives of locked nucleic acids (LNA and 2′-amino-LNA) containing diverse fluorescent tags. Other modified nucleotide analogs have also been reported within SNP sensing settings as more available and less expensive options for the HIV-1 detection (Charts **1**, **2**).

In this chapter, main aspects of modern SNP sensing in HIV and rationale beyond these assays are described. Examples of novel diagnostic assays which: 1) allow studies of HIV-1 genome; 2) the robust detection of SNPs; and 3) rapid adjustment of the treatment of a patient based on the results of testing, are the primary emphasis of this chapter. Overall, giving an overview on existing technologies and promoting further development of rational design strategies, convenient synthesis and robust sensing assays using fluorescent oligonucleotides are the major goals of this chapter.

This chapter starts with a general description of clinically important SNPs in the HIV-1 genome and sources of the viral nucleic acids (cDNA and RNA variants). The reader will also be introduced to the population aspects of HIV infection in different countries. Next, current enzymatic and enzyme-free detection settings are discussed. Fluorescent oligonucleotide probes are applied in most of these assays and are described for each technique. Synthetic nucleotide analogs such as 5-ethynyl-2'-deoxyuridine and diverse locked nucleic acids (LNAs) are introduced as tools when creating SNP sensors for HIV diagnostics [25-40]. Next, imaging of viral nucleic acids is discussed as an emerging research and diagnostic method for HIV-1 nucleic acids. Herein, fluorescent oligonucleotides have additional requirements to properties such as brightness and photostability. Achieving single-molecular level of visualization and possibility of quantification opens up great opportunities for imaging of HIV-1 cDNA and RNA directly in viral capsids and infected cells. A particular attention is paid to the major design considerations for fluorescent oligonucleotide sensors, which efficiently sense SNP in HIV-1 nucleic acids. These aspects of rational design include: sequence of fluorescent oligonucleotide, terminal *vs.* internal dye location within the probe, selection of fluorescent dye, incorporation of additional modifications, currently available oligonucleotide synthesis and fluorescent labeling techniques. The design considerations are given in context of individual assays and with remarks on the price, robustness and efficiency of the obtained probe.

A special case of SNP sensing in HIV protease (PR) gene fragment using rationally designed PAH-LNA/DNA probes is presented. Using novel fluorescent probes, rapid genotyping could be performed after PCR by a simple hybridization assay in full agreement with high-throughput sequencing data. This example is an illustration of the outlined design rules and can be applied as guidance for the development of similar assays. Furthermore, the prepared HIV sensors can be used in imaging experiments or may directly be incorporated in *e.g.,* real-time PCR (RT-PCR) assay.

At the end of this chapter, an overview of emerging technologies for HIV SNP sensing is presented, including new methods of single-molecule imaging, application of nanomaterials, perspective of simultaneous genotyping and gene therapy and co-detection of several infections in one assay.

Drug Resistance and HIV-1

Being a retrovirus with a single-stranded linear RNA genome, HIV-1 converts its RNA into DNA after infecting a suitable host cell. Reverse transcriptase (RT), an RNA-dependent DNA polymerase that transcribes RNA into DNA for further incorporation into the host genome, is an important target for treatment. Reverse transcriptase inhibitors mimic natural nucleotide triphosphates and therefore bind tightly to RT. The nucleotide analogs are designed to block growth of the viral DNA chain (*e.g.,* due to missing of 3'-hydroxyl group as in case of AZT), therefore preventing further replication of the viral genome [1]. The mechanism for resistance to nucleoside reverse transcriptase inhibitors (NRTIs) is discrimination, whereby the RT enzyme can avoid binding of the NRTI, while retaining the ability to recognize the analogs natural deoxynucleoside triphosphate (dNTP) substrate. Examples include virus with the point mutations K65R, L74V, Q151M and M184V, which cause diminished affinity of RT for specific NRTIs with little or no change in affinity for the corresponding dNTP substrate. The consequence is a diminished incorporation of drugs into the DNA chain [2].

Another enzyme of critical importance to HIV-1 life cycle is protease (a protein-cleaving enzyme) which cleaves the large precursor viral proteins into smaller functional molecules. In combinational anti-HIV/AIDS therapy, protease is inhibited in a competitive manner by drugs such as atazanavir and saquinavir. However, multiple mutations occurring during viral replication have adverse consequences for therapy, because the mutated HIV enzymes still bind substrate and function in the presence of inhibitor [2, 3] (Tables **1**, **2**).

Genotyping is an analytical technique which allows the validation of the presence of SNP in viral RNA and/or cDNA leading to mutations in enzymes. Current genotyping techniques include sequencing, microarrays, polymerase-chain reaction (PCR) and one-step hybridization assays. Previously, nearly all publications on HIV-1 genotyping and clinical outcome have described only the results of their analyses. None have published their underlying data, in part, because there have been no resources available for making such data publicly available, at least till now. Today, the obtained genotyping data are summarized in several public databases including Gene Bank and Stanford University HIV Drug Resistance Database. Collected sequences allow the rapid development of new research and clinical assays, as well as comparison of the diverse genotyping approaches.

Table **2** shows an example of HIV-1 genotyping obtained in 2012 by sequencing of patient serum samples at the Moscow AIDS Centre, Russia, in collaboration with World Health Organization (WHO) and Central Institute of Epidemiology of Russia [3]. *HIV Pol* gene fragment includes site 2332-2354 which can contain two mutations leading to resistance of HIV-1 protease to therapy by specific inhibitors. A single replacement G→A at residue 2340 (G2340A) leads to asparagine (N) instead of aspartic acid (D) at residue 30 of HIV-1 protease, which results in the resistance of the enzyme to the protease inhibitor (PI) virasept (nelfinavire). An analogous replacement at position 2346 of *HIV Pol* gene, G2346A, leads to isoleucine (I) instead of valine (V) at residue 32 of HIV-1 PR and causes resistance to all PIs available to date. In addition, the fragment 2332-2354 often contains several polymorphic mutations with a neutral effect on the virus (*neutral polymorphisms*).

According to Stanford University HIV database, "genotyping finds additional applications in HIV-1 diagnostics and research, including the following three fundamental types of correlations: (i) Correlations between genotypic data with treatment of patients from whom sequenced HIV-1 isolates have been obtained (genotype-treatment); (ii) Correlations between genotype and *in vitro* drug susceptibility (genotype-phenotype); and (iii) Correlations between genotype and the clinical response to a new treatment regimen (genotype-outcome)" [5]. The following table summarizes the results of published studies linking clinical response to adjusted PI-containing treatment with HIV-1 genotype (Table **3**) [5-7]. As one can see, switching to new PI after detecting drug resistance resulted in decreased viral RNA concentration for all the cases.

Table 1: Representative data for drug-resistance causing mutations in *HIV Pol*

Number of amino acid in Protease	Wild-type amino acid	Wild-type codone	Mutant amino acid	Mutant codone
30	D	GA[t,c]	N	AA[c,t]
32	V	GT[a,g,t,c]	I	AT[a,c,t]
33	L	CT[agtc] & TT[ag]	F	TT [c,t]
46	M	ATG	I	AT[a,t,c]
			L	CT[agtc] & TT[ag]
47	I	AT[a,t,c]	A	GC[agtc]
			V	GT[a,g,t,c]
50	I	AT[a,t,c]	V	GT[a,g,t,c]
			L	CT[agtc] & TT[ag]
53	F	TT[t, c]	L	CT[agtc] & TT[ag]
82	V	GT[a,g,t,c]	A	GC[agtc]
			T	AC[agct]
			F	TT[t, c]
			S	TC[agct] & AG[ct]
84	I	AT[a,t,c]	V	GT[a,g,t,c]
			A	GC[agtc]
			C	TG[ct]
88	N	AA[tc]	S	TC[agct] & AG[ct]
			D	GA[t,c]
90	L	CT[agtc] & TT[ag]	M	ATG

Thus, rapid reliable genotyping of HIV-1 associated nucleic acids has multiple benefits for patient care, clinical epidemiology, treatment and research on HIV-1 around the world. However, drug-resistance of HIV-1 can be adequately understood only in the context of population studies for each particular country and region where the type of medication applied is taking into account. Table **4** lists percentage of HIV-1/AIDS infected adults in different country groups [4]. A.P. Seltsovsky and co-workers outline the following: "The screening of the population together with national statistical and epidemiological surveillance programs allows virologists to trace with a fair degree of accuracy, all changes of the epidemiological environment in different regions of the country as well as different communities within the country. To achieve this, AIDS professionals draw data that adequately reflect the epidemic process... AIDS specialists in a number of recommendations argue that the system should be improved" [4].

Table 2: Representative sequencing data for *HIV Pol* cDNA fragments 2332-2354 encoding HIV-1 protease [3]. Codons D30 and V32 are indicated in blue and yellow, respectively. Drug resistance-causing SNPs G2340A, G2346A, and neutral polymorphisms are underlined and indicated in red, green and blue, respectively

	Sequence fragment																							
Codon	**G27**			**A28**			**D29**			**D30**			**T31**			**V32**			**L33**			**E34**		
nucleotide #	2332			2335			2338			2341			2344			2347			2350			2353		
Patient #																								
1		G	A	G	C	A	G	A	T	G	A	T	A	C	A	G	T	A	T	T	A	G	A	A
2		G	A	G	C	A	G	A	T	G	A	T	A	C	A	G	T	**G**	T	T	A	G	A	A
3		G	A	G	C	A	G	A	T	G	A	T	A	C	**G**	G	T	A	T	T	A	G	A	A
4		G	A	G	C	A	G	A	T	G	A	T	A	C	A	G	T	A	**C**	T	A	G	A	A
5		G	A	G	C	A	G	A	T	G	A	T	A	C	A	**A**	T	A	T	T	**G**	G	A	A
6		G	A	G	C	A	G	A	T	G	A	T	A	C	A	**A**	T	A	**C**	T	A	G	A	**G**
7		G	A	G	C	A	G	A	T	G	A	T	A	C	A	**A**	T	A	T	T	A	G	A	A
8		G	A	G	C	**G**	G	A	C	G	A	T	A	C	A	G	T	A	**C**	T	A	G	A	A
9		G	A	G	C	A	G	A	T	**A**	A	T	A	C	A	G	T	A	**C**	T	A	G	A	A
10		G	A	G	C	A	G	A	T	**A**	A	T	A	C	**G**	G	T	A	T	T	A	G	A	A
11		G	A	G	C	A	G	A	T	**A**	A	T	A	C	A	G	T	A	T	T	A	G	A	A
12		G	A	G	C	**G**	G	A	T	**A**	A	T	A	C	A	G	T	A	T	T	**G**	G	A	A

Table 3: PI-Resistance causing SNPs and efficiency of adjusted PI-containing treatment for nelfinavir (NFV, NFV/SQV) [5]. Abbreviations: Pts: patients; Rx: regimen; SQV: saquinavir; IDV: indinavir; RTV: ritonavir; BID: twice a day; TID: three times a day; Wk: week

Reference	Previous PI	Follow-up PI	No. Pts	Wk	Effect of SNPs on Drug Response
Lawrence (1999) [6a]	SQV	NFV (750 mg TID)	16	24	No sustained responses were detected. SNP L90M was associated with more rapid virologic failure.
Walmsley (2001) [6b]	Several PIs (SQV, IDV, RTV)	NFV (750 mg TID)	63	24 - 48	41% and 22% of patients had RNA levels declines ≥0.5 logs at 24 and 48 weeks, respectively. SNPs at position 48, 82, 84, and/or 90 were observed in 69% of patients, also corresponding to weak effect of adjusted treatment.
Casado (2001) [7]	IDV ± RTV	NFV/SQV (NFV 750-1250 mg; SQV 600-1000 mg BID-TID)	31	26 - 52	35% and 56% of patients had viral RNA levels <50 logs in 6 and 12 months after adjusted PI treatment, respectively. SNP L90M (0% *vs.* 43%) but not V82A (38% *vs.* 36%) decreased the rate of response.

Control of HIV epidemics strongly depends on effective monitoring, treatment and epidemic prevention system being established in a specific country. In Western Europe, a comparative analysis of the HIV-1/AIDS levels with a special focus on the European capitals is most appropriate since these are the areas most affected by HIV-1/AIDS (Table **4**). On the other hand, due to the high number of HIV-1 infected individuals, less developed countries (mainly located in Africa and Latin America) require simple inexpensive diagnostic techniques in order to efficiently monitor HIV infection in any region of the country.

Finally, in the closely connected world of today, HIV-1 epidemics cannot be dealt with separately for each country or a group of these countries. Diagnostic and research settings aiming at an effective prevention and treatment of HIV-1/AIDS are on demand in every part of the world, especially in big cities and areas with a high risk of infection (Table **4**).

Sources of HIV-1 Nucleic Acids for Testing

As described in Stanford University HIV database, "human plasma is the main source of virus used for clinical testing HIV-1 drug resistance. The sequence of plasma virus represents the species most recently selected for antiretroviral drug therapy since plasma contains only actively replicating virus. Other sources of virus for HIV-1 drug resistance studies include resting T-lymphocytes and macrophages, lymph nodes, cerebrospinal fluid and genital secretions. Virus species harbored in long-lived cells such as resting T lymphocytes and macrophages are the ultimate obstacles to HIV-1 eradication and have been an area of intensive study [8]. In patients with complete virus suppression during therapy (plasma HIV-1 RNA <50 copies/ml), there is generally little or no evidence of virus within long-lived cells [8, 9]. In patients with lapses in therapy, the population of virus within long-lived cells increases and may evolve drug resistant forms [10].

Table 4: Representative adult prevalence rates for HIV-1/AIDS in different countries. Data obtained from the full list of countries available in CIA - The world factbook [4]

Number in the worldwide rating	Country	Percent of HIV infected adults	Year estimated
1	Swaziland	38.80	2003
2	Botswana	37.30	2003
3	Lesotho	28.90	2003
4	Zimbabwe	24.60	2001
5	South Africa	21.50	2003
6	Namibia	21.30	2003
7	Zambia	16.50	2003
8	Malawi	14.20	2003
9	Central African Republic	13.50	2003
10	Mozambique	12.2	2003
49	Thailand	1.50	2003
50	Ukraine	1.40	2003
51	Burma	1.20	2003
52	Gambia	1.20	2003
53	Niger	1.20	2003
54	Jamaica	1.20	2003
55	Estonia	1.10	2001
56	Guatemala	1.10	2003
57	Russia	1.10	2001

Table 4: contd...

77	France	0.40	2003
78	Switzerland	0.40	2001
79	Vietnam	0.40	2003
80	Portugal	0.40	2001
81	Malaysia	0.40	2003
82	Austria	0.30	2003
83	Uruguay	0.30	2001
84	Chile	0.30	2003
85	Mexico	0.30	2003
86	Libya	0.30	2001
87	Canada	0.30	2003
166	Afghanistan	0.01	2001
167	Saudi Arabia	0.01	2001
168	Svalbard	0.00	2001

The concentration of HIV-1 in lymph nodes is usually two to three orders of magnitude greater than the concentration of HIV-1in plasma. Several groups have performed genotyping of HIV-1 protease and RT genes of virus obtained from proviral DNA in peripheral and visceral lymph nodes. This was done in order to determine the effect of antiviral therapy on HIV-1 in these heavily infected parts of the body [11, 12]. Most patients with undetectable levels of virus in the plasma still have detectable virus in lymph nodes, but there is no evidence that mutations develop in lymph nodes and yet remain absent from plasma" [5].

Emerging imaging applications allow monitoring and quantification of HIV-1 nucleic acids directly within the viral capsid and infected host cells [13]. These assays can now be used in research settings and diagnostics, also at the single-molecular level. Major advantage of direct HIV-1 sensing is that no viral RNA purification and enzymatic processing are needed. In that way, overall cost and time of the assay are lower than for *in vitro* clinical methods. Moreover, mistakes during reverse transcription and PCR, along with possible contamination, are avoided. Using single-molecule spectroscopy, important scientific information on viral life cycle can be obtained, as well as dynamic monitoring of its individual steps. In doing this, synthetic nucleotide analogs containing fluorescent dyes are on demand (*e.g.,* 5'-ethynyl-dU, Chart **1**). The field of synthetic nucleotides for imaging HIV-1 is developing rapidly and gives exciting clinically valuable information on the virus.

Finally, there is still a limited knowledge on HIV-1 in the central nervous system (CNS) and its influence on the infection in the brain, and how the levels of HIV-1 in CNS correlate with the viral load in the plasma [14]. Some drugs, especially PIs, penetrate rather slowly into the CNS. Therefore, the HIV virus obtained from CNS was analyzed to verify the fact that CNS permits virus replication during antiretroviral therapy [15-17]. However these studies showed a close correlation between virologic failure and rebound in the CNS and plasma, respectively.

Enzyme-Based Strategies to Sensing HIV-1 Nucleic Acids

A majority of current HIV-1 diagnostic assays require an application of enzymes in order to achieve high sequence specificity and sensitivity. Among enzymatic methods, two major high-throughput assays are represented by HIV-1 RT and protease genotyping by sequencing. These assays start with the extraction of RNA from patient plasma followed by PCR amplification of a fragment including HIV-1protease, part of RT and a shorter fragment of *gag*. The amplified material is subsequently sequenced using next-generation sequencing or pyrosequencing. The latter method has a high sensitivity and represents an ideal method for rapid detection of SNP by sequencing [18]. Using PCR, HIV-1 RNA levels >1,000 copies/mL can be genotyped. PCR assay can be further improved using NESTED assay. By reducing non-specific amplification, NESTED PCR results in increased yields of cDNA, higher specificity and sensitivity of the entire assay. However, NESTED setting also increases the labor and cost of amplification, and introduces a higher risk of sample cross-contamination.

The major advantage of sequencing is the possibility to gain information on the exact nature of a sequence alteration such as SNP. This allows further development of PCR assays and direct methods for any particular mutation [19]. Sequencing data for HIV have been collected in multiple public databases, *e.g.,* Stanford University Database at http://hivdb.stanford.edu/ [5].

HIV-1 genotyping exclusively by PCR is commonly used in HIV diagnostics, owing to its availability, lower cost, and shorter analysis compared to sequencing. [20]. Thus, **allele-specific polymerase-chain reaction (PCR)** is a genotyping technique in which the complexity of target HIV-1 cDNA is reduced by the amplification of a specific region defined by a set of primes [21-24]. The assay begins with purification of total RNA from a sample, followed by reversed transcription and PCR of cDNA. At the end of the preparation step, a single-stranded cDNA is generated by NESTED-PCR step. The specificity is reached using 15-23 nt long primers specific for the region of interest. A sequence of primers is usually determined by sequencing.

Specificity of allele-specific PCR can be improved incorporating synthetic nucleic acid analogs, such as locked nucleic acids (LNA, Chart **1**), into relatively short primers and/or probes (11-15 nt) [25-31]. LNA's bicyclic structure allows it to adopt the RNA mimicking S-type furanose ring conformation. Therefore, the structural and thermodynamic parameters of LNA/DNA oligonucleotides are improved compared to non-modified nucleotides (*e.g.,* high binding affinity and selectivity to DNA and especially RNA targets, and resistance to enzymatic degradation). Several allele-specific LNA/DNA primers and probes have been successfully applied and characterized by thermodynamic and design parameters. However, optimal positioning of LNA units in PCR primers and probes still needs a systematic evaluation. Furthermore, DNA, RNA and LNA nucleotides can be functionalized using *e.g.,* click chemistry, allowing probes to acquire additional advantageous properties such as increased enzymatic stability, fluorescent sensing, *etc*. [32-40].

The genotyping of amplified HIV-1 cDNA targets can be performed by different direct and indirect hybridization strategies including intercalating dyes in allele-specific digital PCR (dPCR) (Fig. **1**) [41], sequence-specific fluorogenic probes [42], electrochemical sensors [43-48] and diagnostic nano-materials [49-55]. In this approach, fluorescent oligonucleotides play an important role as either sequence-specific probes or PCR primers. The typical design of the sequence-specific diagnostic reagent (primer or probe) includes 5'-terminal or internal attachment of fluorescent dye(s) including activated ester or "click" chemistry within a 15-25 nt long sequence. For simultaneous detection of several SNPs in a dPCR or real-time PCR (RT-PCR) setting, a series of probes containing various fluorophores covering a broad excitation/emission region can be applied (Fig. **2**). Such multi-fluorophore approaches are called multiplexing, and have been successfully applied for simultaneous genotyping of diverse nucleic acid targets including HIV-1 gene fragments. The possibility to perform this type of assays favors the use towards fluorescent oligonucleotide probes over intercalating dyes, inspite of the higher price of the former. Importantly, the correct choice of fluorophores plays an important role in the efficiency of any multiplexing assay. A detailed description of this topic is presented later in this chapter.

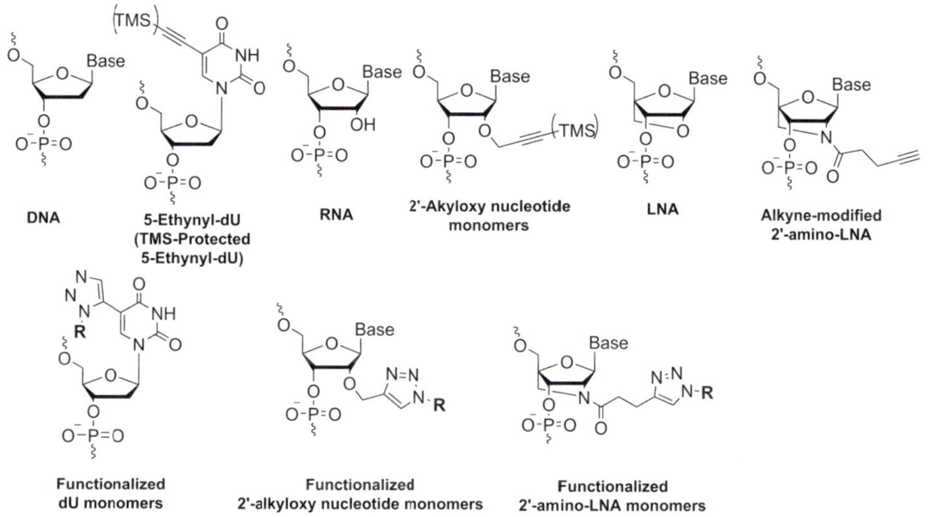

Chart 1: Chemical structures of various DNA, RNA and LNA nucleotides.

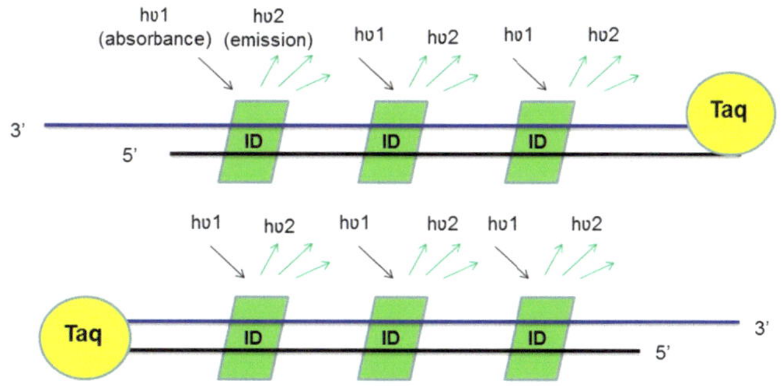

Figure 1: Illustration of intercalating dyes (ID) applied for detection of dsDNA amplified by Taq polymerase (Taq).

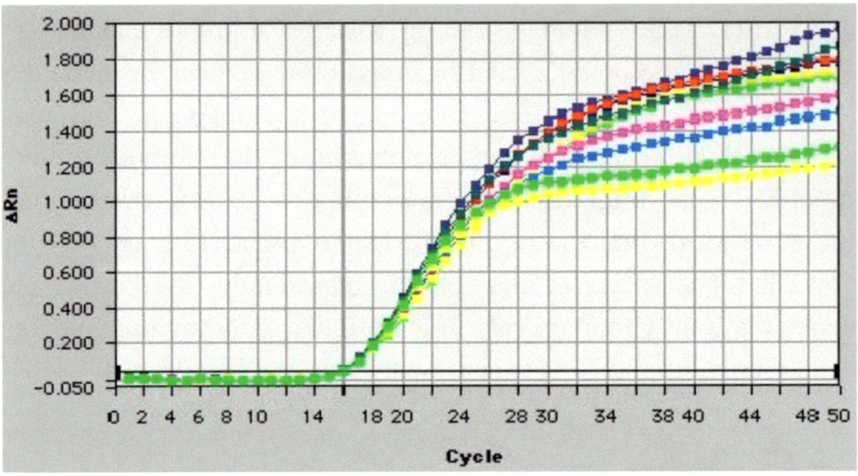

Figure 2: Representative experimental data obtained during multiplex-RT PCR assay. Black line is a threshold which is set empirically or by a statistical calculation at a fluorescence value above background. Reproduced from the web-page of the intracellular pathogen cooperative group: Transcriptomics, St. George's technologies.

The development of *in situ* PCR has enabled researchers to combine the sensitivity of solution based PCR with the target localizing capability of *in situ* hybridization [56-59]. This technique has been instrumental in defining disease states which involve detection of single copy genes in cells and tissues. The use of automated thermal cyclers and so-called slide cyclers has made the *in situ* amplification of genes. However, the detection systems have either been non-specific (direct incorporation of reporters) or difficult to perform (*in situ* hybridization). A novel detection scheme that eliminates hybridization following amplification is developed by Patterson and co-workers [60]. The authors use the 5′-nuclease activity of *Taq* polymerase to cleave *in situ* a 5′-reporter dye from an oligonucleotide probe which hybridizes to the amplified target fragment during amplification. The 5′-reporter dye is disassociated from the 3′-quenching dye and remains localized by charge interactions. Using this technique and rationally designed probes, sensitive and specific detection of HIV-1 DNA has been demonstrated in cells lines and tissues from HIV-1-infected individuals.

Next, a simple method has been developed for measuring proviral HIV-1 DNA in mononuclear cells based on the commercially available **Amplicor(TM) HIV-1 polymerase chain reaction (PCR) assay combined with the limiting dilution**

method [61]. The lowest limit of detection for this method was as low as only four proviral genomes per 10^6 cells. The accuracy was demonstrated by using serial dilutions of infected LAV-8E5 cells. The Amplicor(TM) technique was also used to measure HIV-1 proviral DNA in the PBMCs of 11 patients who had undetectable plasma HIV-1 RNA after being placed on the combination antiretroviral therapy. Although proviral DNA remained detectable in all patients after 36 weeks of treatment, a gradual decrease with an estimated half-life of 21-58 weeks was observed. The reliability of this simple and convenient colorimetric technique indicates its suitability for assessing the effect of current antiretroviral regimens on the latent reservoirs of provirus.

Another approach to SNP genotyping utilizes single-stranded oligonucleotides with a stem-loop structure called **molecular beacons** (MBs; Fig. **3**) [62]. The loop is designed to bind a target sequence, while the stem forms by the hybridization of the arm sequences on either side of the loop sequence. The 5' and 3' termini of MBs are typically labeled with a fluorescent dye and its FRET pair forming second dye, or a quencher of fluorescence. The hybridization of a loop to its target forces opening of MBs and gives increased fluorescence at the certain wavelength, since the fluorophore is moved away from the FRET acceptor/quencher. Main classes of fluorophores incorporated into molecular beacons are shown in Chart **2**. Bright cyanine and xanthene dyes are very often applied in MBs, nevertheless they are rather expensive. Furthermore, some of the dyes are chemically and/or photo unstable. Polyaromatic hydrocarbons (PAHs) have lower molar extinction values compared to cyanines (εmax 45.000-75.000 *vs*. 90.000-250.000, respectively) [63]. However, a high sensitivity of PAHs to microenvironment's structure and polarity, along with their ability to form exciplexes and excimers and remarkable photostability make them promising dyes for the analysis and research on HIV-1 nucleic acids.

As demonstrated by Barreiro and co-authors, a major advantage of MBs is the possibility of multiplexing using up to 30 probes in a high-throughput approach [64]. In doing so, SNP detection using MBs is based on the competition of perfectly-matched and mismatched probes for binding to a PCR template, with each probe containing different fluorescent dyes. Relatively short stem sequence (4-8 nt) has been demonstrated as a beneficial design consideration for genotyping using MBs. Such short stems could be formed in the presence of magnesium within *in vitro* settings. Alternatively, MBs are applied in real-time PCR (RT-PCR), also with a possibility of multiplexing and quantification. The disadvantages of MBs in SNP sensing are complicated sequence design, false signals due to probe degradation and low sensitivity requiring amplification prior to detection [65, 66].

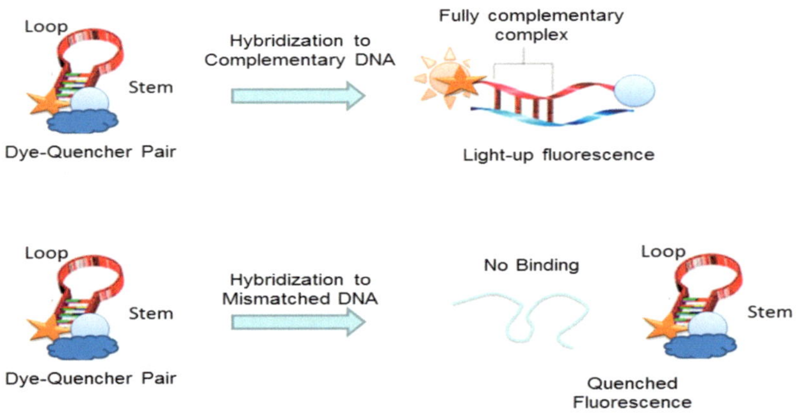

Figure 3: Detection of SNP in viral cDNA by molecular beacon (MB).

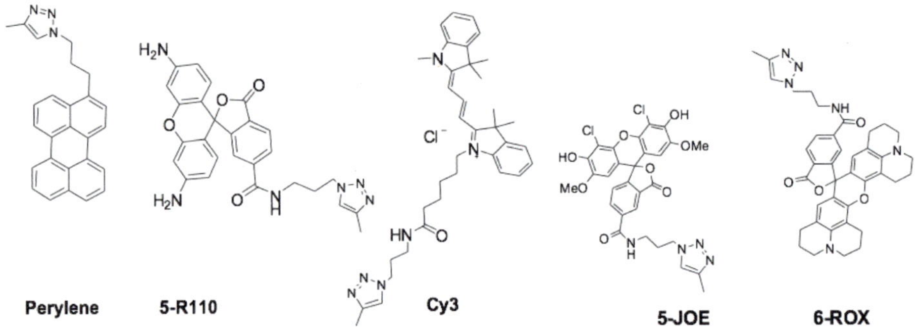

Chart 2: Chemical structures of fluorescent dyes applied in RT-PCR.

As mentioned above, high genomic variability of HIV-1 results in a decreased specificity of standard RT -PCR methods which require long oligonucleotide probes. A decreased hybridization efficiency of complementary oligonucleotides and its negative effect on binding-induced fluorescence signaling result from multiple sequence variations in the HIV-1 genome. The synthetic oligonucleotides containing LNA are useful tools in overcoming these obstacles (Chart **1**). A new application of LNA modified probes is a so-called **Taqman assay** (Fig. **4**). This assay applies a short LNA/ DNA probe which is complementary to the majority of HIV-1 sequences. The probe gets cleaved by nuclease after the extension of a sequence specific primer which results in the release of fluorophore. Using short, ugly specific LNA/DNA probes, the Taqman assay shows a broad dynamic range, remarkable sensitivity and applicability to diverse HIV-1 subtypes. As further outlined by the authors, "this approach to Taqman probe design could be explored further for use in diagnosis and monitoring of HIV- 1 in resource-limited settings, especially where several subtypes co-circulate", owing to the opportunity to create multiplexing settings [67-70].

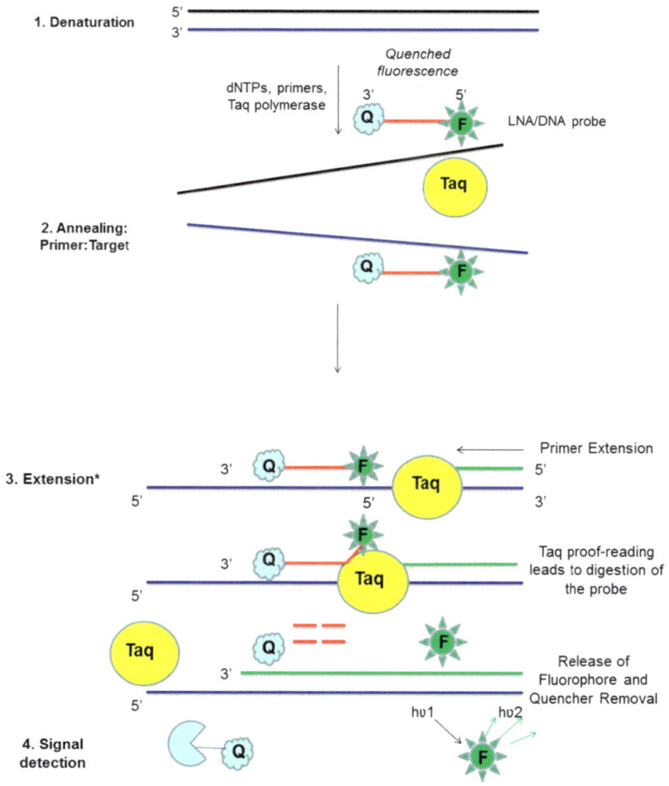

Figure 4: Schematic illustration of LNA-Taqman assay for HIV-1 detection. 3'-Phosphate group on LNA/DNA probe prevents its extension by Taq.

Direct PCR is another technique which is applied in clinical diagnostics of HIV-1 as a faster and less expensive assay than sequencing [71]. A direct PCR is performed in research to investigate the evolution of HIV-1 drug resistance. For both population-based and clonal sequencing, the ability to detect minor variants is inversely related to the proportion of the minor variants within the whole virus population. In direct PCR sequencing, electrophoretic double peaks indicating a nucleotide mixture occur only when the second nucleotide is present in at least 20 % of the total virus population. With either method, unequal amplification of viral variants presents as a mixture because one or more species may be preferentially amplified during PCR due to differences in primer binding. By sequencing multiple clones, one can measure the frequency of distinct variants within HIV-1 and assess the contribution of individual clones to the evolution of drug resistance.

Importantly, in all aforementioned techniques, using amplification to detect HIV-1 RNA or DNA can result in false results and may cause recombination due to template switching. Since *Taq* polymerase lacks proof reading activity, an amplified 2 kb product can contain up to 12 nucleotide changes. Use of a high fidelity DNA polymerase such as *Pfu* in PCR assays can reduce the number of amplification mistakes [72].

Sequencing by Hybridization on Microarray

Recently, several robust and affordable sequencing approaches using a microarray technique have been developed for HIV-1 monitoring. For example, the GeneChip is developed by Affymetrix to sequence the entire HIV-1 protease and the first 1200 nt of HIV-1 RT. Multiple arrays of sequence specific oligonucleotides are packaged in sequencing cartridges acting as hybridization capture probes. During sequencing, cDNA is transcribed into RNA containing fluorescent label and hybridized to capture on the array. Afterwards, laser scanner detects color resulting from binding of RNA to the complementary capture (Fig. **5**). However, information on the expected SNPs in a target gene is required for the design of gene chip. Therefore, this method is called a "re-sequencing". Again, as discussed above, the high genetic variability of HIV-1 is an obstacle for its sequencing by hybridization. According to multiple studies, the Gene Chip technology is less reliable for SNP detection than dideoxynucleotide sequencing. Current sequencing arrays cannot detect insertions and deletions, and are suitable only for HIV-1 subtype B. According to Affymetrix, improved microarrays for sequencing other HIV-1 subtypes and for signaling insertions are under development.

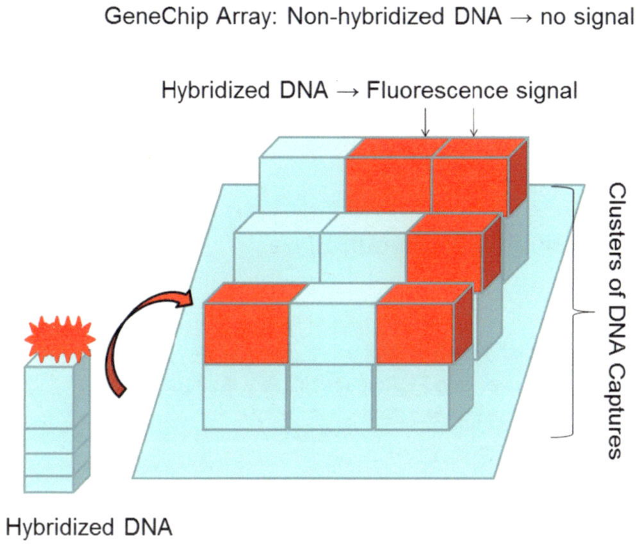

Figure 5: Schematic illustration of GeneChip sequencing assay.

Finally, specific **SNP microarrays** involve hybridization of HIV-1 target to a series of capture probes immobilized on array surface, followed by analysis using a method of choice (*e.g.,* PCR, sequence-specific linear probes or MBs; Fig. **6**). Capture probes have crucial importance for the effective binding of the target DNA or RNA. By including LNA, the performance of the capture probes on microarrays can be dramatically improved. The design rules for highly-specific LNA/DNA capture probes have been recently described by Exiqon TM as follows:

1) Capture probes should be approximately 16-22 nucleotides in length.

2) For SNP detection, 2-3 LNA nucleotides should be positioned at the SNP site and the adjacent nucleotides.

3) No sequential repeats of ≥ 3G or C nucleotides should be created due to the risk of secondary structure formation.

4) No sequential repeats of ≥ 4 LNA nucleotides. LNA hybridizes tightly when several consecutive nucleotides are substituted with LNA units.

5) Self-complementarity of capture probes has to be avoided.

6) GC-content should be approx. 30-60 %.

7) Optimal melting temperature (Tm) of capture and complementary target should be approx. 75 °C.

8) G-C palindromes should not contain LNA.

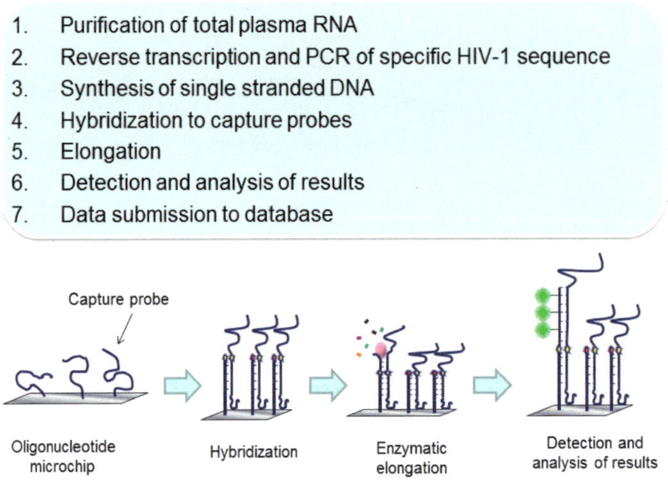

Figure 6: Main steps for HIV-1 genotyping using microarrays.

Imaging HIV-1 Nucleic Acids in Individual Cells

Microarrays and quantitative PCR are powerful tools for gene expression analysis that have facilitated our present understanding of the intricate biology of HIV infected cells and tissues, and have provided an opportunity to diagnose them in clinical settings. Moreover, with recent advances in high-throughput sequencing technologies, transcriptome profiling by RNA sequencing (RNA-sequence) delivers a comprehensive gene expression analysis with a dynamic range [73, 74]. Several recently introduced assays including Nano String Technologies' nCounter gene expression system have similar sensitivity and accuracy as RT-PCR, and include multiplexing capabilities [75]. These technologies provide the ability to understand the function of genes of interest and also to identify gene expression signatures that distinguish altered biological events from normal events. However, most gene expression studies, including those for HIV-1, use bulk measurements from heterogeneous cells and tissues, which can obscure information from rare or specific cell types. By analyzing viral gene expression in individual cells, a more complete picture of the gene expression dynamics within heterogeneous samples can be obtained [76-79]. This is made possible by the development of high-resolution microscopy which gives an opportunity to detect at previously unachievable resolution viral nucleic acids directly within infected cells.

For single-cell microscopy of HIV-1 RNA and cDNA, similar design principles are applied for the probe design as for PCR, sequencing and direct hybridization assays. However, additional requirements for the former are high fluorescence quantum yield and photostability. High-affinity hybridization and excellent fluorescent responses to complementary DNA/RNA targets prompted us to apply multiply labeled PAH-LNA/DNA probes for mRNA imaging *in vitro* and in cell culture (Fig. 7) [80]. In these studies, we used fluorescence microscopy and sequence-specific LNA/DNA oligonucleotides containing photostable perylene dyes attached to 2'-amino-LNA. Using perylene-LNA/DNA probes, we were able to detect the target model mRNA in cell culture with the advantages of high specificity and a perylene excitation wavelength that completely eliminated cell auto fluorescence (λ_{ex} 425 nm). Importantly, fluorescence signaling by the prepared probe was highly dependent on the presence of an SNP in the model target. We believe that owing to such unique combination of biophysical and optical properties, similar PAH-LNA/DNA probes can be applied for monitoring HIV-1 mRNA *in vitro,* in cell culture and *in vivo*.

In another recent study, modified nucleotide analogs were used to visualize HIV-1 genome during HIV- 1 life cycle [81]. Viral RNA within individual cells was monitored using aforementioned 5-ethynyl-2'-deoxyuridine (EU) (Chart **2**). After entry into the core, fluorescent azide molecules of the bright AlexaFluor dye could detect RNA through labeling of already inserted EU by "click" azide-alkyne conjugation. Using *in vitro* labeling of HIV-1 particles by this approach, it was demonstrated that how the amount of the HIV-1 RNA visualized with AlexaFluor-EU decreases after the initial HIV-1 infection of the cells. The authors underline that fluorescent microscopy combined with AlexaFluor-EU labeling technique could also potentially give quantitative information on viral nucleic acids within the host cells and virions [81].

a) **b)**

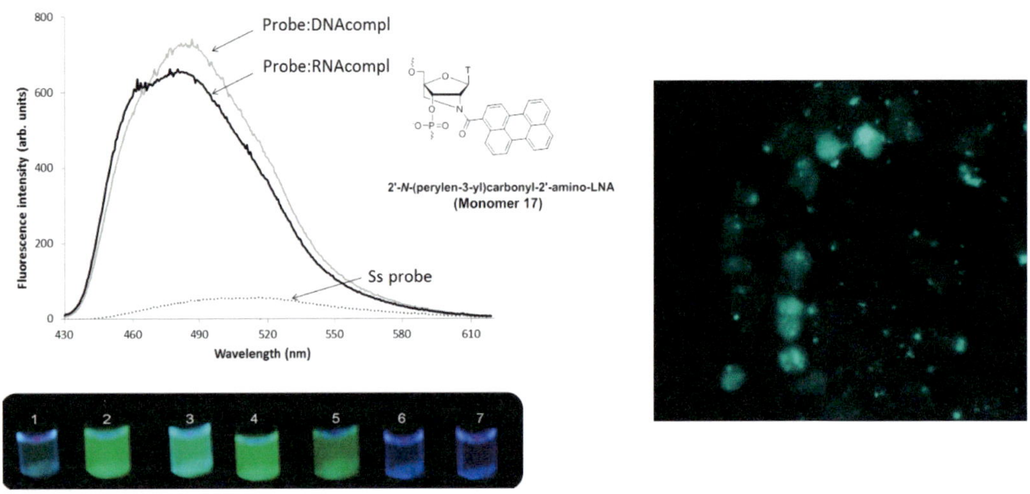

Figure 7: (A) Steady-state fluorescence emission spectra of perylene-LNA modified model probe 5′-d(G(PL-T)G A(PL-T)A (PL-T)GC; (PL-T) = 2′-*N*-(perylen-3-yl)carbonyl-2′-amino-LNA monomer) and the corresponding duplexes with complementary DNA/RNA. Spectra were obtained in a medium salt buffer at 19 °C using an excitation wavelength of 425 nm and 0.1 μM concentration of ONs. Below: photographs of the fluorescence emission in a medium salt buffer: single stranded model probe (vial 1, 1 μM concentration); probe:DNA (vial 2, 1 μM concentration), probe:RNA (vial 3, 1 μM concentration); probe:DNA (vials 4-6, concentrations: 1 μM, 0.5 μM, and 0.1 μM, respectively); medium salt buffer (vial 7). Photographs were taken with a digital camera using a laboratory UV-lamp (λ_{ex} = 365 nm). (B) Images of cell culture observed using fluorescence microscopy: cian fluorescence of the peryle-2'-amino-LNA probe 5'-d(TT^{L}T A(PL-T)A (PL-T)A(PL-T) CA^{Me}C^{L} G) indicated its RNA target (λ_{ex} 425 nm; λ_{em} 480 nm). T^{L} and ^{Me}C^{L} = thymin-1-yl and 5-methylcytosin-1-yl LNA monomers, respectively.

Next, a modified form of branched DNA technology was developed, which allows the visualization of single RNA molecules in cells by image cytometry [82, 83]. Using a similar probe design to image cytometry, Wang and co-workers reported a novel *in situ* hybridization technology platform (RNA Scope) to analyze individual RNA molecules in formalin-fixed, paraffin-embedded tissues [84]. The unique probe design contained paired target probes that formed a z-design platform for signal amplifications promoted by sequential hybridization. This strategy allowed the visualization of single RNA molecules in cells by simultaneous signal amplification of multiple RNA targets. In addition, the described probe design included a unique tail sequence type for each probe in the target probe pair that greatly decreased the possibility of nonspecific hybridizations, yielding superior background suppression.

Another recent report describes a new version of RNA Scope technology applied for the cell analysis in suspension [85]. The RNA Scope technique reported by Hanley and co-workers enables RNA flow cytometry for single cell analysis of intracellular RNAs at high specificity and sensitivity as confirmed by wild-type HIV gag RNA and specific mRNA detection at very low copy numbers.

Fluorescent Oligonucleotide Reagents for HIV-1 Sensing: Design and Synthesis

As exemplified above, the design of fluorescent probes and primers plays a crucial role for the efficacy of the diagnostic assay and research settings on HIV-1 infection. Different design rules have to be applied for oligonucleotides which will be used *in vitro*, in cell culture or *in vivo* assays. General requirements of all the probes/primers are a high target binding affinity and specificity, high sensitivity at low fluorescence background, a robust synthetic route and of a low cost. For *in vivo* imaging, low toxicity and high enzymatic stability of the probes are also important, along with a high photostability and brightness, required for visualization techniques.

General design considerations for all the probes/primers containing covalently attached dye(s) are: length and sequence context number, position and chemical nature of the attached dye(s), additional modifications, and chemistry of the linker. All these parameters have a direct influence on the availability and price of the product. In the case of an intercalating dye, heavily modified probes/primers have to be avoided, since the altered secondary structure of the double-helix forms when a probe binds to its target might decrease the intercalation and may reduce the signal.

Length of Fluorescent Oligonucleotide

In the case of detecting an HIV-1 target in a long genomic RNA or DNA sequence, oligonucleotide lengths of 15-23 nt would ensure the required specificity of binding to the particular target. However, for *in vitro* and cell culture assays, shorter probes have the benefits of lower cost and better performance. With 3-4 LNA modifications, the probes can only be 11-14 nt long. In the presence of a mismatch, such short probes do not form the duplex at a typical temperature of fluorescent analysis (above 19 °C), which results in a very high binding specificity.

Terminal vs. Internal Dye Incorporation

As described by us [86] and others [87-92], an internal incorporation of dyes into oligonucleotides results in probes with a much higher potential for SNP sensing as compared to terminally labeled analogs. Terminally labeled probes are still useful for MBs for RT-PCR, for example, or initial imaging experiments and several clinical settings for HIV-1 testing. However, high signal sensitivity to the local environment can be achieved only when the dye has an ability to interact with nucleic acid components, and this can be achieved most efficiently by internal insertion.

Selection of Fluorescent Dye

A selection of the right dye(s) is crucial for the performance of the product probe/primer and most often for its price. As outlined before, high fluorescence quantum yield and sensitivity to microenvironment are beneficial when selecting the effective dye for any assay (Chart **2**). Currently, there is a broad variety of fluorescent dyes on the market which fulfill these requirements (*e.g.,* xanthenes, cyanines and PAHs). In multiplexing settings, a series of fluorophores with distinctive excitation and emission wavelengths have to be selected. In MB-based studies, a suitable quencher of fluorescence or a FRET pair-forming dye can be selected using design schemes available on the web. Finally, for imaging applications, brightness and photostability of the dye are important. These are the characteristic features of rhodamines, AlexaFluor and ATTO dyes, to name a few.

Additional Modifications

Multiple mutations in the HIV-1 target and internal modifications with bulky fluorophores decrease the affinity of the probe to the target. This can be overcome by additional incorporation of several LNA nucleotides in the strand. Additional benefits of incorporating LNA include improving SNP discrimination and high resistance to nucleases.

Oligonucleotide Synthesis and Fluorescent Labelling

Preparation of oligonucleotide probes can be performed chemically and enzymatically. An enzymatic synthesis has advantages such as the potential for *in situ* labeling followed by the monitoring of a particular stage of viral life cycle (*e.g.,* uncoating and replication). However, most of the fluorescent probes for HIV diagnostics available on the market are prepared by an automated oligonucleotide synthesis method, most often a phosphoramidite method. This method allows for a fully controlled incorporation of modifications and yields 10-70 nt long oligonucleotides of a desired sequence with advantage. When bulky hydrophobic dye(s) have to be incorporated internally, a hand-coupling procedure can be beneficial to obtain a high yield of the product. After synthesis, the product is cleaved from solid support, deprotected and if necessary, purified by HPLC and/or gel electrophoresis.

Notably, several fluorescent dyes can be degraded during oligonucleotide synthesis (numerous rhodamines and cyanine dyes). In this case, the dye can be attached post-synthetically, either on a solid support or in solution. This can be done using activated esters, coupling reactions or click chemistry.

Price, Robustness and Efficiency of the Obtained Probe

Based on our experience, readily available nucleotide scaffolds, short oligonucleotide sequences with additional LNA units, and internally attached bright and sensitive dyes lead to optimal price-performance balance of the resulting probes. Post-synthetic labeling also seems to be a beneficial synthetic route for chemically prepared fluorescent oligonucleotides, presenting an opportunity to incorporate any dye and to use much less of them, often expensive, labeling chemicals than in oligonucleotide synthesis. However, the individual design adjustments of the probes for a particular assay, or the necessity to simultaneously use multiple fluorescent reagents as in RT-PCR, can affect the price and robustness of the probe preparation.

PAH-LNA/DNA Probes for SNP Sensing in HIV-1: A Special Case

The following two examples show how the design rules described above can be successfully applied for the development of new HIV-1 genotyping systems. In our recent research, we apply diverse fluorescent PAH-LNA nucleotide analogs as sensors for HIV-1. In these studies, we show that PAH-LNA units can simultaneously provide increased selectivity and sensitivity when sensing SNPs in highly polymorphic HIV-1 RNA and DNA molecules. Moreover, we demonstrate how additional LNA nucleotides can be combined with fluorescent dyes directly attached to the 2'-amino position of 2'-amino-LNA within a highly effective fluorogenic probe (Charts **1**, **2**) [93-95].

According to our previous research, short fluorescent LNA/DNA probes containing various PAHs such as pyrene [93], (phenylethynyl) pyrenes [94], and perylene [95] represent a class of sensors with advantages of high affinity, specificity and sensitivity in sensing SNPs. In the initial work on PAH-LNA/DNA probes for SNP sensing, Umemoto and co-workers applied pyrene excimer-forming short LNA/DNA oligonucleotides to the SNP detection of a model system [93]. We further developed this system using novel PAH analogs and applied an excimer based design for the genotyping of the HIV-1 protease-encoding gene fragment (Fig. **8**) [94]. The application of novel (phenylethynyl) pyrene dyes, having improved photo physical characteristics from the parent pyrene, resulted in improved sensitivity of the detection with detection limit below 5 nM. As a result of the additional LNAs in our design, we observed an effective detection of SNPs even in the presence of one-two polymorphic mutations located 5-7 nucleotides apart from the position of the drug-resistance causing SNP (Fig. **9a**). We furthermore efficiently applied this system to *in vitro* genotyping of clinical samples amplified by PCR. The resulting data was in full agreement with the sequencing experiments that we performed as controls.

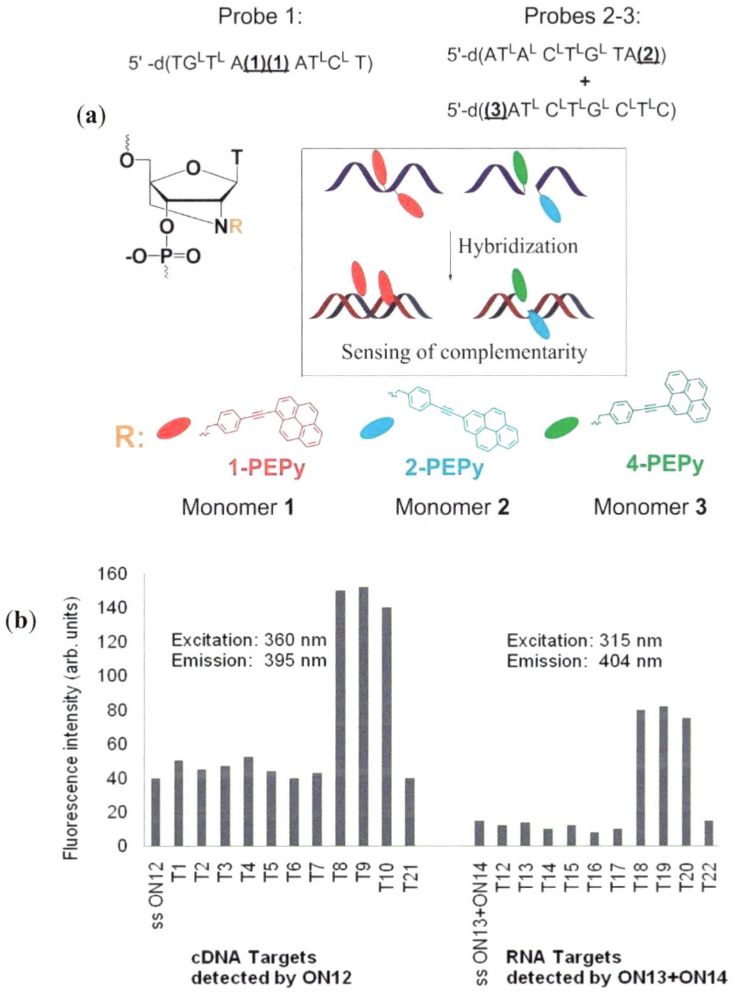

Figure 8: PAH-LNA/DNA probes in colorimetric assays for single-nucleotide polymorphism (SNP) detection [94]. HIV-pol = HIV-1 gene fragment encoding protease. (**a**) Chemical structures and design rules for the PAH-LNA/DNA probes, LNAs are marked with uppercase L; (**b**) Fluorescence spectra of single-stranded probe and its complexes with complementary (mutant) and mismatched (wild-type) DNA targets.

Molecular basis for the achieved SNP sensing is demonstrated in Figs. **9b**, **c**. As seen in the perfectly matched double-stranded complex, two (phenylethynyl) pyrene moieties are in close proximity and simultaneously parallel to each other (Fig. **9b**). This results in excimer formation which gives an additional long-wavelength band in the fluorescence spectrum of the corresponding complex.

When the SNP is located opposite to the PAH-LNA unit, the overall secondary structure is locally disturbed resulting in a (phenylethynyl) pyrene dye positioned further away from the second dye (Fig. **9c**). Therefore, no excimer can be formed when the probe binds to the mutated target, resulting in the absence of the corresponding fluorescence signal in the spectrum [94].

Förster resonance energy transfer (FRET) was also found to be useful for nucleotide-specific genotyping of the HIV PR gene using LNA/DNA probes [95]. It is well known that FRET can take place when two fluorophores with sufficient spectral overlap between the donor fluorescence and acceptor absorbance are in close proximity (distance typically below 7 nm). Importantly, this occurs only provided that the two fluorophores have a favorable donor–acceptor dipole–dipole orientation. FRET can be monitored quantitatively and in real time (*e.g.,* real-time PCR) and has additional possibilities for multiplexing and growing applications for imaging *in vivo*. Multiple FRET pairs have already been applied in SNP diagnostics in different assays which have their own advantages and drawbacks (*e.g.,* Taqman probes, molecular beacons, dye-labeled oligonucleotide ligation and template-directed dye-terminator incorporation). However, these assays mainly applied a dye–quencher design of FRET probes. Recently we explored another important parameter of FRET for SNP sensing, namely a dipole–dipole orientation factor [95]. We also aimed to improve fluorescence properties of the pyrene attached to 2′-amino-LNA by alternating the position of the substitution in the pyrene core from 1 to 4, since this modification has already showed promising results in the labeling of nucleic acids (monomer $\mathbf{M}^2$, Fig. **10**). This was done in double-labeled and dual-probe formats. The performed modification significantly improved photo physical and spectral characteristics of the pyrene with a remarkable effect on its interactions with the commonly used PAH acceptor FRET perylene (monomers $\mathbf{M}^3$–$\mathbf{M}^4$, Fig. **10**). We rationalized these results by molecular modeling studies and furthermore utilized the novel FRET pairs within short LNA/DNA probes for SNP sensing in cDNA fragments obtained from patients currently receiving anti-HIV-1/AIDS therapy (Fig. **11**). We demonstrated that a sequential application of the prepared probes provides exact information on the mismatched nucleotide within the target sequence. This is a result of a conformational change within the double helix when a mismatch is located opposite to the perylene-modified nucleotide. Owing to the high sensitivity of FRET to the dipole-dipole orientation factor between donor and acceptor, such a big change results in a decreased FRET and lowered emission signal of perylene. We speculate that in a similar way other FRET pairs can be attached directly to 2'-amino-LNA, resulting in highly efficient genotyping tools while applying a broad range of excitation/emission wavelengths [95].

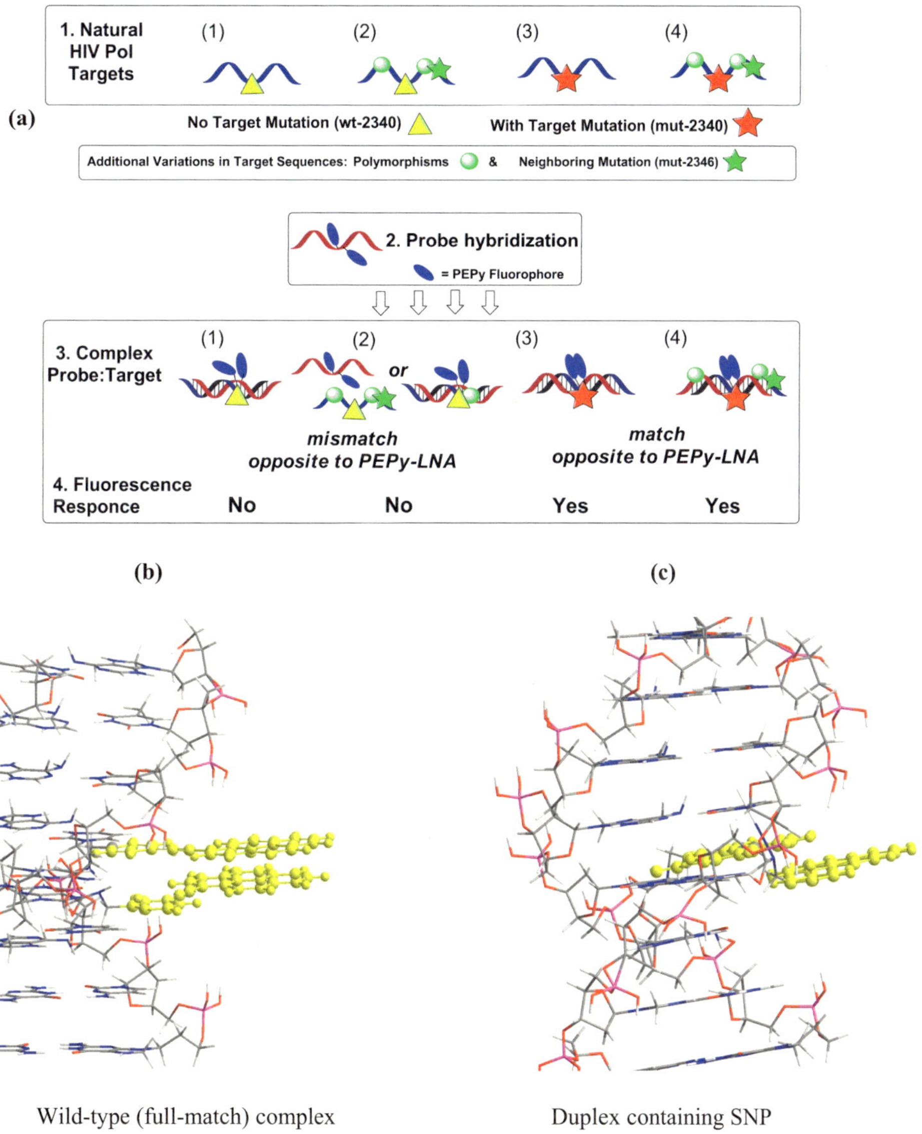

Figure 9: Design of LNA-enhanced PAH-LNA/DNA probes for sensing polymorphic HIV PR gene fragment (**a**); molecular basis for SNP sensing using PAH-LNA/DNA (**b**, **c**).

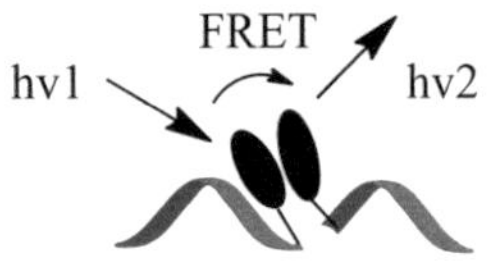

Dual-probe format (DP)

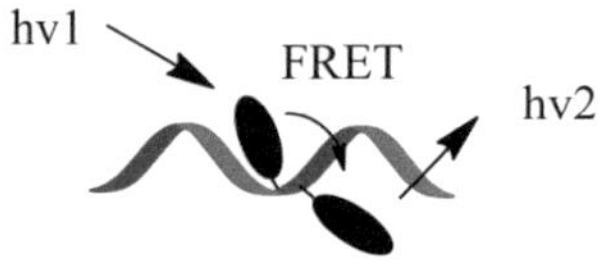

Double-labelled probe format (DLP)

ON1-ON2: 5'-d($\underline{\mathbf{M}}^{1\text{-}2}$CT^{L} TCC AC^{L}A)
+
ON3-ON4: 5'-d(CA^{L}C CAA C$\underline{\mathbf{M}}^{3\text{-}4}$)

ON5-ON8: 5' -d(CA^{L}C CAA C$\underline{\mathbf{M}}^{3\text{-}4}\underline{\mathbf{M}}^{1\text{-}2}$ CT^{L}T CCA C^{L}A)

LNA/DNA Probes:Target cDNA

Mutation G2340A

ON9: 3'-d(C$\underline{T}^{L}\underline{C}^{L}$ $\underline{G}^{L}\underline{T}^{L}\underline{C}^{L}$ $\underline{T}^{L}$A$\underline{\mathbf{M}}^{2}$)
5'-d(GAG CAG AT$\underline{\mathbf{G}}$*ATA CAG TAT TAG AA)
ON11-ON12: 3'-d(($\underline{\mathbf{M}}^{3}$-$\underline{\mathbf{M}}^{4}$)AT $\underline{G}^{L}\underline{T}^{L}\underline{C}^{L}$ $\underline{A}^{L}\underline{T}^{L}\underline{A}^{L}$)

Mutation G2346A

ON10: 3'-d(C$\underline{T}^{L}\underline{A}^{L}$ $\underline{C}^{L}\underline{T}^{L}\underline{A}^{L}$ $\underline{T}^{L}\underline{G}^{L}\underline{\mathbf{M}}^{2}$)
5'-d(GAG CAG ATG ATA CA$\underline{\mathbf{G}}$*TAT TAG AA)
ON13-ON14: 3'-d(($\underline{\mathbf{M}}^{3}$-$\underline{\mathbf{M}}^{4}$)AT $\underline{A}^{L}\underline{A}^{L}\underline{T}^{L}$ $\underline{C}^{L}\underline{T}^{L}\underline{T}^{L}$)

Target cDNA fragments:[1]

Wt (*14*): ...GAGCAGATGATACAGTATTAGAA...
Wt (*18*): ...GAGCAGATGATACAGTATTAGAA...
Wt+pol (*21*): ...GAGCAGATGATA**<u>CG</u>**TATTAGAA...
Wt+pol (*42*): ...GAGCAGAT**<u>r</u>**GATACAGTATTAGAA...
G2340A+pol (*58*): ...GAGCAGAT**<u>A</u>***ATACAGTA**<u>A</u>**TAGAA...
G2346A+pol (*68*): ...GAGCAGATGATACA**<u>A</u>***TATT**<u>G</u>**GAA...

Figure 10: Design of LNA-enhanced PAH-LNA/DNA probes for sensing polymorphic HIV PR gene fragment using FRET between pyrene and perylene dyes. [1] Target sequences obtained by sequencing of DNA from patient samples.

(a)

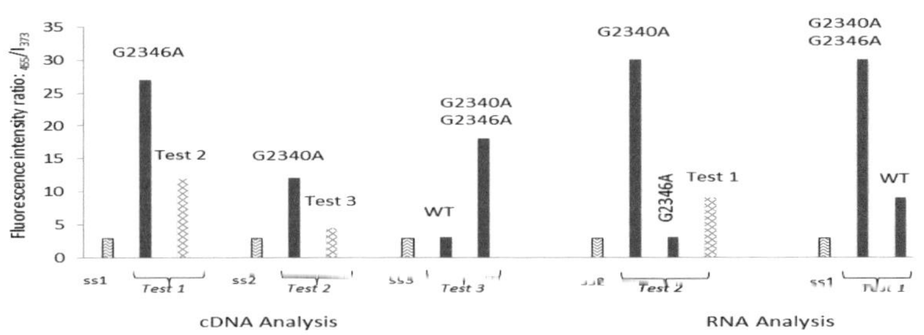

Fig. 11: contd...

(b) **(c)**

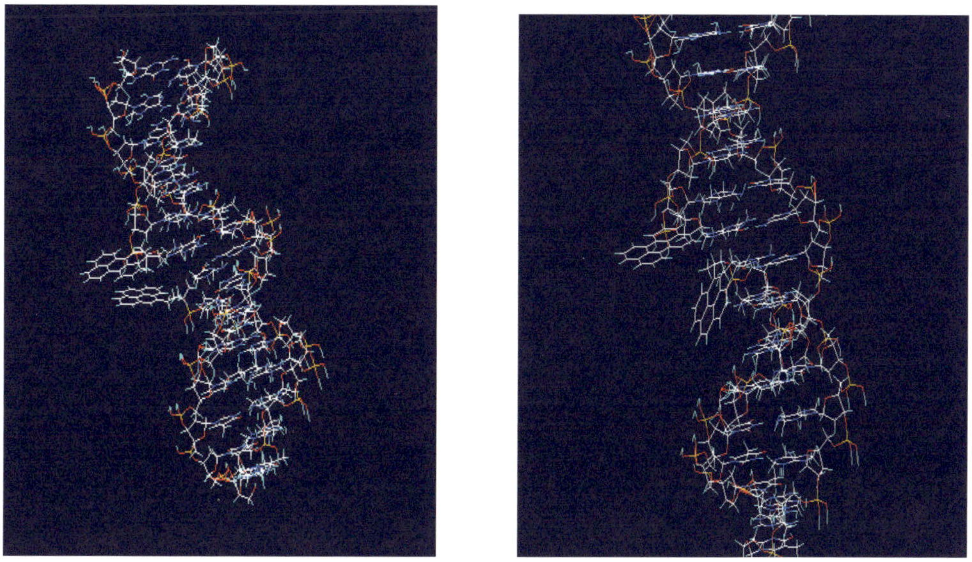

Wild-type (full-match) complex Duplex containing SNP opposite to PAH-LNA

Figure 11: Genotyping of HIV PR gene fragment using FRET PAH-LNA/DNA probes (**a**); molecular basis for SNP sensing using FRET forming PAH-LNA/DNA probes (**b, c**).

Emerging Technologies

Imaging

Major goals for future detection of SNP in HIV-1 nucleic acids are high specificity and affinity of target binding, bright signal, decreased coast for both high-throughput and easy-to-handle assays, along with their high repeatability and robustness. With this respect, non-enzymatic techniques provide advantages of improved repeatability, decreased cost and robustness [96]. Non-enzymatic methods can be also combined with advanced microscopy techniques in order to improve sensitivity of HIV-1 detection. In the very recent paper, fluorescent nucleotide analogs 2-aminopurine and pyrrolo-C have been applied to monitor model DNA and RNA in the real time at the single-molecule level [97]. Clearly, similar assay can be applied for HIV-1 studies and diagnostics.

Another visualization assay for newly synthesized HIV cDNA is a so-called oligo fluorescent *in situ* hybridization (O-FISH) [98]. This technique applies fluorescently labeled sequence specific oligonucleotide (approx. 19-26 nt long), and imaging of the formed duplex by microscopy. The advantage of O-FISH is its high sensitivity. Thus, in a model system O-FISH allowed detection of 1-2 copies of HIV-1 cDNA per individual cell. The authors suggest that O-FISH could potentially be extended for *in situ* visualization of small viral RNA, *e.g.*, scientifically and clinically important microRNA (miRNA) molecules [98].

Simultaneous Diagnostics and Gene Therapy

An important advantage of applying synthetic oligonucleotides to target HIV-1 genome is the possibility to develop a sensing and therapeutic tool simultaneously. By developing SNPs, HIV can develop resistance to currently applied therapeutics rapidly [1-3]. Gene therapy use synthetic oligonucleotides which specifically bind highly conserved regions within the viral genome and are a promising strategy for HIV treatment [99]. For example, synthetic LNA/DNA oligonucleotides binding two highly conserved regions of the HIV-1 genome, packaging signal and trans-activating response regions, have been recently investigated [99]. In this study it was shown that acting as steric block therapeutics, 2'-*O*-methyl/LNA oligonucleotides s inhibit HIV replication efficiently by binding to the selected genomic regions. However, it is still difficult to achieve an effective level of oligonucleotide "diagnostic+therapeutic" oligonucleotide at the appropriate site within the cell. To overcome this obstacle, efficient oligonucleotide delivery approaches have to be developed [100]. Stimulated by constantly growing interest to personalized diagnostics and gene therapy, the field of oligonucleotide delivery is one of the most rapidly developing fields in modern biomedical research and industry.

Impact of Nanotechnology

Non-invasive imaging technologies for the diagnosis of diseases including HIV typically involve the administration of contrast or signal enhancement agents that facilitate the visualization of organs or the state of a particular disease. Nanotechnology, particularly the development of nanoparticles-based agents, has had a tremendous impact on the design of targeted and specific tools with the potential of targeting a particular area and interrogating for normal or disease processes. Thus, diverse nanoparticles, nucleic acid nano-structures and other nanomaterials offer exciting opportunities for future diagnostics of HIV-1 at nanoscale. Major advantages of nanomaterials in diagnostics include improved sensitivity and robustness of detection using much lower amount of target DNA/RNA than in most currently applied methods. For example, only one micro liter of the solution containing the sub-picomole p53 gene DNA samples was sufficient for microscopy based detection using novel colored nanospheres [101]. The oligonucleotides were immobilized on organic nanospheres containing additional fluorescent dyes. In the presence of the single-stranded DNA target that is fully complementary to the immobilized probes, the spheres could aggregate *via* cross-linking. In this way, the resulting colors of the aggregated nanospheres depended on the added DNA sequences and were monitored using an ordinary fluorescent microscope. FRET between the nanospheres also provided information about the SNP in added DNAs.

Next, using synthetic nanoparticles prepared by click chemistry between azido groups of oligo ethylene glycol mecrylate (OEGMA) polymer on the surface of magnetic nanoparticles with a gene-specific probe, the DNA of herpes simplex (HSV) virus was detected without amplification at low picomolar range (*i.e.,* 6 pM in aqueous buffer and 60 pM in fetal bovine serum) by means of fluorescence [102].

Song and co-workers developed colorimetric SNP detection using intrinsic peroxidase-like activity of single-walled carbon nanotubes [103]. Using this enzyme-free assay, SNP has been detected in just 15 min and at 1 nM concentration of DNA 45.

Finally, same detection sensitivity as for PCR (approx. 70 aM) was obtained for magnetic particles modified with capture DNA sequences in a so-called Simoa assay [104]. Remarkably, Simoa technique is a direct diagnostic system and allows a rapid multiplexed detection of nucleic acids and proteins from biologic fluids like blood in a fully automated regimen.

Combined Diagnostics of HIV and Other Infections

An innovative microarray for multiplexed detection of proteins and nucleic acids has been recently developed aiming at monitoring three human viral infections

(HIV, HBV, and HCV) and several associated parameters for diagnosis and therapeutic follow-up [105]. To detect viral antibodies and labeled cDNA in infected sera, purified protein antigens and nucleic acid probes were spotted in 96-well microplates. A reaction buffer had to be optimized so that both hybridization and immunological coupling could be possible under the same experimental conditions, following the same protocol. Specificity was demonstrated by the consecutive addition of each analyte in the same well inducing the coloration of expected spots. Spot density was quantified by software analysis and was related to analyte concentration, demonstrating that the new technique called CombOLISA was suitable for quantitative assays. Notably, results of CombOLISA correlated with values determined using standard commercial immunoassays and were comparable in sensitivity to a standard ELISA.

CONCLUDING REMARKS

To date, multiple strategies have been developed for SNP sensing in HIV-1 DNA and RNA. Generally, these strategies can be classified as sophisticated, high-throughput methods, portable and having easy-to-use settings. Both groups of methods are based on specific binding of the target viral RNA/cDNA and its sensing by the method of choice. Although enzymatic strategies such as PCR, sequencing and SNP microarrays are well-established in research and clinical laboratories, they are more time consuming and expensive for applications in all the areas where HIV-1 spreads. Moreover, SNP diagnostic methods which rely on protein enzymes, such as sequencing and PCR, often lack specificity and reproducibility. These disadvantages can be solved by the development of non-enzymatic rapid SNP sensing methods and by single-molecule imaging techniques. As described in this chapter, the novel promising SNP probe designs include direct imaging at the single-molecule level, nanoparticles and other biopolymers, modified nucleic acid analogs, including LNA and PAH-LNA analogs. Although most of amplification-free assays *in vitro* are still less sensitive than classic enzyme-based methods, they already have a great advantage of high specificity, low cost and a robust detection technique. Further development of fluorogenic ultra-bright probes for enzyme-free SNP sensing and especially single-molecule imaging might benefit from new chemical substances, biophysical and biotechnological approaches. Future sensor probes for SNP diagnostics in HIV-1 could be based on recently introduced super-bright photostable BODIPY dyes [106], bioorthogonal nucleic acid analogs for *in vivo* incorporation and monitoring [36], and diverse nanomaterials modified with PAH-LNA/DNA probes [86, 107].

ACKNOWLEDGEMENTS

The author would like to acknowledge financial support from The Sapere Aude programme of The Danish Council for Independent Research (Grant No. FNU 11-115447) and Augustinus Foundation (Grant No. 95 305 73949). The author also acknowledges Laura Miotke, Paul Zakrevsky, Per Trolle Jørgensen and Lars Lønstrup for help in the preparation of this chapter.

CONFLICT OF INTEREST

The authors confirm that this chapter contents have no conflict of interest.

REFERENCES

[1] Kuriyan J, Konforti B, Wemmer D. In "The Molecules of life". Garland Science, 2012.

[2] Marcelin AG. Resistance to nucleoside reverse transcriptase inhibitors. In Antiretroviral resistance in clinical practice 2006. London: Mediscript, ch. 1.

[3] Astakhova IK, Samokhina E, Babu BR, Wengel J. Novel (phenylethynyl)pyrene-LNA constructs for fluorescence SNP sensing in polymorphic nucleic acid targets. ChemBioChem 2012; 13: 1509-19.

[4] A.P. Seltsovsky, S.V. Polyakov, A.I. Mazus, E.M. Kozhokin A.Y. Olshansky. NetLogo. http: //www.spid.ru/09/pic/090304.pdf. Moscow Healthcare Department, Russia's Institute of Strategic studies, 2005, Moscow.

[5] Rhee SY, Gonzales MJ, Kantor R, Betts BJ, Ravela J, Shafer RW. Human immunodeficiency virus reverse transcriptase and protease sequence database. Nucleic Acids Res 2003; 31: 298-303.

[6] (a) Lawrence J *et al.* Clinical resistance patterns and responses to two sequential protease inhibitor regimens in saquinavir and reverse transcriptase inhibitor-experienced persons. J Infect Dis 1999; 179: 1356-64; (b) Walmsley SL, Becker MI, Zhang M, Humar A, Harrigan PR. Predictors of virological response in HIV-infected patients to salvage antiretroviral therapy that includes nelfinavir. Antivir Ther 2001; 6: 47-54

[7] Casado JL *et al.* Efficacy, tolerance, and pharmacokinetics of the combination of stavudine, nevirapine, nelfinavir, and saquinavir as salvage regimen after ritonavir or indinavir failure. AIDS Res Hum Retroviruses 2001; 17: 93-8.

[8] Zhang L *et al.* Genetic characterization of rebounding HIV-1 after cessation of highly active antiretroviral therapy. J Clin Invest 2000; 106: 839-45.

[9] Ramratnam B *et al.* The decay of the latent reservoir of replication-competent HIV-1 is inversely correlated with the extent of residual viral replication during prolonged anti-retroviral therapy. Nat Med 2000; 6: 82-5.

[10] Zhang L *et al.* Quantifying residual HIV-1 replication in patients receiving combination antiretroviral therapy. N Engl J Med 2000; 340: 1605-13.

[11] Haddad DN, Birch C, Middleton T, Dwyer DE, Cunningham AL, Saksena NK. Evidence for late stage compartmentalization of HIV-1 resistance mutations between lymph node and peripheral blood mononuclear cells. AIDS 2000; 14: 2273-81.

[12] Wong JK, Ignacio CC, Torriani F, Havlir D, Fitch NJ, Richman DD. *In vivo* compartmentalization of human immunodeficiency virus: evidence from the examination of pol sequences from autopsy tissues. J Virol 1997; 71: 2059-71.

[13] Bann DV, Parent LJ. Application of Live-Cell RNA Imaging Techniques to the Studyof Retroviral RNA Trafficking. Viruses 2012; 4: 963-979.

[14] Daar ES Does the human immunodeficiency virus (HIV) RNA concentration in cerebrospinal fluid help clinicians diagnose or understand HIV-induced neurological disease? Clin Infect Dis 1998; 26: 1074-5.

[15] Cunningham PH, Smith DG, Satchell C, Cooper DA, Brew B. Evidence for independent development of resistance to HIV-1 reverse transcriptase inhibitors in the cerebrospinal fluid. AIDS 2000; 14: 1949-54.

[16] Gunthard HF *et al.* Residual human immunodeficiency virus (hiv) type 1 rna and dna in lymph nodes and hiv rna in genital secretions and in cerebrospinal fluid after suppression of viremia for 2 years. J Infect Dis 2001; 183: 1318-27.

[17] Venturi G, Catucci M, Romano L, Corsi P, Leoncini F, Valensin PE, Zazzi M. Antiretroviral resistance mutations in human immunodeficiency virus type 1 reverse transcriptase and protease from paired cerebrospinal fluid and plasma samples. J Infect Dis 2000; 181: 740-5.

[18] Larsen BB *et al.* Improved Detection of Rare HIV-1 Variants using 454 Pyrosequencing. Plos One 2013; DOI: 10.1371/journal.pone.0076502.

[19] Altmann A, Weber P, Bader D, Preuss M, Binder EB, Müller-Myhsok B. A beginners guide to SNP calling from high-throughput DNA-sequencing data. Hum Genet 2012; 131: 1541-54.

[20] Haubrich R, Demeter L. Clinical utility of resistance testing: retrospective and prospective data supporting use and current recommendations. J Acquir Immune Defic Syndr 2001; 26: S51-9.

[21] Gaudet M, Fara AG, Beritognolo I, Sabatti M. Allele-specific PCR in SNP genotyping. Methods Mol Biol 2009; 578: 415-24.

[22] Said EA *et al.* Association of single-nucleotide polymorphisms in TLR7 (Gln11Leu) and TLR9 (1635A/G) with a higher CD4T cell count during HIV infection. Immunol Lett 2014; 160: 58-64.

[23] Iyer S, Bouzek H, Deng W, Larsen B, Casey E, Mullins JI. Quality score based identification and correction of pyrosequencing errors. PLoS One 2013; 8: e73015.

[24] Madlala P *et al.* Association of polymorphisms in the LEDGF/p75 gene (PSIP1) with susceptibility to HIV-1 infection and disease progression. AIDS 2011; 25: 1711-9.

[25] Koshkin A, Rajwanshi VK, Wengel J. Novel Convenient Syntheses of LNA [2.2.1] Bicyclo Nucleosides. Tetrahedron Lett 1998; 39: 4381-4.

[26] Hari Y, Obika S, Sasaki M. Effective synthesis of C-nucleosides with 2'-4'-BNA modification. Tetrahedron 2002; 58: 3051-63.

[27] Latorra D, Arar K, Hurley JM. Design considerations and effects of LNA in PCR primers. Mol Cell Probes 2003; 17: 253-9.

[28] Di Giusto DA, King GC. Strong positional preference in the interaction of LNA oligonucleotides with DNA polymerase and proofreading exonuclease activities: implications for genotying assays. Nucleic Acids Res 2004; 32. e32.

[29] Levin JD *et al.* Position-dependent effects of locked nucleic acid (LNA) on DNA sequencing and PCR primers. Nucleic Acids Res 2006; 34: e142.

[30] Rupp J, Solbach W, Gieffers J. Single-nucleotide-polymorphism-specific PCR for quantifcation and discrimination of Chlamydia pneumoniae genotypes by use of a "locked" nucleic acid. Appl Environ Microbiol 2006; 72: 3785-7.

[31] Johnson MP, Haupt LM, Griffiths LR. Locked nucleic acid (LNA) single nucleotide polymorphism (SNP) genotype analysis and validation using real-time PCR. Nucleic Acids Res 2004; 32: e55.

[32] Spiteri C, Moses JE. Copper-catalyzed azide-alkyne cycloaddition: regioselective synthesis of 1,4,5-trisubstituted 1,2,3-triazoles. Angew Chem Int Ed 2010; 49: 31-3, and articles cited therein.

[33] Ustinov AV, Stepanova IA, Dubnyakova VV, Zatsepin TS, Nozhevnikova EV, Korshun VA. Modification of nucleic acids using [3+2] dipolar cycloaddition of azides and alkynes. Rus J Bioorg Chem 2010; 36: 437-81, and references therein.

[34] El-Sagheer AH, Brown T. Click chemistry with DNA. Chem Soc Rev 2010; 39: 1388-405, and references therein.

[35] El-Sagheer AH, Brown T. Click nucleic acid ligation: applications in biology and nanotechnology. Acc Chem Res 2012, 45, 1258-67, and references therein.

[36] Rieder U, Luedtke NW. Alkene-tetrazine ligation for imaging cellular DNA. Angew Chem Int Ed 2014; doi: 10.1002/anie.201403580.

[37] Neef AB, Luedtke NW. An azide-modified nucleoside for metabolic labeling of DNA. ChemBioChem 2014; 15: 789-93.

[38] Astakhova IK, Wengel J. Interfacing click chemistry with automated oligonucleotide synthesis for the preparation of fluorescent DNA probes containing internal xanthene and cyanine dyes. Chem Eur J 2013; 19: 1112-22.

[39] Astakhova IK, Hansen LH, Vester B, Wengel J. Peptide-LNA oligonucleotide conjugates. Org Biomol Chem 2013; 11: 4240-9.

[40] Jørgensen AS, Gupta P, Wengel J, Astakhova IK. "Clickable" LNA/DNA Probes for Fluorescence Sensing of Nucleic Acids and Autoimmune Antibodies. Chem Commun 2013; 49: 10751-3.

[41] Didelot A *et al.* Multiplex picoliter-droplet digital PCR for quantitative assessment of DNA integrity in clinical samples. Clin Chem 2012; doi: 10.1373/clinchem.2012.193409.

[42] Østergaard ME, Hrdlicka PJ. Pyrene-functionalized oligonucleotides and locked nucleic acids (LNAs): Tools for fundamental research, diagnostics, and nanotechnology. Chem Soc Rev 2011; 40: 5771-8.

[43] Rodrigo MAM *et al.* HIV Biosensors - the potential of the electrochemical way. Int J Electrochem Sci. 2014; 9: 3449-57.

[44] Zhang H. Devices and methods for detecting analytes using electrosensor having capture reagent. WO2001038873 A2, 2001.

[45] Niu SY, Li F, Zhang SS, Wang L, Li XM, Wang SY. Studies on the interaction mechanism of 1,10-phenanthroline cobalt(II) complex with DNA and preparation of electrochemical DNA biosensor. Sensors 2006; 6: 1234-44.

[46] Niu SY, Zhang SS, Wang L, Li XM. Hybridization biosensor using di(1,10-phenanthroline) (imidazo[f]1,10-phenanthroline)cobalt(II) as electrochemical indicator for detection of human immunodeficiency virus DNA. J Electroanal Chem 2006; 597: 111-8.

[47] Kerman K, Mahmoud KA, Kraatz HB. An electrochemical approach for the detection of HIV-1 protease. Chem Commun 2007; 37: 3829-31.

[48] Liu ZM, Li ZJ, Shen GL, Yu RQ. Label-free detection of DNA hybridization based on MnO 2 nano-particles. Anal Lett 2009; 42: 3046-57.

[49] Astakhova IK, Kumar TS, Campbell MA, Ustinov AV, Korshun VA, Wengel J. Branched DNA nanostructures efficiently stabilised and monitored by novel pyrene-perylene 2'-α-L-amino-LNA FRET pairs. Chem Commun 2013; 49: 511-3.

[50] Astakhova IV, Kumar TS, Wengel J. Fluorescent oligonucleotides containing a novel perylene 2′-amino-α-L-LNA monomer: Synthesis and analytical potential. Coll. Czeck. Chem Commun 2011; 76: 1347-60.

[51] Murphy D, O'Brien P, Redmond G. Sub-picomole colorimetric single nucleotide polymorphism discrimination using oligonucleotide-nanoparticle conjugates. Analyst 2004; 129: 970-4.

[52] Jian JW, Huang CC. Colorimetric detection of DNA by modulation of thrombin activity on gold nanoparticles. Chem Eur J 2011; 17: 2374-80.

[53] Bao YP, Huber M, Wei TF, Marla SS, Storhoff JJ, Müller UR. SNP identification in unamplified human genomic DNA with gold nanoparticle probes. Nucleic Acids Res 2005; 33: e15.

[54] Kitamura Y, Ihara T, Tsujimura Y, Osawa Y, Jyo A. Colorimetric allele analysis based on the DNA-directed cooperative formation of luminous lanthanide complexes. Nucleic Acids Symp Ser 2006; 105-6.

[55] Mirkin CA, Letsinger RL, Mucic RC, Storhoff JJ. A DNA-Based Method for Rationally Assembling Nanoparticles into Macroscopic Materials. Nature 1996; 382: 607-9.

[56] Komminoth P, Long AA. In-situ polymerase chain reaction. An overview of methods, applications and limitations of a new molecular technique. Virchows Arch B Cell Pathol Incl Mol Pathol 1993; 64: 67-73.

[57] Naif H, Cunningham A. *In situ* PCR for detection of HIV using digoxigenin-labeled oligonucleotides. Biochemica 1995; 3: 23-4.

[58] Bagasra O. Protocols for the *in situ* PCR-amplification and detection of mRNA and DNA sequences. Nature Protocols 2007; 2: 2782-95.

[59] Chen RH, Fuggle SV. *In situ* PCR amplification of intracellular mRNA. Methods Mol Biol 1996; 71: 123-32.

[60] Patterson BK, Jiyamapa D, Mayrand E, Hoff B, Abramson R, Garcia PM. Detection of HIV-1 Dna in Cells and Tissue by Fluorescent *in Situ* 5′-Nuclease Assay (FISNA). Nucleic Acids Res 1996; 24: 3656-8.

[61] Belinda Y-L. NetLogo. http: //www.medscape.com/viewarticle/410196. Medscape Multispeciality, 2001.

[62] Marras SA, Kramer FR, Tyagi S. Genotyping SNPs with molecular beacons. Methods Mol Biol 2002; 212: 111-28.

[63] Lakowicz JR. Principles of Fluorescence Spectroscopy. 3rd ed., 2006, Springer Science+Business Media, LLC, Singapore, KYO.

[64] Barreiro LB, Henriques R, Mhlanga MM. High-throughput SNP genotyping: combining tag SNPs and molecular beacons. Methods Mol Biol 2009; 578: 255-76.

[65] Kannegård KK, Okholm AH, Kjems J, Wengel J. A quencher-free molecular beacon design based on pyrene excimer fluorescence using pyrene-labeled UNA (unlocked nucleic acid). Bioorg Med Chem 2013; 21: 6186-90.

[66] Brown LJ, Cummins J, Hamilton A, Brown T. Molecular beacons attached to glass beads fluoresce upon hybridisation to target DNA. Chem Commun 2000; 621-2.

[67] Erali M, Hillyard DR. Evaluation of the ultrasensitive Roche Amplicor HIV-1 Monitor assay for quantitation of human immunodeficiency virus type 1 RNA. J Clin Microbiol 1999; 37: 792-5.

[68] Perrin L, Pawlotsky JM, Bouvier-Alias M, Sarrazin C, Zeuzem S, Colucci G. Multicenter performance evaluation of a new TaqMan PCR assay for monitoring human immunodeficiency virus RNA load. J Clin Microbiol 2006; 44: 4371-5.

[69] Damond F *et al.* Human immunodeficiency virus type 1 (HIV-1) plasma load discrepancies between the Roche Cobas Amplicor HIV-1 Monitor version 1.5 and the Roche Cobas AmpliPrep/Cobas TaqMan HIV-1 assays. J Clin Microbiol 2007; 45: 3436-8.

[70] Li P *et al.* Novel application of Locked Nucleic Acid chemistry for a Taqman assay for measuring diverse human immunodeficiency virus type 1 subtypes. J Virol Methods 2010; 170: 115-20.

[71] Shafer RW, Dupnik K, Winters MA, Eshleman SH. A Guide to HIV-1 Reverse Transcriptase and Protease Sequencing for Drug Resistance Studies. NetLogo. http: //hivdb.stanford.edu/pages/pdf/sequencingGuide.pdf. HIV-1 RT and Protease Sequencing for Drug Resistance Studies.

[72] a) Cline J, Braman JC, Hogrefe HH. PCR fidelity of pfu DNA polymerase and other thermostable DNA polymerases. Nucleic Acids Res 1996; 24: 3546-51; b) Brown AJL, Simmonds P. Sequence analysis of virus variability based on the polymerase chain reaction (PCR). In HIV A Practical Approach Virol Immunol 1995; 1: 161-86.

[73] Iacobucci I *et al.* Application of the whole-transcriptome shotgun sequencing approach to the study of Philadelphia-positive acute lymphoblastic leukemia. Blood Cancer J 2012; 2: e61.

[74] Wang Z, Gerstein M, Snyder M. RNA-Seq: a revolutionary tool for transcriptomics. Nat Rev Genet 2009; 10: 57-63.

[75] Geiss GK *et al.* Direct multiplexed measurement of gene expression with color-coded probe pairs. Nat Biotechnol 2008; 26: 317-25.

[76] Di Carlo D, Tse HT, Gossett DR. Introduction: why analyze single cells? Methods Mol Biol 2012; 853: 1-10.

[77] Narsinh KH *et al.* Single cell transcriptional profiling reveals heterogeneity of human induced pluripotent stem cells. J Clin Invest 2011; 121: 1217-21.

[78] Raj A, Tyagi S. Detection of individual endogenous RNA transcripts *in situ* using multiple singly labeled probes. Methods Enzymol 2010; 472: 365-86.

[79] Bengtsson M, Stahlberg A, Rorsman P, Kubista M. Gene expression profiling in single cells from the pancreatic islets of Langerhans reveals lognormal distribution of mRNA levels. Genome Res 2005; 15: 1388-92.

[80] Astakhova I, Korshun VA, Jahn K, Kjems J, Wengel, J. Perylene attached to 2'-amino-LNA: Synthesis, incorporation into oligonucleotides, and remarkable fluorescence properties in vitro and in cell culture. Bioconjugate Chem 2008; 19: 1995-2007.

[81] Xu H *et al.* Evidence for biphasic uncoating during HIV-1 infection from a novel imaging assay. Retrovirology 2013; 10: 70.

[82] Lalmansingh AS, Arora K, DeMarco RA, Hager GL, Nagaich AK. High-Throughput RNA FISH Analysis by Imaging Flow Cytometry Reveals That Pioneer Factor Foxa1 Reduces Transcriptional Stochasticity. PLoS One 2013; 8: e76043.

[83] Raj A, van Oudenaarden A. Single-molecule approaches to stochastic gene expression. Annu Rev Biophys 2009; 38: 255-70.

[84] NetLogo. http: //www.acdbio.com/products/rnascope-assays/rnascope-fl/

[85] Hanley MB, Lomas W, Mittar D, Maino V, Park E. Detection of Low Abundance RNA Molecules in Individual Cells by Flow Cytometry. PLoS One 2013; 8: e57002.

[86] Astakhova IK, Wengel J. Scaffolding along Nucleic Acid Duplexes Using 2′-Amino-Locked Nucleic Acids. Acc Chem Res 2014; 47: 1768-77.

[87] Sau SP, Hrdlicka PJ. C2′-Pyrene-functionalized. Triazole-linked DNA: Universal DNA/RNA Hybridization Probes. J Org Chem 2012; 77: 5-16.

[88] Holzhauser C, Wagenknecht H-A. DNA and RNA "Traffic Lights": Synthetic Wavelength-Shifting Fluorescent Probes Based on Nucleic Acid Base Substitutes for Molecular Imaging. J Org Chem 2013; 78: 7373-9.

[89] Demchenko A. Advanced Fluorescence Reporters in Chemistry and Biology I: Fundamentals and Molecular Design. Springer Science & Business Media, 2010.

[90] Iwase R, Mahara A, Yamana K, Yamaoka T, Murakami A. Study on RNA structure by pyrene-labeled 2'-O-methyloligoribonucleotides. Nucleic Acids Symp Ser 1999; 42: 115-6.

[91] Johansson MK, Fidder H, Dick D, Cook RM. Intramolecular Dimers: A New Strategy to Fluorescence Quenching in Dual-Labeled Oligonucleotide Probes. J Am Chem Soc 2002; 124: 6950-6.

[92] Vendrell M, Zhai D, Er JC, Chang Y-T. Combinatorial Strategies in Fluorescent Probe Development. Chem Rev 2012; 112: 4391-420.

[93] Umemoto T, Hrdlicka P, Babu BR, Wengel J. Sensitive SNP Dual-Probe Assays Based on Pyrene-Functionalized 2′-Amino-LNA: Lessons To Be Learned. ChemBioChem 2007; 8: 2240-8.

[94] Astakhova IK, Samokhina E, Babu BR, Wengel J. Novel (Phenylethynyl)pyrene-LNA Constructs for Fluorescence SNP Sensing in Polymorphic Nucleic Acid Targets. ChemBioChem 2012; 13: 1509-19.

[95] Kumar TS, Myznikova A, Samokhina E, Astakhova IK. Rapid genotyping using pyrene-perylene locked nucleic acid complexes. Artif XNA DNA PNA 2013; 4: 58-68.

[96] Zhang H, DeConinck AJ, Slimmer SC, Doyle PS, Lewis JA, Nuzzo RG. Genotyping by Alkaline Dehybridization Using Graphically Encoded Particles. Chemistry 2011; 17: 2867-73.

[97] Alemán EA, de Silva C, Patrick EM, Musier-Forsyth K, Rueda D. Single-Molecule Fluorescence Using Nucleotide Analogs: A Proof-of-Principle. J Phys Chem Lett 2014; 5: 777-81.

[98] Jones KL *et al*. Visualising single molecules of HIV-1 and miRNA nucleic acids. BMC Cell Biology 2013, 14: 21.

[99] Brown DE, Arzumanov A, Syed S, Gait MJ, Lever AM. Inhibition of HIV-1 replication by oligonucleotide analogues directed to the packaging signal and trans-activating response region. Antivir Chem Chemother 2006; 17: 1-9.

[100] Jewell CM, Jung J-M, Atukorale PU, Carney RP, Stellacci F, Irvine DJ. Oligonucleotide Delivery by Cell-Penetrating "Striped" Nanoparticles. Angew Chem Int Ed 2011; 50: 12312-5.

[101] Ihara T, Tanaka S, Chikaura Y, Jyo A. Preparation of DNA-modified nanoparticles and preliminary study for colorimetric SNP analysis using their selective aggregations. Nucleic Acids Res 2004; 32: e105.

[102] Thomson DAC, Tee EH-L, Tran NTD, Monteiro MJ, Cooper MA. Oligonucleotide and polymer functionalized nanoparticles for amplification-free detection of DNA. Biomacromolecules 2012; 13: 1981-9.

[103] Song Y, Wang X, Zhao C, Qu K, Ren J, Qu X. Label-Free Colorimetric Detection of Single Nucleotide Polymorphism by Using Single-Walled Carbon Nanotube Intrinsic Peroxidase- Like Activity. Chem Eur J 2010; 16: 3617-21.

[104] ELISA-inspired technology developed in so-called Simoa instrument by Quanterix, founded in 2007 by D. Walt and N. Naclerio.

[105] Perrin A, Duracher D, Perret M, Cleuziat P, Mandrand B. A combined oligonucleotide and protein microarray for the codetection of nucleic acids and antibodies associated with human immunodeficiency virus, hepatitis B virus, and hepatitis C virus infections. Anal Biochem 2003; 322: 148-55.

[106] Loudet A, Burgess K. BODIPY dyes and their derivatives: syntheses and spectroscopic properties. Chem Rev 2007; 107: 4891-932.

[107] Tian H, Sakmar TP, Huber T. Site-specific labeling of genetically encoded azido groups for multicolor, single-molecule fluorescence imaging of GPCRs. Methods Cell Biol 2013; 117: 267-303.

Frontiers in Clinical Drug Research: HIV, Vol. 1, **2015, 123-184**

CHAPTER 5

Next Generation Anti-HIV Agent 4′-Ethynylstavudine: From the Bench to the Clinic

Kazuhiro Haraguchi[1,*], Shingo Takeda[2], Yutaka Kubota[2], Hiroki Kumamoto[2], Hiromichi Tanaka[2], Takayuki Hamasaki[3], Masanori Baba[3], Elijah Paintsil[4], Yung-Chi Cheng[5] and Yasuo Urata[6]

[1]Department of Pharmaceutical Sciences, Nihon Pharmaceutical University, Saitama 362-0806, Japan; [2]School of Pharmacy, Showa University, Tokyo 142-8555, Japan; [3]Division of Antiviral Chemotherapy, Center for Chronic Viral Diseases, Graduate School of Medical and Dental Sciences, Kagoshima University, Kagoshima 890-8544, Japan; [4]Department of Pediatrics, School of Medicine, Yale University, New Haven, CT 06520, USA; [5]Department of Pharmacology, School of Medicine, Yale University, New Haven, CT 06520, USA and [6]Oncolys BioPharma Inc., 4-1-28 Toranomon, Minato-ku, Tokyo 105-0001, Japan

Abstract: Much attention has been paid to branched-sugar nucleosides due to their biological activities. During our ongoing research project utilizing unsaturated-sugar nucleosides, epoxy-sugar derivatives were found to be useful precursor for the stereo-selective synthesis of these nucleoside derivatives on the basis of their ring opening with organoaluminum or organosilicon reagents. In this chapter, we describe novel synthetic methods for 1′ and 4′-branched-sugar nucleosides. During this research, a novel anti-HIV agent, 4′-ethynylstavudine (4′-Ed4T) has emerged.

4′-Ed4T possessed more potent anti-HIV activity than the parent compound stavudine (d4T). Other characteristic biological properties of 4′-Ed4T are as follows: 1) much less toxic to various cells and also to mitochondorial DNA synthesis than d4T, 2) better substrate for human thymidine kinase than d4T, 3) resistant not only to chemical glycosidic bond cleavage but also to catabolism by thymidine phosphorylase, 4) the activity improves in the presence of a major mutation, K103N, associated with resistance to non-nucleoside reverse transcriptase inhibitors (NNRTIs). The detailed antiviral activities, pharmacology and clinical developments (Phase I and Phase IIa) of 4′-Ed4T are described.

***Corresponding author Kazuhiro Haraguchi:** Department of Pharmaceutical Sciences, Nihon Pharmaceutical University, 10281 Komuro, Inamachi, Kita-adachi-gun, Saitama 362-0806, Japan; Tel: 81-48-721-7294; Fax: 81-48-721-6208; E-mail: harakazu@nichiyaku.ac.jp

Atta-ur-Rahman (Ed)

Keywords: 4′-ethynylstavudine (4′-Ed4T), anti-HIV-1 agent, clinical development, epoxide, NRTIs, nucleoside, organoaluminum reagent, organosilicon reagent, stavudine.

INTRODUCTION

Nucleoside reverse transcriptase inhibitors (NRTIs) occupy the mainstream of combination antiretroviral therapy (cART) for treatment of HIV patients. Guidelines for major HIV-1 treatment recommend that cART should be started with two NRTIs plus one other active agent, a non-nucleoside reverse transcriptase inhibitor (NNRTI), a protease inhibitor or an integrase inhibitor [1-3]. NRTIs have been widely used in first-line regimens. However, there are remained problems such as potential long-term toxicities and the evolution of cross-resistance to members of this class of drugs. Some of NRTIs are not routinely used due to their toxicities, which include mitochondrial toxicity, namely peripheral neuropathy [4, 5], lipoatrophy [6, 7], metabolic acidosis [8], anemia and pancreatitis [2, 9, 10].

Despite the favorable toxicity profiles of lamivudine (3TC) and emtricitabine (FTC), their use in combination is not recommended due to their minimal additive anti-HIV activity and similar resistance profiles [2]. FTC combined with tenofovir disoproxil fumarate (TDF) or 3TC combined with abacavir (ABC) is recommended by current treatment guidelines [1-3]. Among these combinations, TDF combined with FTC is preferred, based on its overall efficacy, safety, tolerability, and convenient dosing regimen. However, there are problems concerning nephrotoxicity, decreased bone mineral density, and increased risk of fractures with TDF [1-3, 11, 12]. ABC is associated with hypersensitivity reaction in HLA-B*5701-positive patients and has been linked to an increased risk of myocardial infarction and cardiovascular disease [13, 14].

Under the present circumstances such as increasing duration of antiviral therapy and convenience of treatment regimens becoming an important factor in improving adherence, important considerations for developing novel antiretroviral agents are long-term toxicity and tolerability and pharmacokinetic (PK) profiles. Upcoming NRTIs have to possess important profiles such as potent anti-HIV activity, a tolerability profile that is similar to or better than currently available antiretroviral agents, a favorable long-term safety profile in terms of bone mineral density and decline in renal function, with a high genetic barrier to HIV drug resistance/limited cross-resistance to existing NRTIs.

4′-Ethynylstavudine (4′-Ed4T) is a thymidine-based NRTI that shows the following significant profiles.

1) 4′-Ed4T has demonstrated greater *in vitro* potency, reduced *in vitro* mitochondrial toxicity and evidence of a higher genetic barrier to resistance compared with other thymidine analogs [15-17].

2) 4′-Ed4T reduced inhibition of host DNA polymerases [16] and minimal cytotoxicity or effect upon mitochondrial DNA (mtDNA) content was seen in cultures of human proximal tubule epithelium, skeletal muscle, or differentiated adipocytes [18]. This is in contrast to stavudine, adefovir and ABC, which caused cytotoxicity and reductions in mtDNA [18].

3) Preclinical studies have also demonstrated a favorable safety profile for 4′-Ed4T, with no evidence of renal or bone toxicity observed in rats and cynomolgus monkeys receiving chronic high doses of 4′-Ed4T [19]. This is in contrast to reports of renal and bone toxicity in monkeys, rats, and mice following treatment with high-doses of tenofovir [20-25].

4) 4′-Ed4T has also demonstrated activity against some NRTI-resistant HIV-1 mutants, and a number of HIV-1 subtypes [26, 27].

The aim of this chapter is a review of chemistry, virology, pharmacology and clinical development of 4′-Ed4T.

Chemistry of Epoxysugar Nucleosides and Synthesis of 2′,3′-Didehydro-3′-Deoxy-4′-Ethynylthymidine (4′-Ethynylstavudine)

3′-Azido-3′-deoxythymidne (AZT) was the first anti-HIV drug, which is a NRTI (Fig. **1**). The emergency of AZT as anti-HIV drug stimulated the synthesis of sugar-modified nucleosides and the evaluation of their anti-viral activity. Since then, other clinically used anti-HIV derivatives such as zalcitabine (ddC), didanosine (ddI) and stavudine (d4T) have been approved. However, the long-term usage of these anti-HIV drugs led to delayed toxicity in patients and/or emergence of drug resistant HIV variants. These circumstances necessitated novel anti-HIV agent with lower toxicity and wider anti-viral spectrum. The fact has accelerated the extensive synthetic research for developing novel anti-HIV sugar-modified nucleosides [28-34].

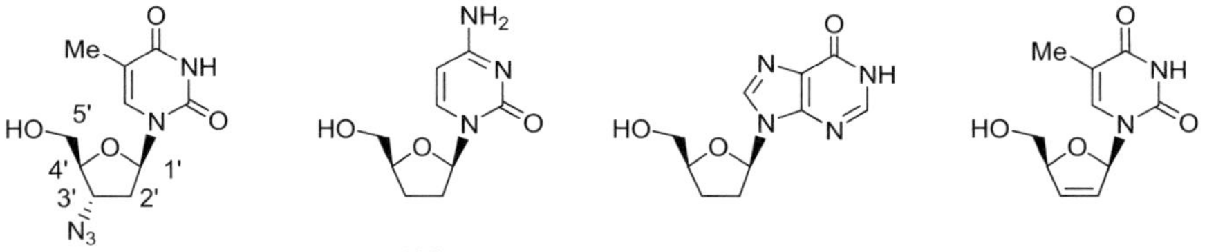

Figure 1: Anti-HIV drugs: nucleoside reverse transcriptase inhibitors (NRTIs) [28].

Among the sugar-modified nucleosides, there have been known branched-sugar nucleosides, which have pentose-moiety branched with carbon-substituent at the 1′-, 2′-, 3′-, 4′-or 5′-position. Anti-tumor and anti-viral branched-sugar derivatives are shown in Fig. **2**. Nucleoside antibiotic angustmycin C, which is branched with hydroxymethyl group at the anomeric position of adenosine, shows anti-tumor activity [35]. 2′-Methylcytidine shows inhibitory activity against HCV [36]. On the other hand, 3′-ethynylcytidine exhibits anti-tumor activity [37]. Moreover, 4′-cyanothymidine exhibits significant anti-HIV activity [38].

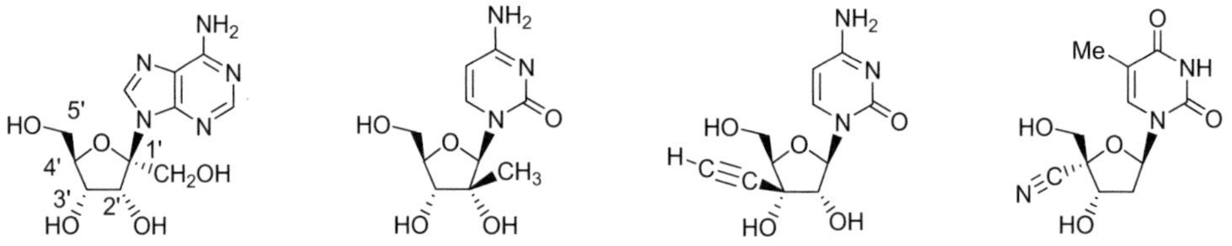

Figure 2: Biologically-active branched-sugar nucleosides [35-38].

2′-Branched ribonucleosides such as 2′-methylcytidine could be synthesized by 1,2-addition of carbon nucleophile to 2′-keto compound available from the oxidation of 2′-hydroxyl group of naturally occurring ribonucleosides (Fig. **3**). Likewise, 3′-ketonucleoside has been utilized for the synthesis of 3′-branched nucleosides such as 3′-ethynylcytidine.

On the contrary for the above synthesis, introduction of carbon-substituent to the 1′ or 4′-position are difficult because no functional groups are present at the position.

Therefore, the development of the efficient method leading to the synthesis of these nucleosides has been challenging study in the nucleoside chemistry.

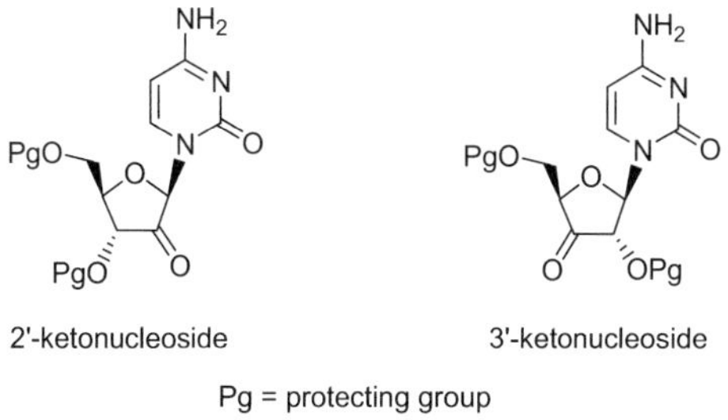

Figure 3: 2'-Keto and 3'-ketonucleosides utilizing for the synthesis of 2'-and 3'-branched derivatives [36, 37].

The first synthesis of the 1′-branched derivatives starting from naturally occurring nucleoside has been performed by means of nucleophilic substitution of **1**, which was prepared from bromo-pivaloyloxylation of 1′,2′-unsaturated nucleosides, with organosilicon or organoaluminum reagents (Scheme **1**) [39]. In the synthetic transformation, the desired 1′-α-carbon-substituted nucleoside **2** was obtained *via* neighboring group participation exerted by 2′-β-bromine atom of the anomeric carbenium ion **I**. Compound **2** could be converted into 2′-deoxy-and arabinofuranosyl nucleosides **3**, but the corresponding ribofuranosyl counterpart was not available.

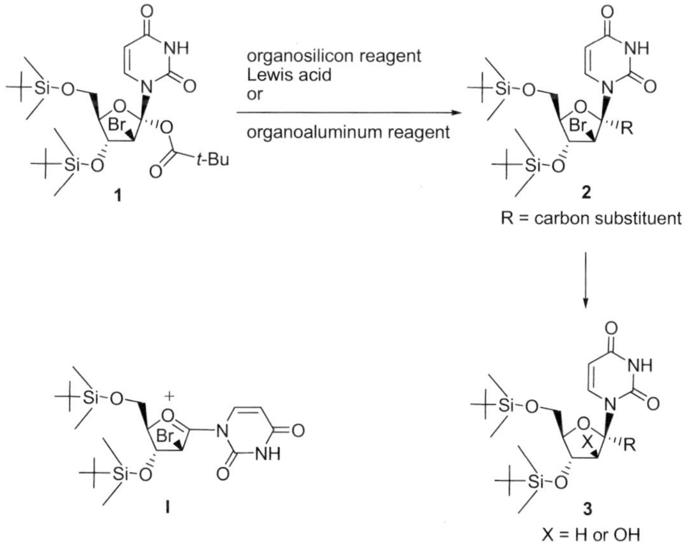

Scheme 1: Synthesis of 1'-branched nucleosides **3** from **2** prepared by nucleophilc substitution of **1** [39].

In this context, reaction of 2′-*O*-samarium enolate **II**, generated by SmI_2-mediated reduction of α-ketophenylselenide **4**, with carbon electrophile has been reported (Scheme **2**) [40]. Thus, reaction of **4** with SmI_2 and subsequent nucleophilic addition to aldehyde provided the aldol product **5**, followed by β-face-selective hydride reduction of **5** to give ribonucleoside **6** branched at the anomeric position.

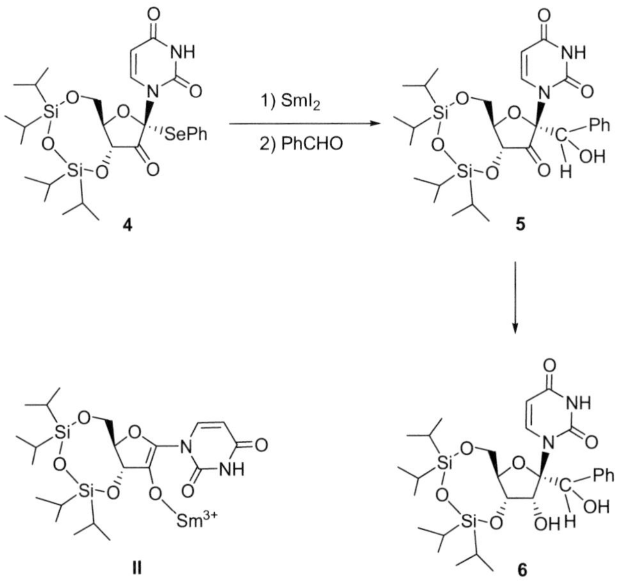

Scheme 2: Synthesis of 1'-branched nucleosides on the basis of electrophilic substitution [40].

As another synthetic method for 1′-branched nucleosides, the reaction of the anomeric radical with radical acceptor has also been utilized. The first report dealing with this methodology is shown in Scheme **3** [41]. Thus, when 2′-bromo-1′-*O*-pivaloy-2′-deoxy-α-uridine derivative **7** was treated with tributyltin radical, the incipient 2′-carbon radical **III** was rearranged to anomeric radical **IV** through 1,2-acyloxy migration and subsequent reaction of **IV** with allyltributyltin gave 1′-*C*-allyl-arabinofuranosyluracil nucleoside **8**. In this case, sp^2-hybridized anomeric radical reacted at the α-face to give β-anomer as a sole product.

The other methods utilizing the anomeric radical are shown in Schemes **4** and **5**. The reaction illustrated in Scheme **4** is the reaction of the radical precursor 1′-phenylsulfanyl-2′-deoxyuridine **9** with allyltributyltin to give 1′-*C*-allyl-2′-

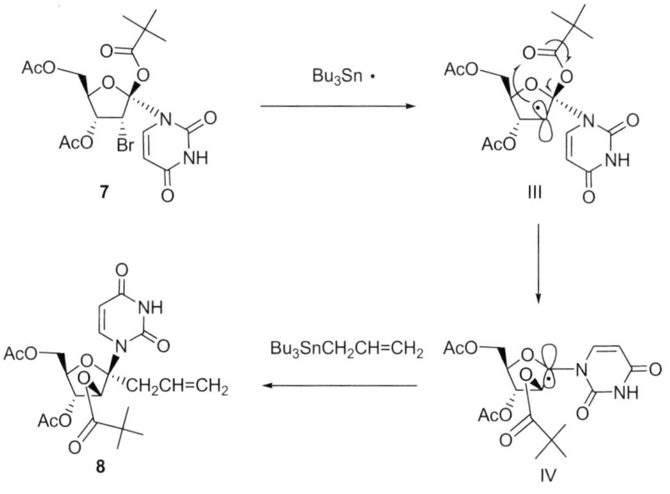

Scheme 3: Synthesis of 1'-branched nucleosides utilizing nucleoside anomeric radical [41].

deoxynucleoside (**10**) [42]. The other method is intramolecular radical cyclization of **11** (Scheme **5**) [43]. The resulting bicyclic product **12** was transformed into 1′-*C*-vinyluridine derivative (**13**) by means of fluoride ion-mediated E2-elimination. These above synthetic method for 1′-branched nucleosides have some drawbacks such as limited substituent to be introduced or difficulty of selective synthesis of the β-anomers.

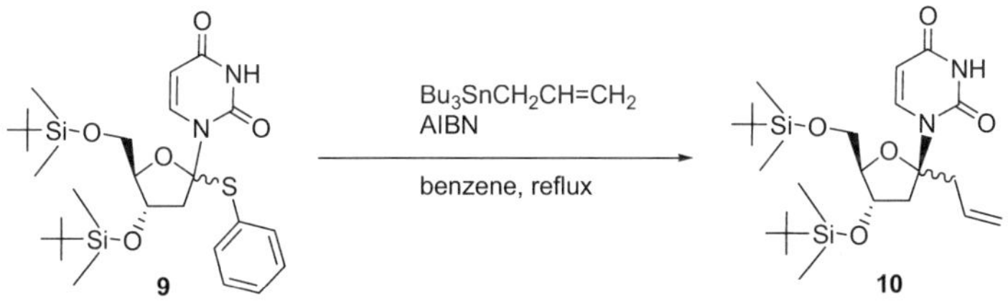

Scheme 4: Radical reaction of 1'-phenylsulfanyl nucleoside **9** under radical reaction leading to 1'-allyl-2'-deoxyuridine **10** [42].

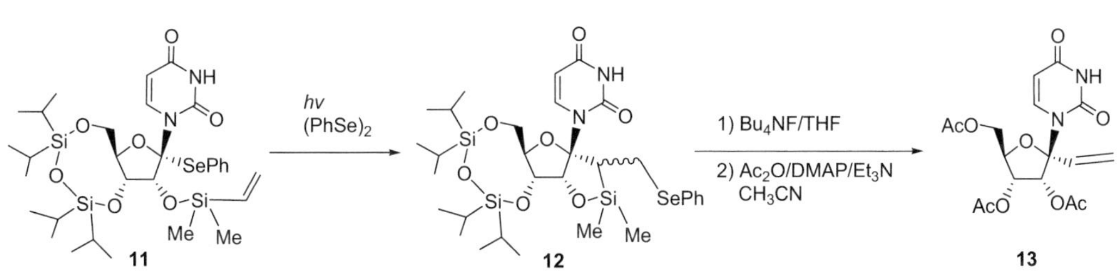

Scheme 5: Intramolecular radical cyclization of **11** and subsequent transformation of **12** to 1'-vinyl udidine **13** [43].

In the meantime, 4′-branched nucleosides such as 4′-cyanothymidine have been primarily synthesized from common key intermediate 4′-hydroxymethyl-nucleoside **16** (Scheme **6**) [44]. Thus, aldol-Cannizzaro reaction of thymidine 5′-aldehyde **14** gave **15**. Selective tritylation of α-hydroxyl group, silylation of β-hydroxyl group of **15** and subsequent removal of the trityl group of the resulting bis-*O*-protected product

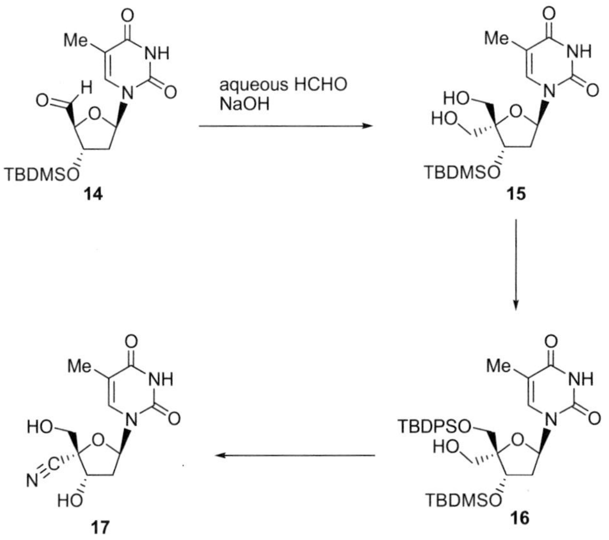

Scheme 6: Synthesis of 4'-branched nucleosides on the basis of aldol-Cannizzaro reaction [44].

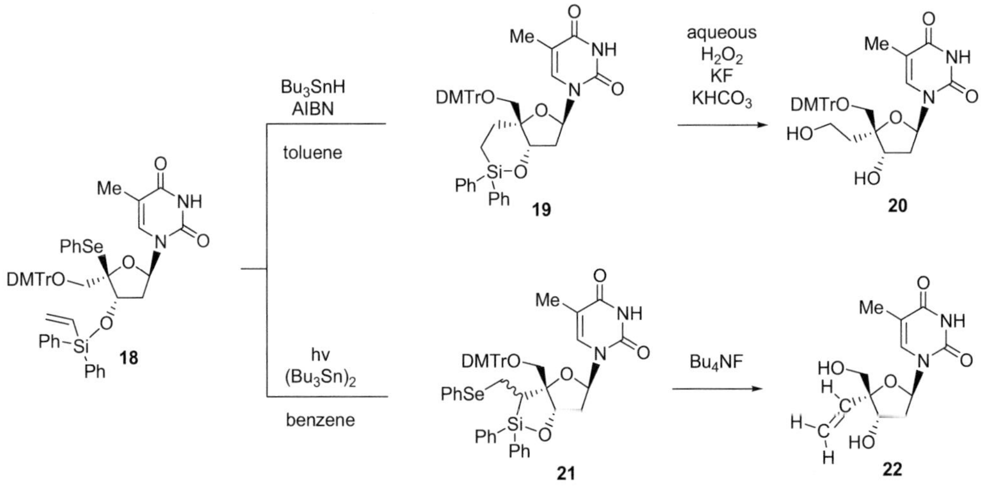

Scheme 7: Synthetic sequence for 4'-branched nucleosides by means of intramolecular cyclization of nucleoside C4′-radical [45].

provided the key 4′-α-hydroxymethyl nucleoside **16**. The key nucleoside **16** was transformed into **17** after conventional synthetic sequence. Drawbacks of this method required tedious steps for obtaining the hydroxymethyl derivative **16** and the introduction of 4′-substituent has been limited. Recently, novel methods have been developed, which were intramolecular radical cyclization of a 3′-*O*-silicon-tethered nucleoside C4′-dadical (**18→19→20/18→21→22**) (Scheme **7**) [45] and electrophilic substitution of the enolate **24** derived from nucleoside 5′-esters **23** with alkyl halides to lead to the respective 4′-*C*-allyl-and 4′-*C*-methyl thymidine derivatives **25a** along with its epimers **25b** (Scheme **8**) [46].

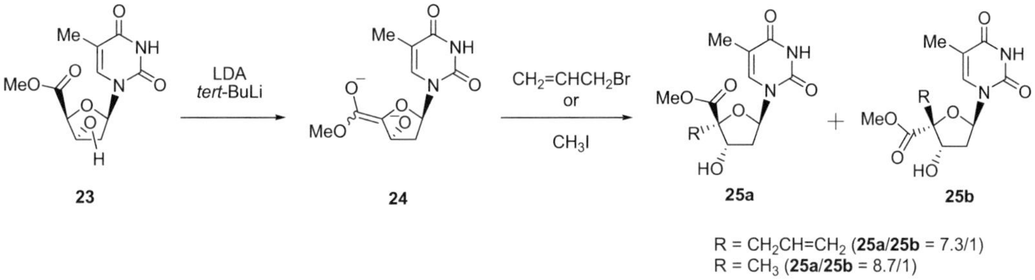

Scheme 8: Synthetic sequence for 4'-branched nucleosides by means of electrophilic substitution of nucleoside 5′-esters [46].

Synthetic Chemistry of Epoxy-Sugar Nucleoside

Reaction of epoxides with carbon nucleophile has occupied one of the major methods for construction of carbon-carbon bond [47]. Epoxy-sugar nucleosides include four derivatives; 1′,2′-, 2′,3′-, 3′,4′-, and 4′,5′-epoxides (Fig. **4**). Of these, reaction of 2′,3′-epoxy derivative has been only precedent. Thus, 2′,3′-lyxo-epoxyuracil nucleoside **26** underwent regioselective ring opening by the reaction with LiC≡CH to provide 3′-deoxy-3′-ethynylarabinofuranosyluracil nucleoside **27** (Scheme **9**) [48].

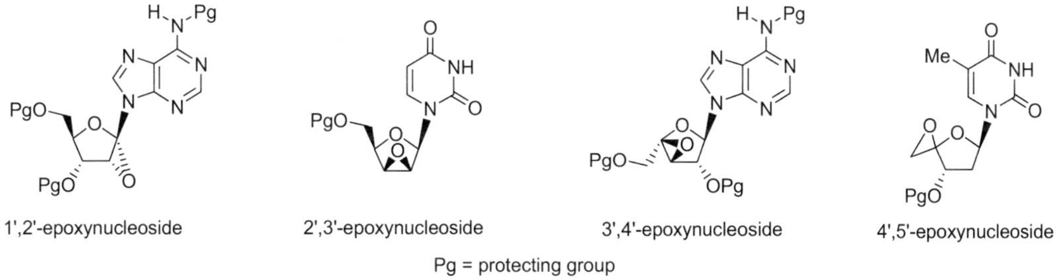

Figure 4: Structures of four possible epoxy-sugar nucleosides [77].

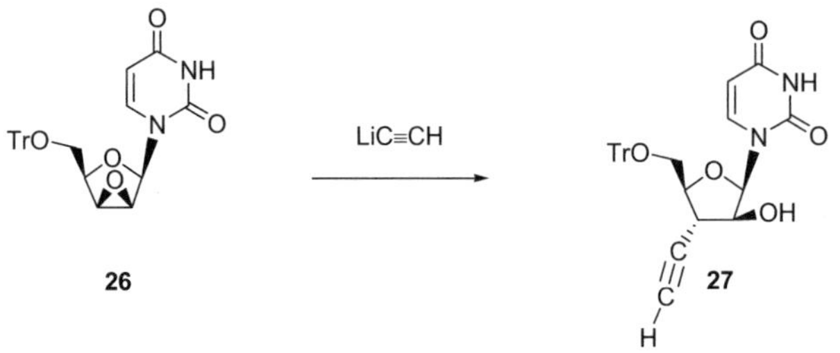

Scheme 9: Synthesis of 3'-branched uracil nucleoside **27** from 2',3'-lyxo-epoxide **26** by reaction with LiC≡CH [48].

The other three epoxy-sugar nucleosides have characteristic structure in that the carbon bonded to the furanose ring oxygen is directly attached to the epoxide ring. Therefore, these epoxides are expected to readily undergo regioselective nucleophilic ring opening because of concomitant formation of oxonium ion. By the same reason, the preparation of these epoxides from the corresponding unsaturated-sugar nucleosides has to be performed under non-nucleophilic conditions. In fact, 1′,2′-epoxynucleoside **28** exists as an equilibrium mixture with oxonium ion **29**. Under aqueous conditions, **29** is readily converted into uracil and ribonolactone *via* hemiacetal **30** (Scheme **10**).

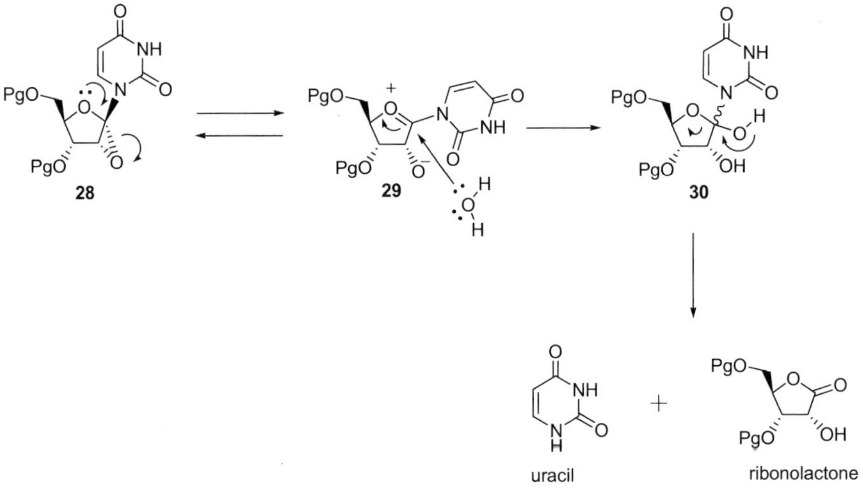

Scheme 10: Characteristic instability of 1',2'-epocynucleoside **28** [52].

In this circumstances, we have envisioned that dimethyldioxirane (DMDO) would be suitable oxidizing reagent for the preparation of the above unstable 1′,2′-, 3′,4′-, and 4′,5′-epoxides because DMDO is able to transform an alkene into the respective epoxide in aprotic solvent under neutral conditions. DMDO is prepared by oxidation of acetone by potassium peroxomonosulfate (Oxone) (Scheme **11**) [49-51].

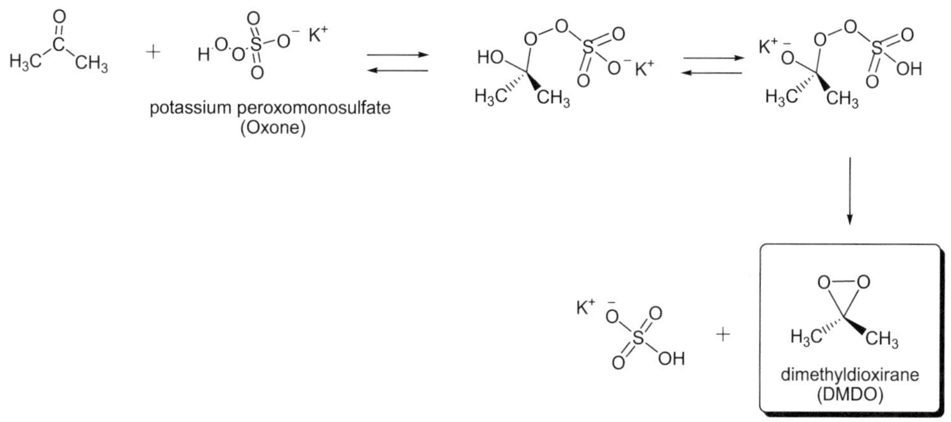

Scheme 11: Preparation of dimethyldioxirane (DMDO) from acetone and Oxone [49-51].

As anticipated, 1′,2′-, 3′,4′-and 4′,5′-epoxynucleosides could be prepared by DMDO-mediated oxidation of the corresponding unsaturated nucleosides (Scheme **12**). Reaction of 1′,2′-epoxynucleoside with organoaluminum reagent gave "*syn*-opened" product stereoselectively. On the contrary, "*anti*-opened" product was obtained as a major product from the reaction of 3′,4′-epoxynucleoside with trimethylaluminum reagent. Interestingly, stereoselective 4′-α-carbon-carbon bond formation occurred in the $SnCl_4$-initiated ring opening of 4′,5′-epoxynucleoside with organosilicon reagent.

In this section, stereo-controlled synthesis of 1′-α-and 4′-α-branched nucleosides by means of ring opening of epoxy-sugar nucleosides are described. During this study, we have discovered an anti-HIV agent, 4′-ethnynylstavudine (4′-Ed4T). The structure-activity relationship study of 4′-Ed4T and development of the large-scale synthetic methods aiming at the clinical studies will also be disclosed.

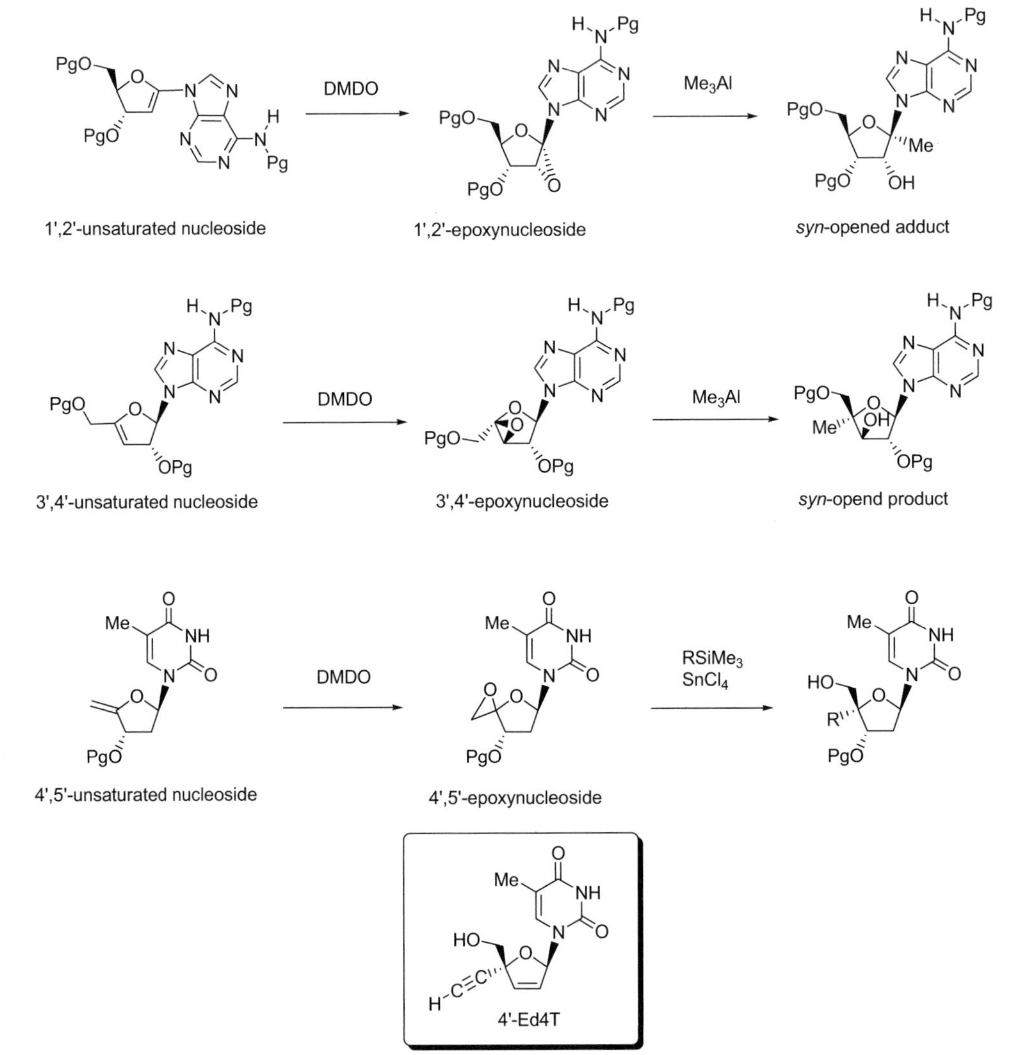

Scheme 12: Summry for preparation and ring-openig of epoxy-sugar nucleosides (Pg = protecting group).

Reaction of Nucleoside 1′,2′-epoxides with Organoaluminum Reagents: Stereoselective Synthesis of Ribonucleosides Branched at the Anomeric Position [52]

Reaction of TBDMS-protected 1′,2′-unsaturated uridine (**31**) with DMDO in CH_2Cl_2 at –30 °C, the epoxidation reaction was completed for 30 min (Scheme **13**). Because the resulting epoxy-nucleoside **32** was found to be unstable, the structure of the epoxide could not be assigned by ^1H NMR. Therefore, the reaction mixture was subsequently reacted with Me_3Al to provide 1′-*C*-methyluracil nucleoside (**33α**) as a sole product. The depicted structure of **33α** was determined by NOE correlation between H-6/H-4′, CH_3-1′/H-3 and H-2′/H-4′. On the basis of the configuration of 2′-OH of **33α**, the epoxidation of **31** gave 1′,2′-"up"-epoxide **32** selectively. Likewise, Me_3Al-mediated ring opening of the epoxide derived from the epoxidation of 1,1,3,3-(tetraisopropyldisiloxane-1,3-diyl) (TIPDS)-protected **34** provided **35α** as a major isomer. These stereochemical outcome revealed that the DMDO-mediated epoxidation of TBDMS-and TIPDS-protected 1′,2′-unsaturated uracil nucleosides proceeded at the β-face predominantly.

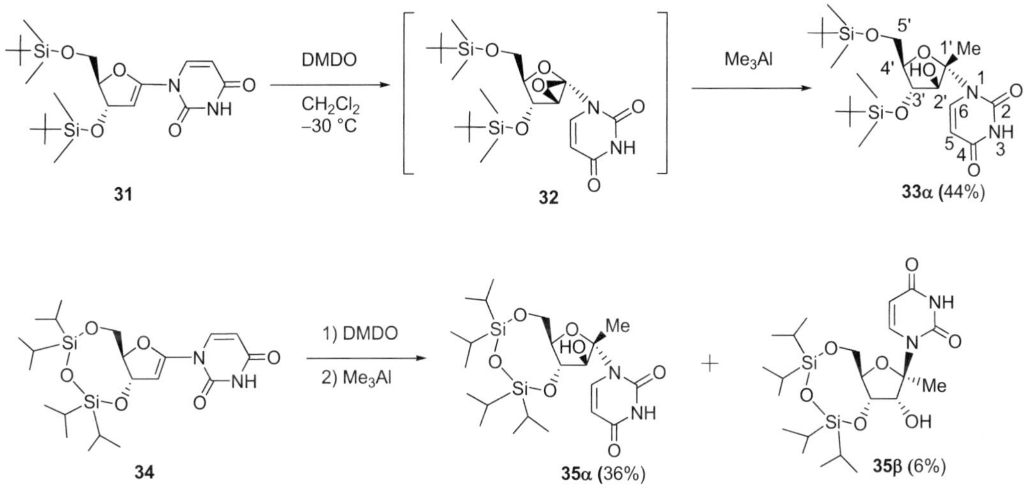

Scheme 13: Epoxidation of 1',2'-unsaturated uracil nucleosides **31**/**34** and ring opening of the resuting1',2'-epoxynucleosides with Me_3Al [52].

On the contrary, di-*tert*-butylsilylene (DTBS)-protected epoxide **37** obtained from **36** was found to be stable for its structure determination by ^1H NMR measurement (Scheme **14**). The NOE experimental data revealed that the epoxide **37** has 1′,2′-"down"-configuration. Upon reacting the epoxide **37** with Me_3Al, the desired *syn*-adduct **38β** was obtained along with its epimer *anti*-adduct **38α** in a ratio of 5: 1 in 86% isolated yield. On the basis of the molecular modeling study and the value of the coupling constant $J_{3',4'}$ (11.0 Hz) of **36**, its Newman projection formulae of the sugar portion could be proposed (Fig. **5**) [53]. As can be seen in Fig. **5**, the hydrogen atom at the 3′-position occupies a pseudo-axial position. When DMDO is reacting from its β-face of the enol ether, steric repulsion between the 3′-hydrogen and DMDO is inevitable. Therefore, the epoxidation proceeded at the α-face to furnish **37** as a sole product. In the case of TBDMS-protected **31** and TIPDS-protected **34**, these coupling constant $J_{3',4'}$ values are 2.6 and 4.4 Hz, respectively. These values suggest that the 3′-hydrogen occupy the pseudo-equatorial position. These conformational features made DMDO to epoxidize the double bond from the β-face due to predominant steric hindrance of 3′-silyloxy-substituent leading to the formation of 1′,2′-"up"-epoxide **32** as a major product.

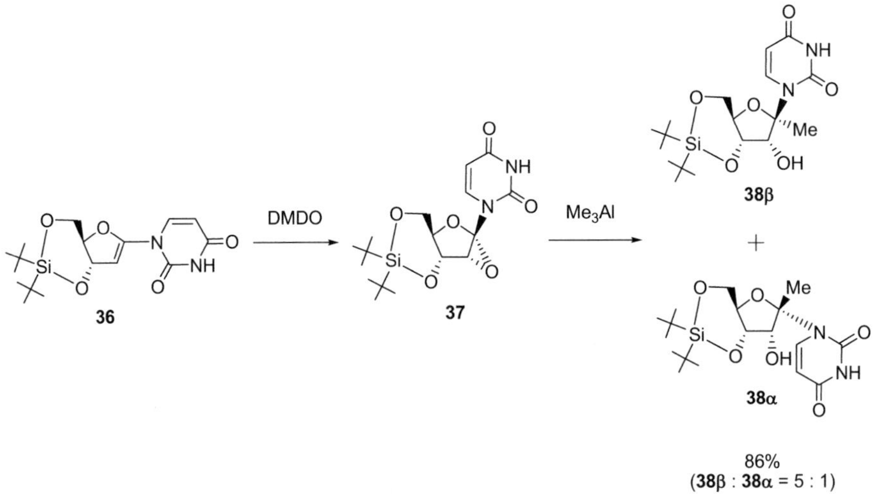

Scheme 14: DMDO-mediated epoxidation of DTBS-protected 1',2'-unsaturated uracil nucleoside **36** and ring opening of 1',2'-"down"-epoxynucleoside **37** leading to **38** [52].

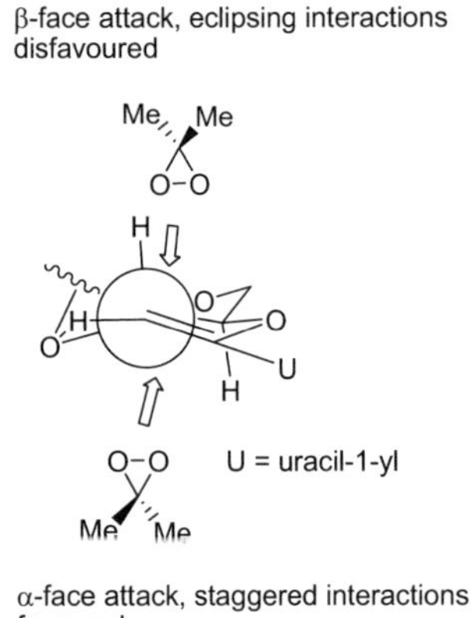

Figure 5: Plausible elucidation for α-face-selectivity of DMDO-mediated epoxidation of DTBS-protected **36** [53].

Next, the reaction of **37** with other organoaluminum reagents was examined (Scheme **15**) and these results are shown in Table **1**, which includes the result of the reaction with Me_3Al in entry 1. Except for the result with triisobutylaluminum shown in entry 3, in which the isolated yield of 1′-*C*-isobutyl derivative (**40**) decreased to 32% due to concomitant hydride reduction, 1′-*C*-ethyl-(**39**), 1′-*C*-ethynyl-(**41**), 1′-*C*-vinyl-(**42**) and 1′-*C*-phenyluridine derivative (**43**) could be obtained in moderate to good yields (entries 2 and 4-6). As can be seen in the ratio of β-and α-anomers, the expected *syn*-ring-opened β-anomer was always accompanied with the *anti*-ring-opened α-uridine derivatives, except for the reaction of Ph_3Al.

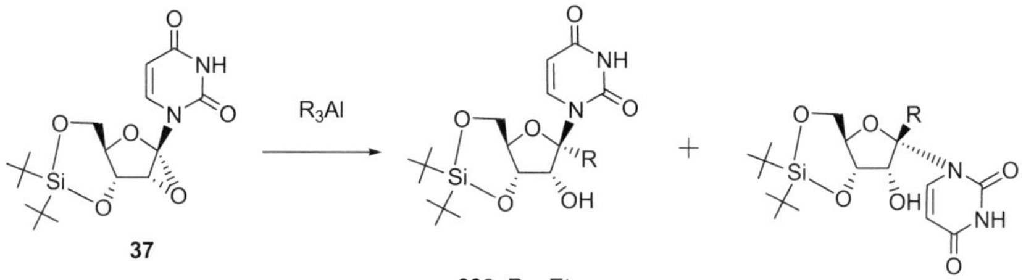

37

39β: R = Et
40β: R = *i*-Bu
41β: R = C≡CH
42β: R = C=CH2
43β: R = Ph

39α: R = Et
40α: R = *i*-Bu
41α: R = C≡CH
42α: R = C=CH2

Scheme 15: Ring opening of 1',2'-epoxynucleoside **37** with organoaluminum reagents [52].

Table 1: Reaction of 1',2'-epoxynucleoside **37** with organoaluminum reagents [52]

Entry	R3Al (Equiv)	Products	İsolated Yield (%)	Ratio of β/α
1	Me_3Al (3)	38β/38α	86	5/1
2	Et_3Al (3)	39β/39α	90	4/1
3	*i*-Bu_3Al (3)	40β/40α	35	9/1
4	$(HC{\equiv}C)_3Al$ (3)	41β/41α	64	4/1
5	$(H_2C{=}CH)_3Al$ (3)	42β/42α	90	32/1
6	Ph_3Al (3)	43β	55	-

To elucidate these stereochemical results, we proposed a plausible mechanism for the ring opening of **37** with R_3Al (Scheme **16**). Initially, dissociation of N^3-H of **37** with R_3Al give **V** and subsequent coordination to the oxygen atom of the epoxide ring as well as to that of the C2-carbonyl of **V** would furnish **VI**, which then forms the oxonium intermediate **VII**. At this stage, when the transfer of the aluminum ligand R takes place from the 2′-*O*-aluminate (path a), β-uridine derivatives **38β-43β** should be formed, whereas such attack from the base moiety (path b) results in the formation of α-uridine derivatives **38α-42α** or β-uridine derivatives depending upon the comformation about the glycoside bond. The exclusive formation of **43β** in the reaction of Ph_3Al would be explicable in terms of inability of this bulky reagent to coordinate to the C^2-carbonyl oxygen.

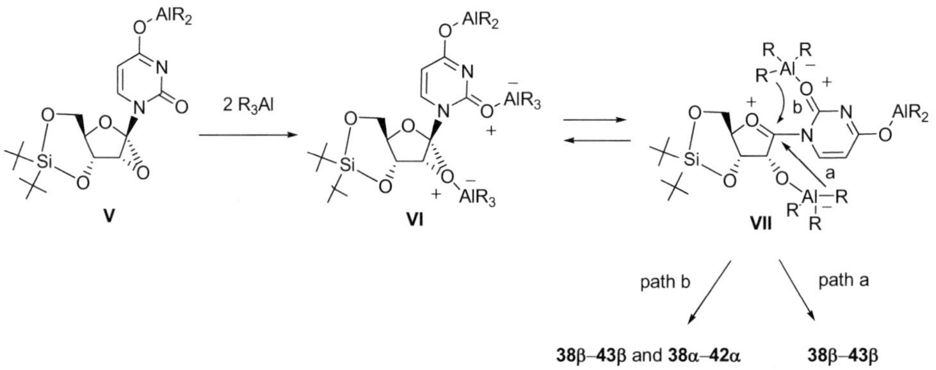

Scheme 16: Possible reaction mechanism for the reaction of 1',2'-epoxynucleoside **34** with organoaluminum reagents [52].

On the basis of this mechanism, one would anticipate that the presence of a bulky protecting group at the N^3-position would avoid the coordination of R_3Al to the C^2-carbonyl oxygen. Therefore, reactions employing the N^3-protected substrates **44** and **45** were carried out to give the *syn*-ring-opened product β-uridine derivatives **46-51** as a sole product (Scheme **17**). Removal of N^3-BOM group of **46-48** and N^3-benzoyl group of **49-51** could be performed by catalytic hydrogenolysis or treatment with NH_3/MeOH, respectively.

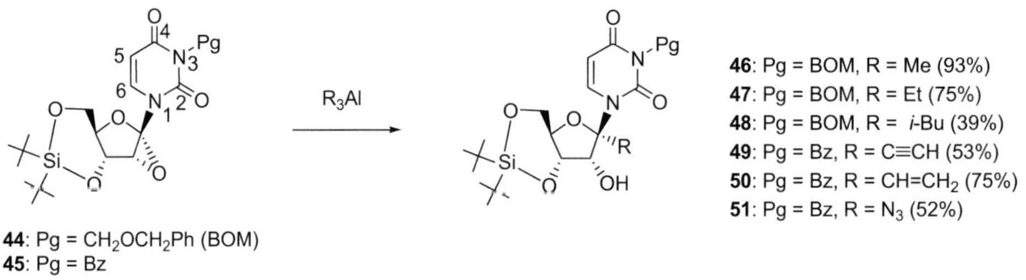

Scheme 17: Reaction of N^3-protected 1',2'-epoxyuridine derivatives **44** and **45** with organoaluminum reagents [52].

Finally, we have explored ring-opening of 1′,2′-epoxyadenine derivative with organoaluminum reagents (Scheme **18**). Ring opening of 1′,2′-α-epoxide **52** with Me_3Al gave 1′-*C*-methyladenosine derivative **53** in 80% isolated yield. Likewise, 1′-*C*-ethyl-(**54**), 1′-*C*-isobutyl-(**55**), 1′-*C*-ethynyl-(**56**) and 1′-*C*-vinyl-(**57**) adenine nucleosides could be synthesized as single stereoisomer. 1′-*C*-Vinyladenosine **57** could be transformed into protected angustmycin C **58** by OsO_4-mediatde oxidative cleavage of the vinyl group and subsequent hydride reduction of the resulting 1′-*C*-aldehyde. This is the first example that angustmycin C was synthesized from adenosine.

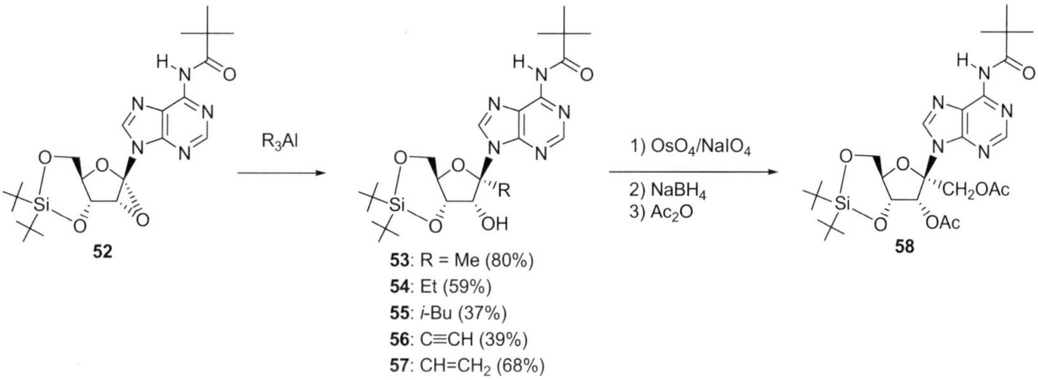

Scheme 18: Ring opening of 1',2'-α-epoxyadenine derivative **52** with organoaluminum reagents to lead to **53-57** and synthesis of protected angustmycin C [52].

As described above, we have developed a novel method for the synthesis of 1′-branched uridine and adenosine derivatives through DMDO-mediated α-face-selective-epoxidation of the respective DTBS-protected 1′,2′-unsaturated nucleosides and subsequent *syn*-ring-opening of the resulting 1′,2′-α-epoxides with organoaluminum reagents. These novel 1′-branched nucleosides did not show any anti-viral activities.

Anti-Ring Opening of the Epoxides Derived from 3′,4′-Unsaturated Adenosine with Me₃Al: Stereoselective Synthesis of 1′-C-methylxylofuranosyl Adenosine [54]

Although epoxides derived from simple alkene react with Me_3Al in a mode of *anti*-ring-opening, the epoxides derived from cyclic enol ethers such as glycals give *syn*-ring-opened products. In this context, by employing 3′,4′-β-epoxy nucleoside **60** derived from the DMDO-mediated epoxidation of 3′,4′-unsaturated adenine nucleoside **59**, we investigated factors governing the stereoselectivity of its ring-opening of the epoxide (*anti-vs. syn*-opening) with Me_3Al.

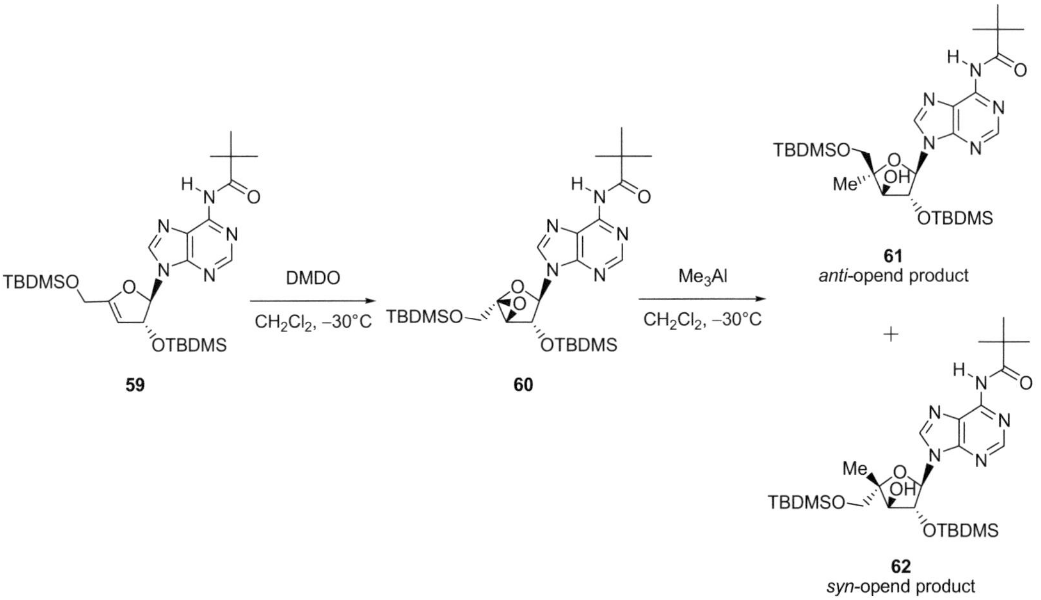

Scheme 19: Epoxidation of 3',4'-unsaturated adenine nucleoside **59** and ring-opening of the epoxy nucleoside **60** with Me_3Al [54].

Although **60** belongs to glycal-derived epoxide, unexpected preferential formation of the *anti*-opened **61** was observed when the reaction was performed in CH_2Cl_2 (Scheme **19**). Also, it was found that the ratio of **61** (*anti*-opened)/**62** (*syn*-opened) varied significantly (from 2/1 to 6/1) by increasing the amount of Me_3Al (from 1.0 equiv. to 10 equiv.) (Table **2**). On the contrary to these results, when the same reaction was carried out in THF, Et_2O, or 1,4-dioxane by using 6.0 equiv. of Me_3Al the exclusive formation of the *syn*-opened product **62** was observed (Table **2**, entry 6). To see if the presence of the N^6-pivaloyladenine base has any influence on the stereochemistry, the corresponding sugar epoxide **64** was prepared from **63** and reacted with Me_3Al (6.0 equiv.). As can be seen in Scheme **20**, the sole formation of the *syn*-opened product **65** was observed although this reaction was carried out in CH_2Cl_2.

Table 2: Ring opening of **60** with Me_3Al by varying the amount of reagent [54]

Entry	Equiv of Me_3Al	Combined Yield (%) of 61 and 62	Ratio of 61/62
1	1.0	69	2/1
2	3.0	76	2/1
3	4.0	80	3/1
4	6.0	90	5/1
5	10	93	6/1
6 [a]	6.0	59	only **62**

[a] The Me_3Al used in this entry was prepared by reacting a THF solution of MeMgCl with $AlCl_3$.

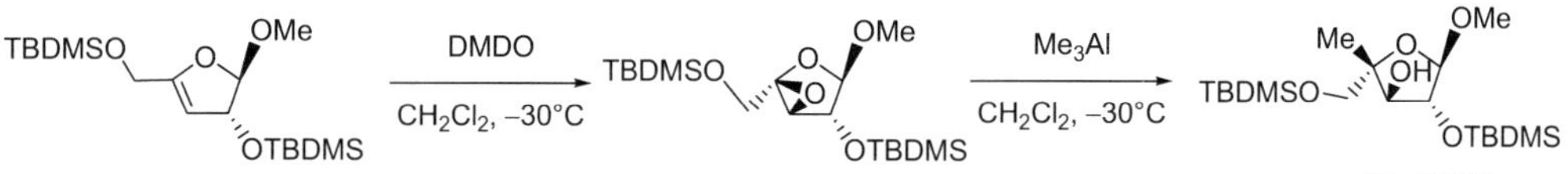

63 **64** **65** (90%) *syn*-opened product

Scheme 20: Epoxidation of **63** and ring-opening of the sugar epoxide **64** with Me_3Al leading to *syn*-ring-opened **65** [54].

On the basis of these results obtained from the above experiments, we could propose a plausible mechanism of the ring opening between **60** and Me_3Al (Scheme **21**). Due to its highly oxygenophilic character, the organoaluminum reagent would coordinate to the oxygen atom in the 3′,4′-epoxy structure of **60** to provide **VIII**, which subsequently undergoes the epoxide ring opening to form an oxonium ion that carries an alkoxyaluminate at the 3′-position. Two extreme conformers can be illustrated for the oxonium ions (**IX** and **X**) as a result of the rotation of the 3′-*O*-Al bond. In one conformer **IX**, aluminum atom is occupied above the furanose ring, and in the other conformer **XI**, it is outside the ring avoiding either steric or electronic repulsion with the adenine base.

When the amount of the remaining Me_3Al is limited or it is co-ordinated to an ethereal solvent, intramolecular attack of the methyl ligand from **IX** would take place to give **XII** (*syn*-opening), which is converted to **62**. When trimethylaluminum is sufficiently available in CH_2Cl_2, it is a favorable situation for **X** to transfer its methyl ligand to trimethylaluminum, yielding tetramethylaluminate and **XI**. Under such circumstances, the adenine base as well as the 3′-alkoxyaluminum substituent in **XI** would make the aluminate to attack from α-face to lead to the dominant formation of **XIII** (*anti*-opening), which furnishes **61**. Such transfer of the methyl ligand from **X** to Me_3Al would also be affected by the concentration of trimethylaluminum in the reaction medium. In fact, when the reaction was carried out in a 50-fold diluted reaction medium, the ratio of **61**/**62** was changed from 5/1 to 1.5/1.

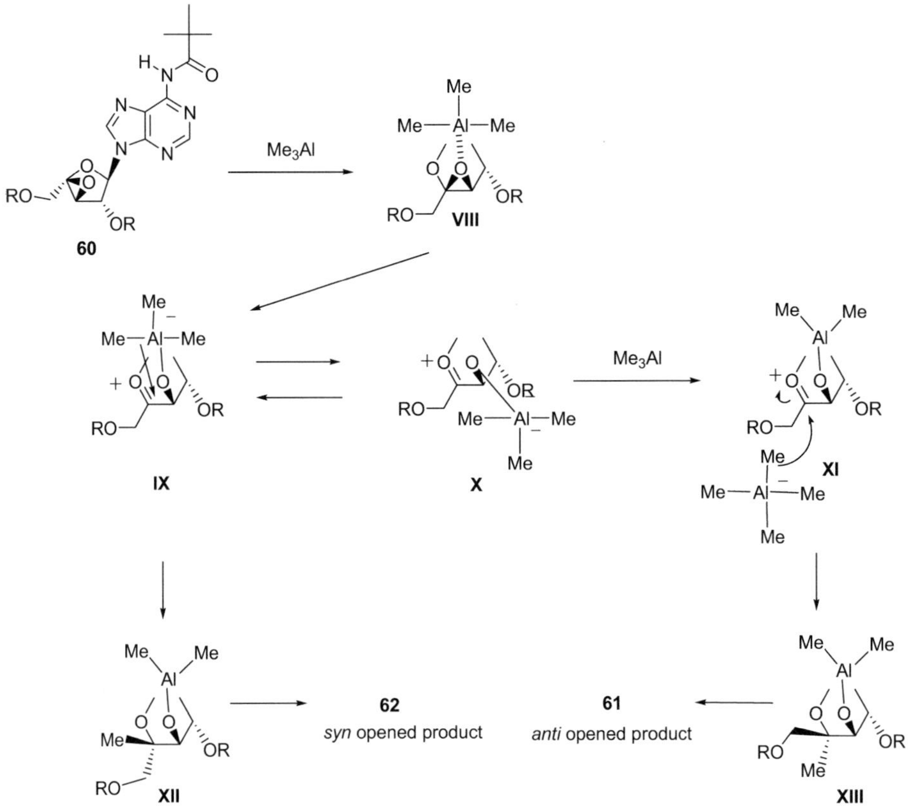

Scheme 21: Proposed reaction mechanism for the ring opening of epoxide **60** [54].

One would anticipate that the stereochemical outcome of this ring opening reaction also would be affected by the bulkiness of the 2′-*O*-silyl protecting group. The ratio of **67**/**68** = 5/1 in the reaction of **66** became 10/1 when the corresponding TES (triethylsilyl)-protected epoxide was utilized (Scheme **22** and Table **3**). It was unexpected result for us that the TBDPS (*tert*-butyldiphenylsilyl)-protected epoxide **69** gave the reversed stereoselectivity (**70**/**71** = 1/7).

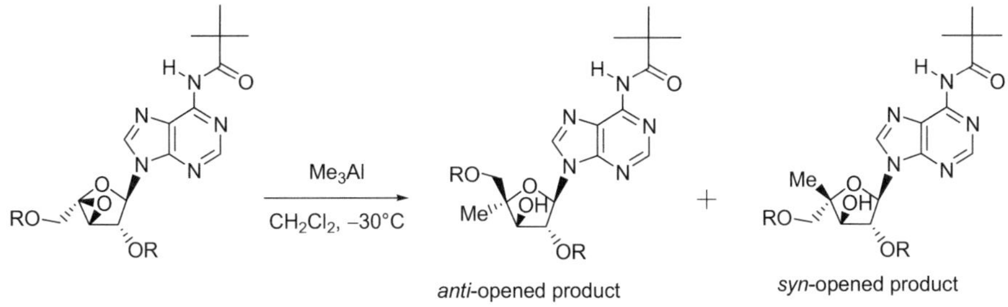

59: R = TBDMS
66: R = SiEt$_3$
69: R = TBDPS

61: R = TBDMS
67: R = SiEt$_3$
70: R = TBDPS

62: R = TBDMS
68: R = SiEt$_3$
71: R = TBDPS

Scheme 22: Effect of bulkiness of the protecting groups for the ratio of *anti*-opened/*syn*-opened products [54].

Table 3: Reaction of **59**, **66** and **69** with Me$_3$Al [54].

Entry	Epoxide	Products	Combined Yield (%)	β-D-isomer/α-L-İsomer
1	**59**	**61** and **62**	90	**61** and **62** = 5/1
2	**66**	**67** and **68**	89	**61** and **62** = 10/1
3	**69**	**70** and **71**	94	**70** and **71** = 1/7

A significant change of the ratio was also observed by varying the reaction temperature. At a higher temperature, almost equal amounts of **61** and **62** were formed (at room temperature, 0.7/1). At a lower temperature of –80 °C, the ratio was inverted and became 30/1. On the basis of combining the results obtained from the above experiment, the highest stereoselectivity (**67**/**68** = 50/1, combined yield 90%) was attained by performing the ring opening reaction of **66** at –80 °C in CH_2Cl_2. (Scheme **23**).

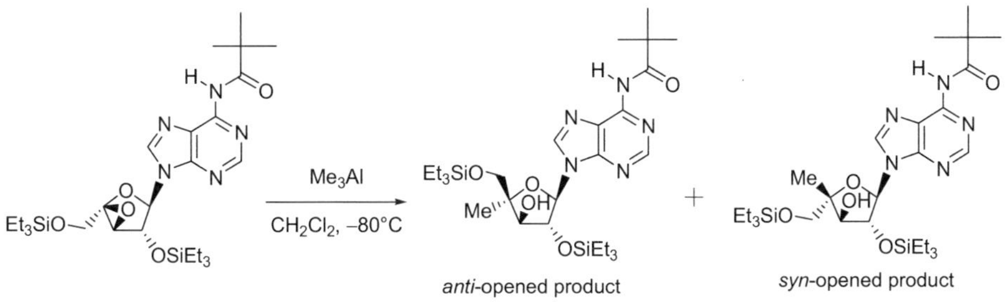

66 **67** 90% (50 : 1) **68**

Scheme 23: Optomized reaction conditions leading to *anti*-opened product **67** [54].

Ring Opening of 4′,5′-Epoxy Thymine Nucleosides: Highly Stereoselective Synthesis of 4′-α-Branched Nucleosides and Finding of a Promising Anti-HIV-1 Agent 4′-Ethynylstavudine (4′-Ed4T)

The research described in this chapter was initiated by the recent reports that 4′-substituted nucleosides exhibit significant inhibitory activity against HIV proliferation [38, 44, 55-58]. As mentioned above, the most commonly utilized method for the synthesis of these nucleoside derivatives is manipulation of 4′-hydroxymethyl derivatives of nucleosides prepared *via* aldol-Cannizzaro reaction [57, 59]. This fact made us to intend to develop a new and general method. In this section, we describe development of novel method for the stereoselective synthesis of 4′-α-carbon-substituted nucleosides based on epoxidation of 4′, 5′-unsaturated nucleosides followed by ring opening with organosilicon reagents in the presence of $SnCl_4$ as a Lewis acid.

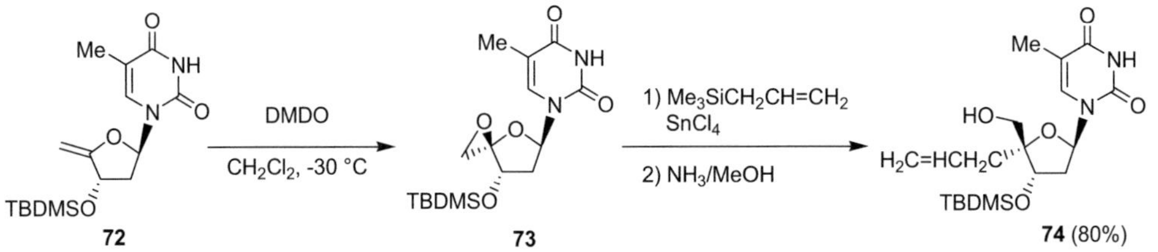

Scheme 24: DMDO-mediated epoxidation of **72** and subsequent ring-opening of **73** leading to **74** [60].

Reaction of 3′-*O*-TBDMS-4′,5′-unsaturated thymidine (**72**) with DMDO gave the respective 4′, 5′-epoxynucleoside **73** (a single isomer, evidenced by ^{1}H NMR) (Scheme **24**) [60]. The depicted stereochemistry of **73** was assigned on the basis of the observed NOE correlation between H-5′/Si-*t-Bu* (0.9%) as well as the assumption that the α-face of the 4′, 5′-double bond would be shielded by the TBDMS group. DMDO has been known to oxidize the pyrimidine moiety of nucleosides but no such side reaction was observed in the epoxidation of **72**. When **72** was reacted with allyltrimethylsilane (3 equiv.) in the presence of $SnCl_4$ (3 equiv.), the two products were obtained. Their ^{1}H NMR spectra showed that the more polar product was the expected 4′-α-*C*-allylthymidine **74** [NOE data: H-5′/H-3′ (5.3%) and H-1′/CH_2=CH*CH_2*-4′ (0.8%)] while the less polar one was its 5′-*O*-trimethylsilyl derivative. After simple extractive workup of the reaction mixture followed by treatment with NH_3/MeOH, **74** could be obtained in 80%

yield. The use of other Lewis acids, such as $TiCl_4$ or $EtAlCl_2$, gave rise to the cleavage of the glycoside bond to lead to the formation of thymine, and **71** was obtained only in very low yields (5-7%).

The above stereoselective allylation at the 4′-position also worked with 4′,5′-epoxides **76** and **79** derived from uracil-**75** and adenine ribonucleoside **78** (Fig. **6**). Thus, allylation of the epoxide prepared from **75** gave 4′-α-*C*-allyluridine **77** in 90% yield after NH_3/MeOH treatment of the reaction mixture. In the case of **78**, to avoid N^1-oxidation by DMDO, it was necessary to acylate the 6-NH_2 group. By using the N^6-pivaloyl derivative **78**, 4′-α-*C*-allyladenosine **80** was obtained in 52% overall yield through the epoxide **79**.

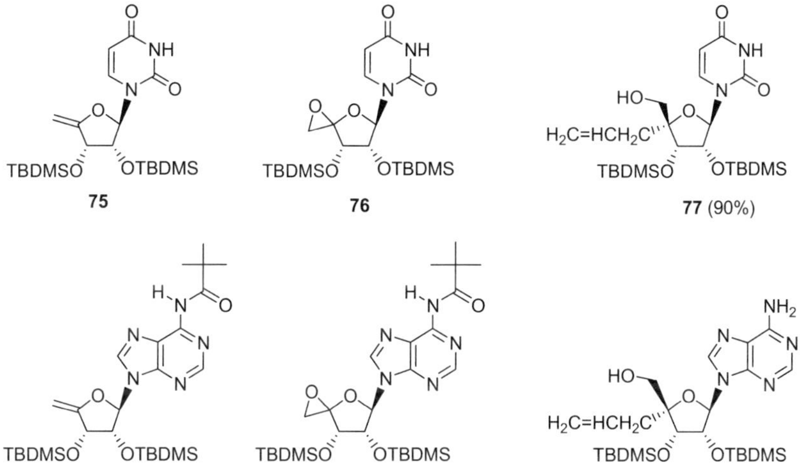

75 **76** **77** (90%)

78 **79** **80** (52%)

Figure 6: Epoxidation and subsequent ring-openinf starting from uridine-**75** and adenosine **78** derivatives [60].

To clarify the mechanism of the highly α-stereoselective allylation at the 4′-position, the above reactions utilizing **75** were studied in detail. Reaction of **75** with DMDO gave a 4′,5′-epoxide **76** as a single isomer, although its stereochemistry could not be determined using NOE experiment. When this epoxide was reacted solely with $SnCl_4$ in CH_2Cl_2, two 4′-chlorinated products (**82** and **84**) were isolated. The stereochemistry was established on the basis of NOE experiment. Analysis of their $J_{1',2'}$ and $J_{2',3'}$ values revealed that **82** and **84** would take the conformations as depicted in Scheme **25**, respectively. Independent treatment of **82** and **84** with $SnCl_4$ resulted in isomerization, forming both compounds. Although no reaction occurred by adding allyltrimethylsilane to a CH_2Cl_2 solution of **82**, addition of a catalytic amount of $SnCl_4$ (0.5 equiv.) to this mixture caused an instantaneous reaction to give the spiro intermediate **86** (a mixture of two diastereomers) that was isolated by HPLC and fully characterized. In the reaction medium, **86** was found to be converted slowly to **77** and **88**. Compound **84** behaved exactly in the same manner as **82**. These experimental observations led us to propose the reaction mechanism as shown in Scheme **25**. The 4′-β-(**83**) and 4′-α-chloro (**85**) derivatives exist in equilibrium, and are interconvertible through the oxonium ion **81**. For the $SnCl_4$-assisted reaction with allyltrimethylsilane,

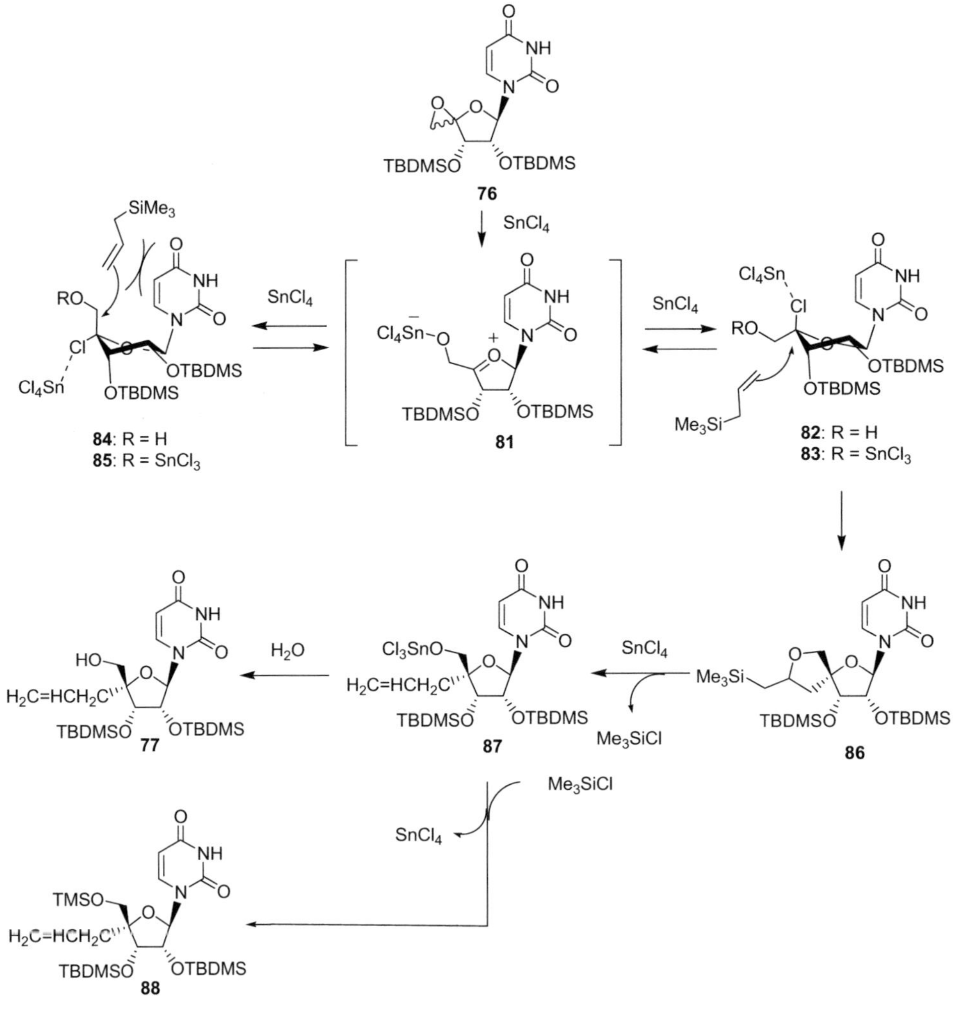

Scheme 25: The proposed reaction mechanism of $SnCl_4$-mediated ring-opening of 4',5'-epoxyuridine **76** with allyltrimethylsilane [60].

85 would be kinetically less favored because of the pseudo-equatorial orientation of the chlorine atom, and presumably also due to steric hindrance exerted by the base moiety. On the other hand, the pseudo-axial chlorine atom in **83** as well as the sterically less encumbered α-face permit its ready S_N2 reaction with allyltrimethylsilane to furnish the intermediate **86**. The β-effect of the silicon atom ensures regioselective opening of the spiro ring to yield **87**. Trapping of **87** with TMSCl gives rise to **88**, whereas quenching with H_2O furnishes **77**.

Finally, the scope of the $SnCl_4$-mediated ring opening reaction was briefly examined by reacting 4′,5′-epoxythymidine derivative **73** with other organosilicon reagents (Fig. 7). Compounds **89** (47%) and **90** (32%) could be obtained as a single isomer by utilizing (2-bromoallyl) trimethylsilane and (cyclopentenyl) trimethylsilane, respectively, under the above reaction conditions. It would be worthy to mention that the present method provides an access to a potent anti-HIV agent, 4′-α-cyanothymidine by using cyanotrimethylsilane to yield **91** (45%).

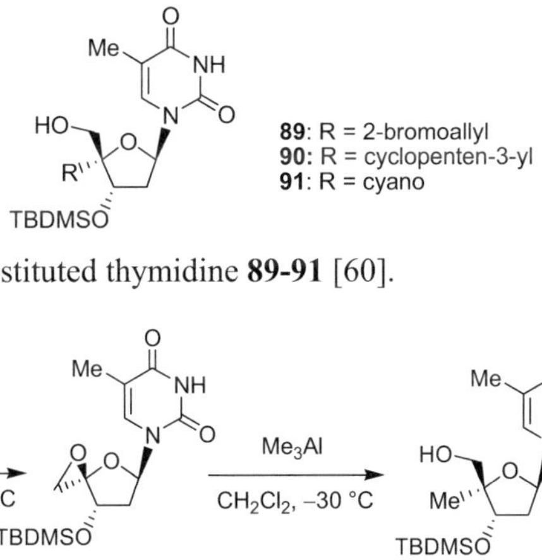

Figure 7: Structure of 4'-substituted thymidine **89-91** [60].

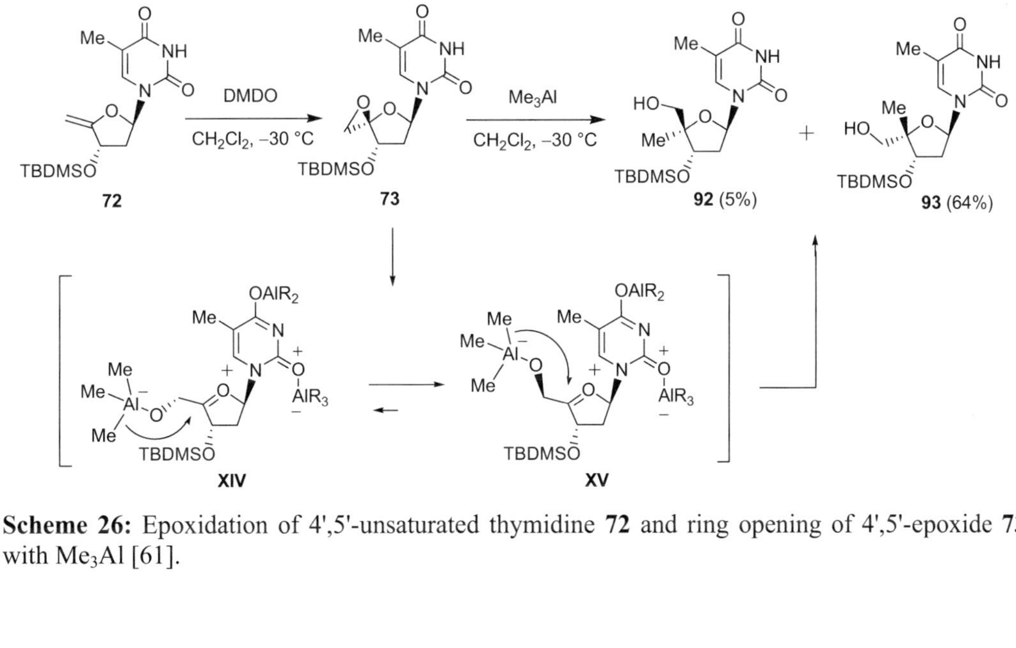

Scheme 26: Epoxidation of 4',5'-unsaturated thymidine **72** and ring opening of 4',5'-epoxide **73** with Me_3Al [61].

We have turned our attention to the ring opening of the epoxide **73** derived from **72** with Me_3Al (Scheme **26**) [61]. The reaction provided the 4′-*C*-methyl-α-L-isomer **93** as major isomer, the desired β-D-isomer **92** being formed only in 5% yield. This stereochemical outcome is rationalized to be due to conformational preference of the oxonium intermediate illustrated as **XV**, which can avoid the steric repulsion between the 5′-*O*-aluminate and the 3′-*O*-TBDMS group. In fact, the 4′,5′-epoxide **94** having the opposite 3′-configuration to **72** (Scheme **27**), upon reacting with Me_3Al, gave solely the 4′-*C*-methyl-β-D-isomer **95** (72%) through the aluminate **XVI**. By utilizing this method, the 4′-*C*-vinyl **96** and 4′-*C*-ethynyl **97** derivatives could be also synthesized.

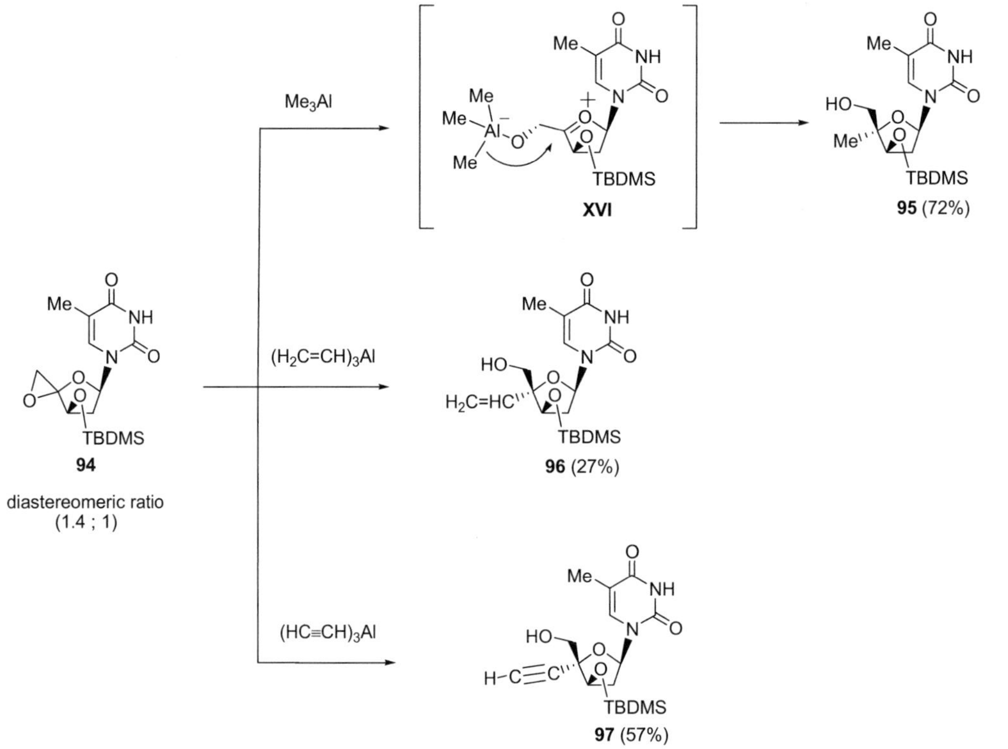

Scheme 27: Ring opening of 4',5'-epoxythymidine derivative **94** with organoaluminum reagents [61].

To invert the 3′-hydroxyl group of these 4′-branched products **95-97** by substitution reaction, 4′-*C*-methyl derivative **95** was converted into the respective 3′,5′-bis-*O*-chloromesyl derivative **98** through 2 steps (Scheme **28**). When **98** was reacted with cesium acetate in the presence of 18-crown-6 in benzene under reflux conditions, the expected thymidine derivative **99** could not be obtained but the elimination product 4′-*C*-methyl derivative **100** of clinically used anti-HIV drug d4T (stavudine) (**104**) was formed. Therefore, these 4′-branched products **95-97** were transformed into the respective d4T derivatives **101-103** (Scheme **29**).

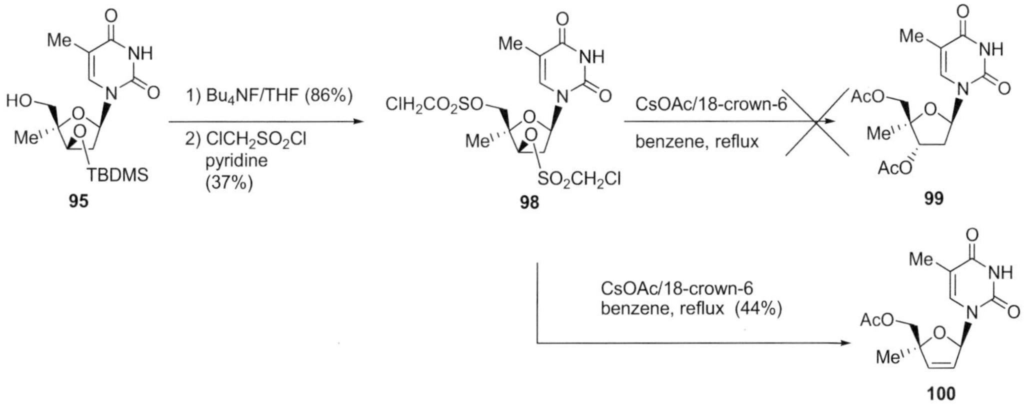

Scheme 28: Attempts to perform inversion at the 3'-position of **95** and unexpected formation of elimination product **100** [61].

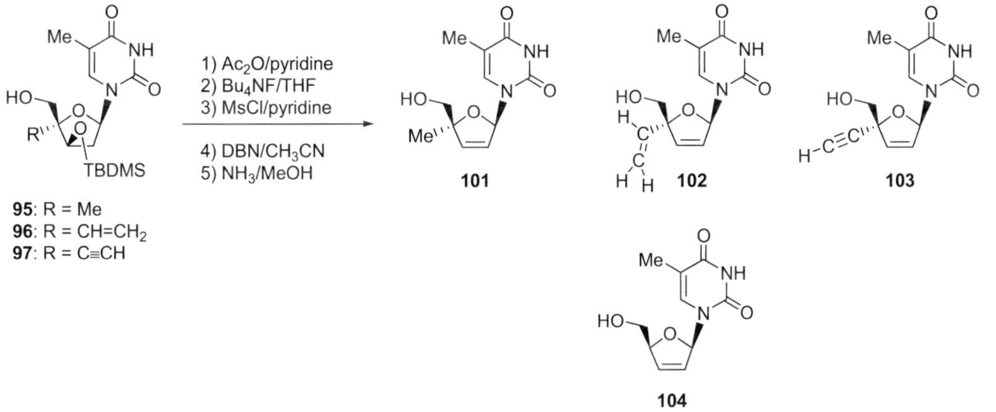

Scheme 29: Synthesis of 4'-substituted derivatives **101-103** of d4T (**104**) [61].

Among the synthesized d4T derivatives, 2′,3′-didehydro-3′-deoxy-4′-ethynylthymidine (**103**, 4′-Ed4T) was found to be more inhibitory against HIV-1 than the parent compound d4T (**104**), and much less toxic to various cells and also to mitochondrial DNA synthesis (Table **4**) [15, 61]. This finding was quite unexpected, since it has been reported that removal of the 3′-hydroxyl group in the anti-HIV active 4′-azidothymidine (**105**) leads to complete loss of the activity: 4′-azido-3′-deoxythymidine **106** and 2′,3′-didehydro-3′-deoxy-4′-azido-thymidine **107** are devoid of the activity (Fig. **8**)[55]. This compound has several additional advantages as a promising anti-HIV-1 agent: 1) it is a better substrate for human thymidine kinase than stavudine [62, 63], 2) it is very much more resistant to catabolism by thymidine phosphorylase [15], and 3) its anti-HIV activity is enhanced in the presence of a major mutation K103N [63], associated with resistance non-nucleoside reverse transcriptase inhibitors.

Table 4: Anti-HIV-1_{IIIB} activity of 4'-carbon-substituted stavudines **101-103** [61]

Compound	IC_{50} (μM)[a]	CC_{50} (μM)[b]
101	> 100	> 100
102	> 100	> 100
103 (4'-Ed4T)	0.20	> 100
104 (d4T)	2.8	100

[a] Inhibitory concentration required to achieve 50% protection of MT-2 cells against the cytopathic effect of HIV-1 III_B.
[b] Cytotoxic concentration required to reduce the viability of mock-infected MT-2 cells by 50%.

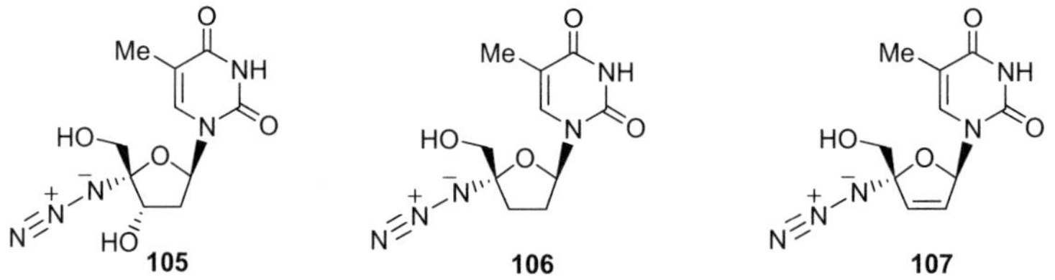

Figure 8: Structure of **105-107** [61].

Structure-Activity Relationship Study of Anti-HIV-1 Agent 4′-Ed4T

To study the structure-activity relationship for 4′-Ed4T (**103**), 4′-allyl-(**112**), 4′-methylethynyl-(**114**), 4′-chloroethynyl-(**115**), 4′-cyano-(**123**) were synthesized. Moreover, synthesis of the respective carbocyclic (**135** and **145**) and 4′-thio counterpart (**158**) were also carried out.

Synthesis of 4′-Allyl-and Terminally-Substituted Ethynylstavudine [60, 63]

3′-*O*-TBDMS-4′-*C*-allylthymidine (**74**) was subjected to acetylation of the 5′-hydroxyl group and the resulting **108** was desilylated by reacting with Bu_4NF in

THF to give **109** (Scheme **30**). Mesylation of **109** and subsequent β-elimination of **110** furnished d4 nucleoside **111**. Finally, deprotection of **111** provided the target 4′-allyl-d4T **112**.

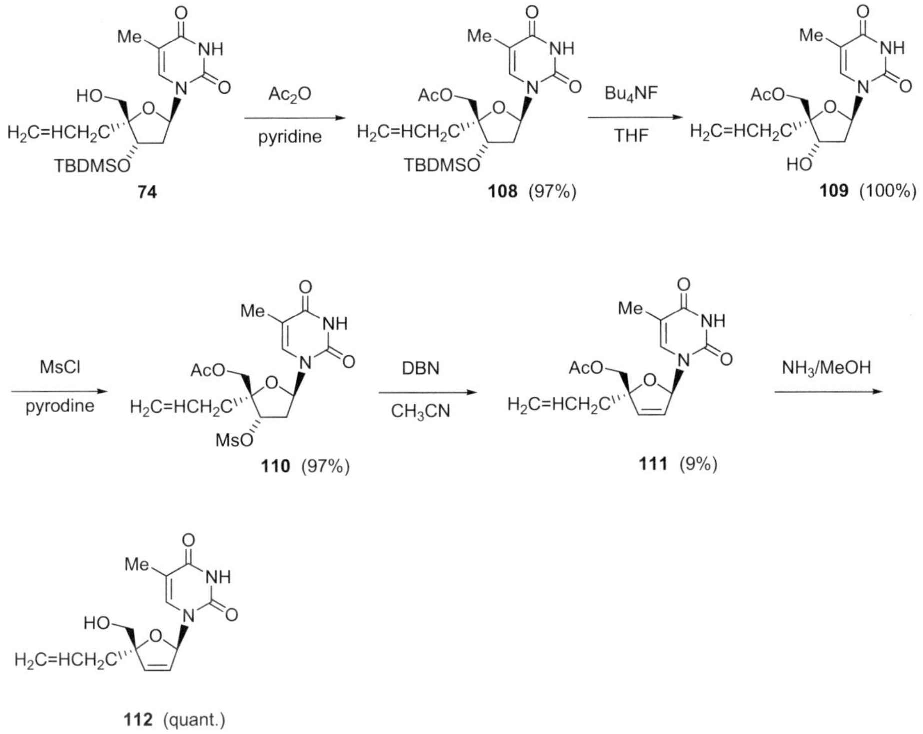

Scheme 30: Synthesis of 4'-allyl-d4T **112** [60].

4′-Methylethynyl-(**114**) and 4′-chloroethynyl (**115**) d4T were synthesized from 4′-Ed4T **103** as follows (Scheme **31**). Thus, **103** was protected with triethylsily group to give **113**. Compound **113** was transformed into the respective lithium acetylide by treatment with lithium hexamethyldisilazide (LiHMDS) followed by reacting with CH_3I or *N*-chlorosuccimide (NCS) gave **114** and **115** after deprotection.

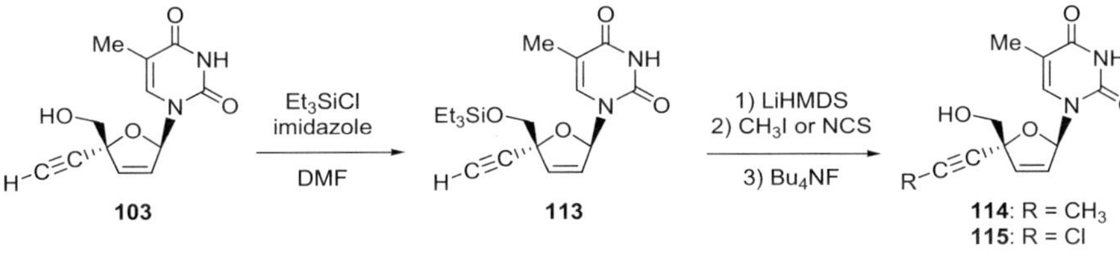

Scheme 31: Synthesis of 4'-methylethynyl-(**114**) and 4'-chloroethynyl-d4T (**115**) [63].

Synthesis of 4′-Cyano-d4T [64]

Synthetic route for the substrate 3′,4′-unsaturated thymine nucleoside **120** for this study is shown in Scheme **32**. Cleavage of the epoxide ring of the 2′,3′-epoxide **116**, prepared from 1-(β-D-ribofuranosyl)thymine according the published procedure, was carried out by reacting with a phenylselenide anion prepared from $(PhSe)_2$ and $LiAlH_4$ to give the desired 3′-phenylseleno derivative (**117**, 56%) as well as its 2′-isomer (**118**, 42%). The 5′-*O*-trityl group of **117** was replaced with TBDPS group from the expectation that the anisotropic effect of this silyl protecting group would serve as a stereochemical determinant of the 4′-substituted products at a later stage. Further acetylation of the 2′-hydroxyl group gave **119**.

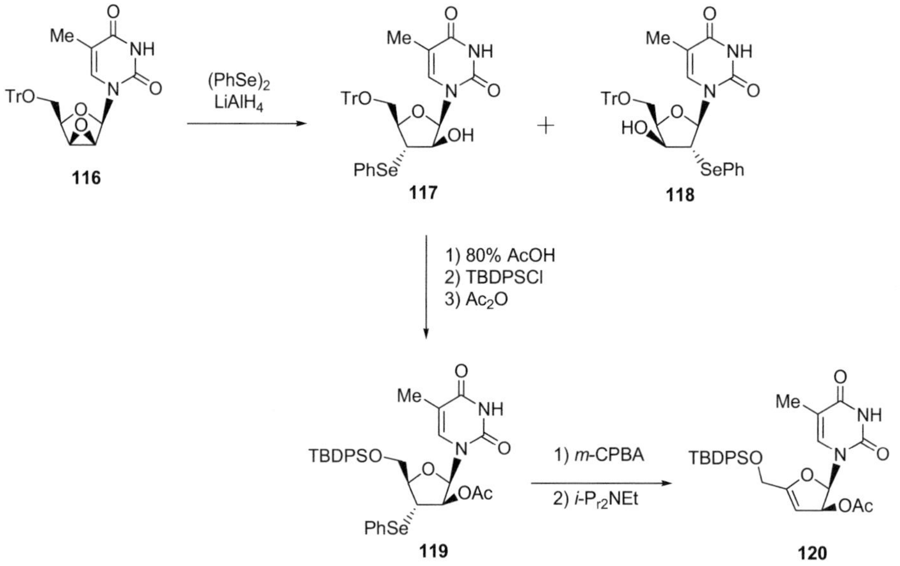

Scheme 32: Preparation of 3',4'-unsaturated thymidine derivative **120** [64].

Reaction of **119** with *m*-CPBA gave the corresponding selenoxide in 70% yield. Subsequent *syn*-elimination was conducted in THF at 70 °C for 1 h in the presence of *i*-Pr_2NEt. Despite the presence of two *syn*-hydrogens (H-2′ and H-4′) available for the elimination, exclusive removal of the H-4′ was observed in this reaction to give the substrate 3′,4′-unsaturated derivative **120** as the sole product in 67% yield.

When **120** was reacted with TMSCN in the presence of $SnCl_4$ in CH_2Cl_2, two isomeric products **121** (48%) and **121** (43%) resulting from allylic substitution were isolated as shown in Scheme **33**. The stereochemistry of **121** at the 4′-position was deduced from the ^{1}H NMR observation that its 5-Me resonance appeared at a significantly higher field of δ 1.53 when compared with that of **122** (δ 1.95) or **120** (δ 1.92), due to the anisotropic effect of the phenyl ring in the 5′-*O*-TBDPS group. Finally, deprotection of the 5′-*O*-silyl group in **121** was performed by reacting with Bu_4NF to give the desired 4′-cyano analogue **123** in quantitative yield.

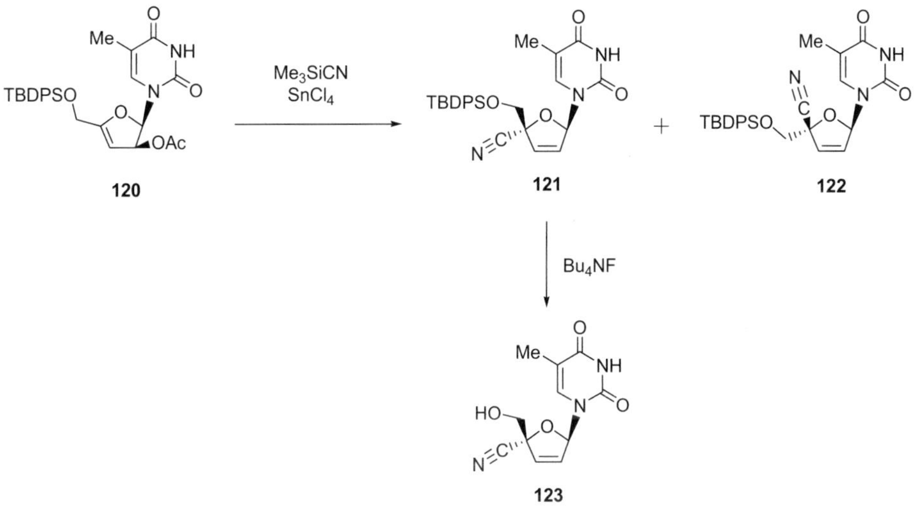

Scheme 33: Synthesis of 4'-cyano-d4T **123** [64].

Synthesis of Carbocyclic Analogue of 4′-Ethynylstavudine [65]

Carbocyclic nucleosides, in which the furanose ring oxygen atom is replaced with methylene functionality, have attracted much attention due to its remarkable anti-tumor and anti-viral activities. Among these nucleoside analogues, carbovir and its cyclopropylamino derivative abacavir, which have cyclopentene structure in the aglycon moiety, have been known to act as potent anti-HIV agent. In this context, we have intended to synthesize the carbocyclic counterparts **135** of 4′-Ed4T **103** as racemates.

The synthetic route was illustrated in Scheme **34**. We initiated the present synthesis with the introduction of a hydroxymethyl group to **124**. The target alcohol **125** was obtained in 77% yield by converting to its tin enolate (Bu_3SnCl/HMPA-THF/0 °C/0.5 h) and then reacting with paraformaldehyde. It was found, however, that direct treatment of **125** simply with 37% aqueous HCHO in the presence of AcOH gave **125** in excellent yield.

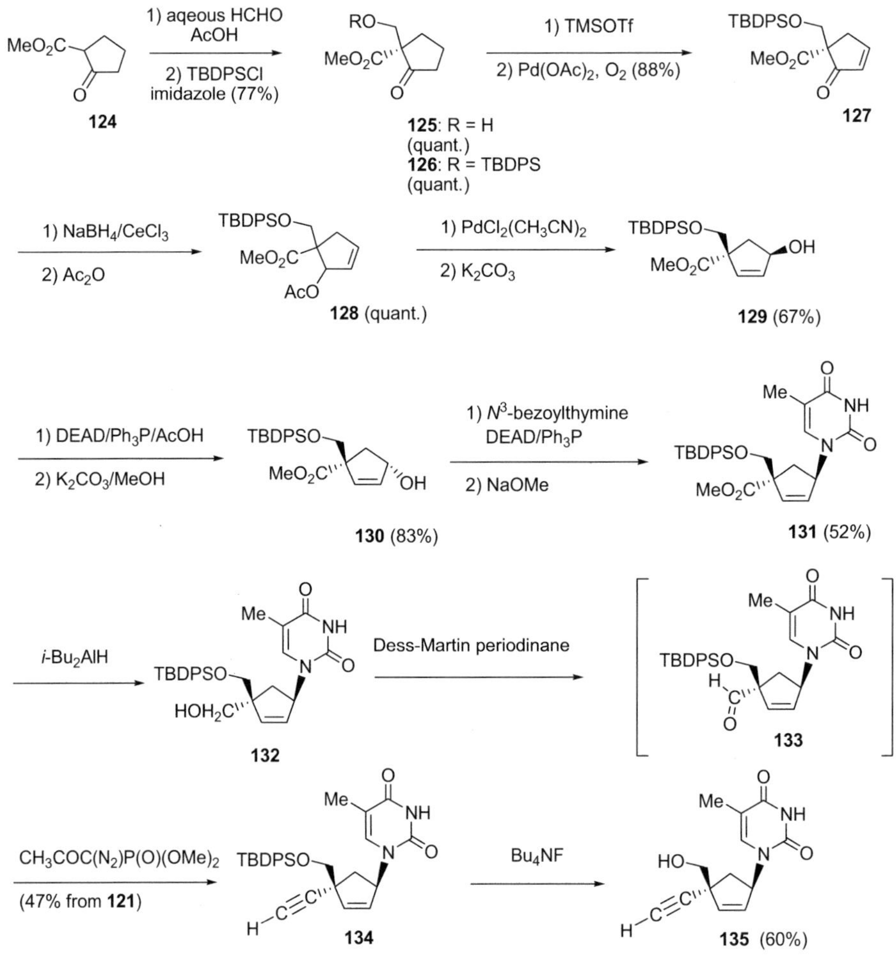

Scheme 34: Synthesis of carbocyclic analogue **135** of 4'-Ed4T **103** [65].

Protection of the primary hydroxyl group of **125** with TBDPSCl gave **126** in 77% yield. Conversion of **126** to the respective enone **127** was conducted by palladium catalyst-mediated dehydrogenation through the corresponding silyl-enolate to give the enone **127** in 88% yield. The Luche reduction of **127** followed by acetylation gave the allyl acetate **128** in quantitative yield as a single isomer. Compound **128**, upon $PdCl_2(CH_3CN)_2$-catalyzed allylic rearrangement followed by deacetylation, gave the allyl alcohol **129** in 67% yield. The stereochemistry of **129** could be assigned on the basis of the results of NOE experiments. The desired carbocyclic unit **130** was prepared in 83% yield by the Mitsunobu inversion of **129** and subsequent deacetylation.

Glycosidation between **130** and N^3-benzoylthymine was conducted under the Mitsunobu conditions. The resulting reaction mixture was treated with NaOMe in MeOH to provide the respective carbocyclic nucleoside **131** in 52% yield. The HMBC spectrum of **131** gave a cross peak between H-6 and C-1′, which confirmed the desired N^1-glycoside.

Reduction of the ester function of **131** was carried out with *i*-Bu_2AlH. However, it turned out that, even at low temperature (−70 °C in CH_2Cl_2), only a small amount of the desired aldehyde **133** was formed, the main product being the hydroxymethyl derivative **132**. The fact led us to reoxidize **132** with Dess-Martin periodinane in CH_2Cl_2 and the resulting aldehyde **133** was used for further transformations without structure determination.

Finally, the preparation of the 4′-ethynyl derivative (**134**) was examined Thus, treatment of **133** with a diazophosphonate $CH_3COC(N_2)P(O)(OMe)_2$ (Ohira-Bestman reagent) in MeOH in the presence of K_2CO_3 furnished **134** in 47% yield. Its ^{13}CNMR spectrum showed the presence of two ^{13}C-resonances apparently derived from carbon atoms of the ethynyl group: d 71.1 ($\underline{C}$≡CH) and 84.8 (C≡$\underline{C}$H). In addition, an NOE enhancement (0.5%) was observed between H-6 and CH_2-6′ of **134**, supporting the depicted β-nucleoside. Desilylation of **134** was carried out by conventional procedure (Bu_4NF in THF) to furnish the target molecule **135** (60%).

Synthesis of 4′-Difluoromethylene Analogue of 4′-Ethynylstavudine [66]

As another furanose ring modified analogue of 4′-Ed4T **103**, we synthesized **145**, in which the furanose ring oxygen of **103** is replaced with a geminal-difluoromethylidene (CF_2) group, because the CF_2 group has been suggested to work as an isopolar and isosteric substituent for oxygen.

For the preparation of the *gem*-difluoro carbocyclic unit **139**, the cyclopentenol **129** described in Scheme **34**, was utilized (Scheme **35**). Oxidation of **129** with PDC gave the cyclopentenone **136**. To introduce the fluorine atom, the ketone **136** was first converted to the corresponding silyl enol ether, and then reacted with

Selectfluor®. This procedure gave the monofluorinated ketone **137**. By repeating this fluorination procedure for **137**, the difluorocyclopentenone **138** was obtained in 76% yield from **136**. The Luche reduction of **138** proceeded stereoselectively to give the desired alcohol **139** as the sole product. The stereochemistry of **139** was confirmed by NOE experiments.

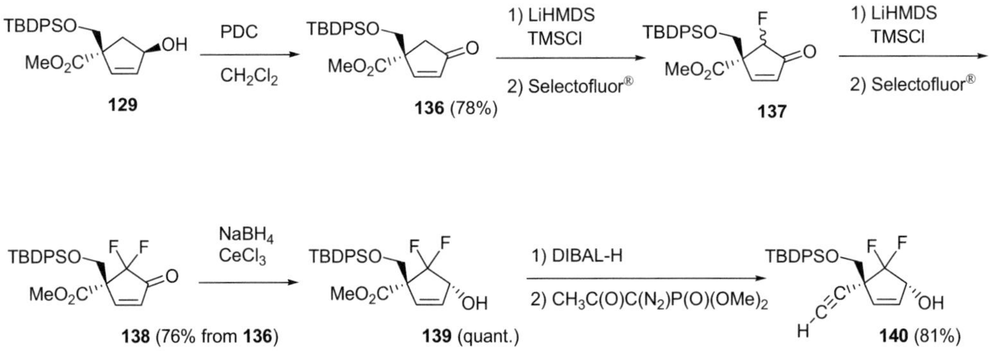

Scheme 35: Synthesis of geminally-difluorinated cyclopentenyl precursor **139** and **140** [66].

Transformation of the ester function of **139** to an ethynyl group was carried out by partial reduction with DIBAL-H, which was followed by treatment with the Ohira-Bestman reagent. This protocol gave the desired cyclopentenol **140** in 81% yield for two steps.

Introduction of thymine base was next examined (Scheme **36**). Compound **140** was reacted with N^3-benzoylthymine under the conventional Mitsunobu conditions. After removal of the N^3-benzoyl group, there were formed three N^1-alkyled products: one was the desired S_N2-product **141** and the others were S_N2'-products **142α** and **143β**. The depicted stereochemistry of these products was confirmed by NOE experiments. The regiochemistry of these glycosides **141**, **142α** and **142β** was assigned on the basis of HMBC spectra: **141** showed the correlation was observed between H-6′ protons (δ 3.90 and 3.94) and sp^2-hybridized carbon (C-3′, δ 136.6); **142α** and **142β** have the correlation between H-6′ protons and sp^3-hybridized carbon (C-3′, δ 62.1 and 65.1, respectively).

After screening the substituents (-CH_2OTBDPS, CN and-CO_2Me) at the 4-position of the cyclopentenol, the highest S_N2-selectivity was observed in the reaction of the 4-methoxycarbonyl derivative **139**, forming **143** as the sole product in 58% yield.

The 4′-methoxycarbonyl carbocyclic nucleoside **143** was reduced with DIBAL-H and then reacted with Ohira-Bestman reagent to give **144** in 80% yield. The target molecule **145** could be obtained in good yield after desilylation with Bu_4NF/THF in the presence of AcOH. The structural confirmation of **145** came from its X-ray crystallographic analysis. The glycosyl tortional angle of **145** showed its *anti*-orientation, which is similar to that of the parent compound stavudine (**104**). However, the orientation of the hydroxylmethyl group at the C-4′ position adopted *trans*, *gauche* ($\gamma = -144.8°$) conformation, which was completely different from that of **104** ($\gamma = -52.8°$). Moreover, the cyclopentene ring of **145** has an envelope type puckering, due to sticking out of the CF_2 group from the cyclopentene plane toward the thymine base: the C-5′ of **145** deviates ca. 0.44 Å from the plane consisting of C1′, C2′, C3′ and C4′. Presumably due to these conformational differences, **145** did not show the inhibitory activity against HIV-1.

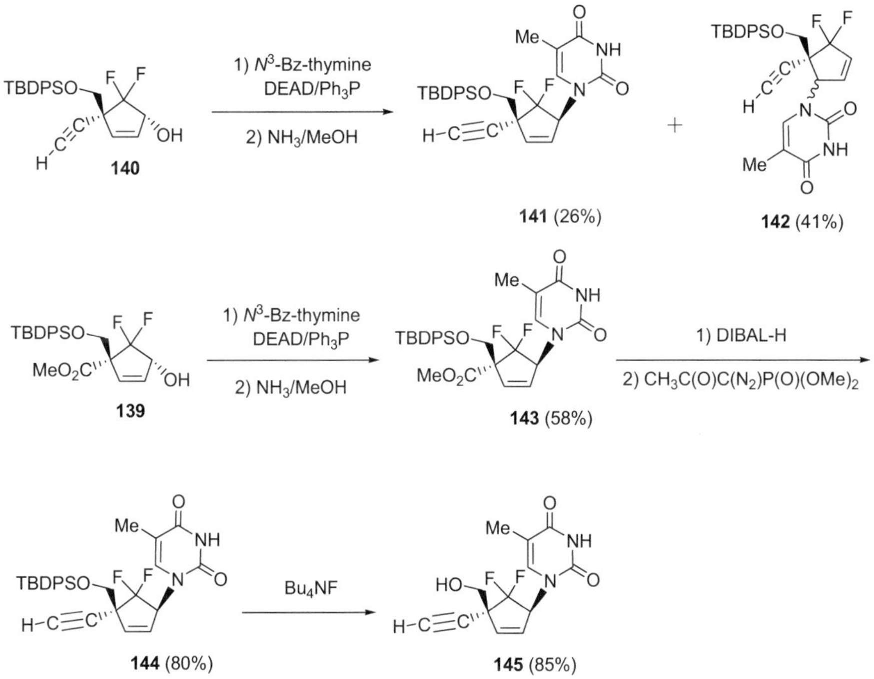

Scheme 36: Synthesis of geminally-difluorinated derivative **145** of 4'-Ed4T **103** [66].

Synthesis of 4′-Thio Analogue of 4′-Ed4T [67]

Nucleosides in which the furanose ring oxygen is replaced with a sulfur atom have been known as 4′-thionucleosides. Extensive synthetic studies of 4′-

thionucleosides started in 1991 because potent anti-viral and anti-tumor activities of 4′-thiothymidine and 2′-deoxy-4′-thiocytidine were reported. Through the synthetic studies, several biologically interesting compounds have been discovered. This fact led us to synthesize the 4′-thio-counterpart of 4′-Ed4T **103**.

The synthetic sequences were illustrated in Scheme **37** and **38**. An aldol reaction between **146** and formaldehyde gave **147** (95%), which was then *O*-silylated to yield **148** in 89% yield. Transformation of **148** to the enone **149** (92%) was performed by Pummerer-type reaction by reacting with *N*-chlorosuccinimide. Luche reduction of **149** gave a mixture of **150** and its epimer with a ratio of *ca.* 10/1 (89% combined yield). The depicted stereochemistry of **150** was confirmed on the basis of NOE experiment. The stereoselectivity observed in the 1,2-reduction of **149** has a precedent in the case of methyl 1-methyl-2-oxo-3-cyclopentenecarboxylate [68]. Benzoylation of **150** gave the glycosyl donor **151** in 94% yield.

For the introduction of a thymine base, electrophilic glycosidation was examined. Electrophilic glycosylation using thiofuranoid glycals has previously been reported from our laboratory [69-72]. When the benzoylated thiofuranoid glycal **151** was reacted with bis-*O*-(trimethylsilyl)thymine (1.5 equiv) in the presence of *N*-iodosuccinimide (1.5 equiv) in CH_3CN, a mixture of the target β-anomer (**152**) and α-anomer (**153**) (**152**: **153** = 10: 1) was formed in 98% combined yield (Scheme **37**). In this case, the desired β-anomer **152** was isolated from the anomeric mixture simply by crystallization. The stereochemistry of **152** was confirmed on the basis of its NOE data [H-2′/H-5′ (1.2%) and H-3′/H-1′ (2.9%)], while the structure of the α-anomer (**153**) was determined on the basis of X-ray crystallographic analysis.

Compound **152** was found to readily undergo reductive elimination with activated Zn to give the 4′-carbomethoxy derivative (**154**) of 4′-thiostavudine in 99% yield (Scheme **38**). Attempted direct transformation of **154** to its 4′-formyl derivative (*e.g.*, *i*-Bu_2AlH in CH_2Cl_2 or THF) all met with concomitant formation of the 4′-hydroxymethyl derivative (**155**). Therefore, **154** was converted to **155** (98%) by reacting with an excess amount of $NaBH_4$ in MeOH/THF, and then the resulting **155** was reoxidized with $(CF_3CO)_2O$/DMSO in CH_2Cl_2 at −80 °C to give the aldehyde **156** in 97% yield.

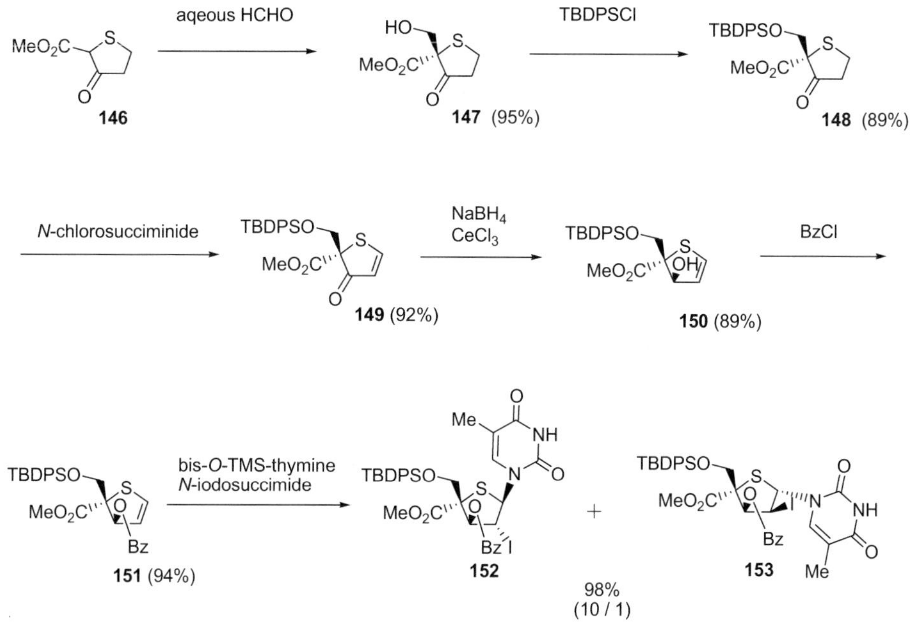

Scheme 37: Synthesis of the glycoside **152** [67].

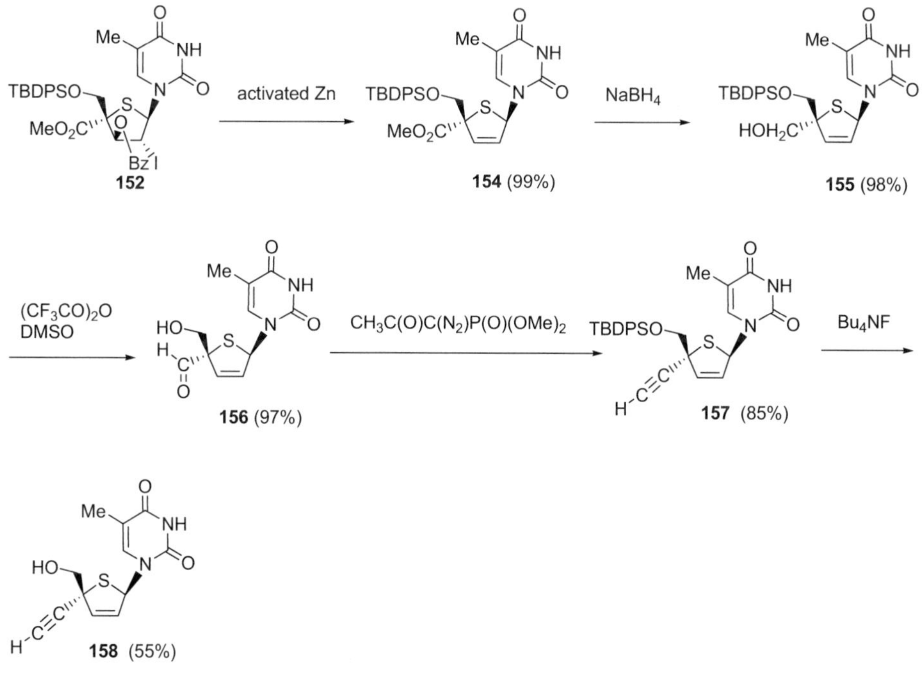

Scheme 38: Synthesis of 4'-thio derivaive **158** of 4'-Ed4T [67].

With the aldehyde **156** in hand, preparation of the 4′-ethynyl derivative (**157**) from **156** was examined. The reaction between **156** and Me_3SiCHN_2/lithium diisopropyl amide (LDA) gave several unknown byproducts, and the desired **157** was isolated only in 20% yield. This result presumably originates in the highly basic nature of LDA, which is needed to generate an anionic species from Me_3SiCHN_2. In fact, the use of Ohira-Bestman reagent in combination with K_2CO_3 in MeOH gave **157** in a higher yield of 85%. Finally, **157** was deprotected to yield the corresponding free (±)-4′-thio counterpart **158** of 4′-Ed4T **103**. Its optical resolution was carried out as follows. After esterification of **158** with (-)-camphanic chloride, HPLC separation ($CHCl_3$/MeOH = 200/1) enabled us to isolate the two diastereomers. Each diastereomer was then treated with K_2CO_3/MeOH to give the respective optically active **158**.

Summary of Anti-HIV-1 Activity of the Analogue of 4′-Ed4T [63]

Anti-HIV-1 activity and its cytotoxixity of the 4′-carbon-substituted d4T derivatives as well as its carbocyclic and 4′-thio counterpart thus far prepared were summarized in Tables **5** and **6**. As a result of our brief examination of structure-activity relationship (SAR) of 4′-carbon-substituted 2′,3′-didehydro-3′-deoxythymidine derivatives, it became apparent that the introduction of a methyl (**101**), or vinyl (**102**) or allyl (**112**) group at the 4′-position leads to complete loss of the activity (entries 2, 3 and 5) and that methylation (**114**) or halogenation (**115**) of the ethynyl group of **103** is also discouraging (entries 6 and 7). Although the 4′-cyano analogue (**123**) was found to be active as we anticipated, its activity is almost five times lower than that of stavudine (**104**) (entry 8).

Unfortunately, carbocyclic (**135**) and difluoromethylene analogue (**145**) of **103** resulted in total loss of the activity (entries 9 and 10). It has been proposed that planarity of the furanose ring of **104** plays one important role for the recognition cellular kinase. Presumably due to these conformational differences, **135** and **145** were not inhibitory against HIV-1 proliferation.

(±)-4′-Ethynyl-4′-thiostavudine (**158**), showed EC_{50} of 0.74 μM, which is almost comparable to that of stavudine (**104**). It should be noted that 4′-thiostavudine itself has been reported not to be inhibitory against HIV-1. Optical resolution of **158** revealed that its levo-enantiomer((–)-**158**) is the active component. Although the actual configuration of (–)-**158** is not known at the moment, it may be possible to assume that this compound has D-configuration, since the L-isomer of stavudine has been reported not to be inhibitory against HIV-1.

Table 5: Anti-HIV-1 (IIIB strain) activity and cytotoxicity of 4'-carbon-substituted stavudine analogues in MT-2 cells [63]

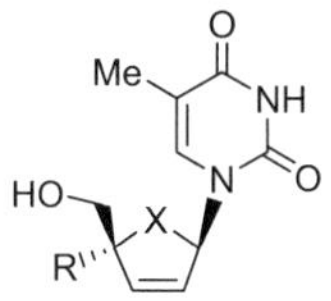

104: X = O, R = H
101: X = O, R = Me
102: X = O, R = CH=CH_2
103: X = O, R = C≡CH
112: X = O, R = CH_2CH=CH_2
114: X = O, R = C≡CMe
115: X = O, R = C≡CCl
123: X = O, R = C≡N
135: X = CH_2, R = C≡CH
145: X = CF_2, R = C≡CH

Entry	Compound	X	R	EC_{50} (μM)[a]	CC_{50} (μM)[b]
1	d4T (**104**)	O	H	1.3 ± 0.4	98.0 ±10.8
2	4'-methyl-d4T (**101**)	O	Me	> 100	> 100
3	4'-vinyl-d4T (**102**)	O	CH_2=CH_2	> 100	> 100
4	4'-ethynyl-d4T (**103**)	O	C≡CH	0.25 ± 0.14	> 256[c]
5	4'-allyl-d4T (**112**)	O	CH_2CH=CH_2	> 100	> 100
6	4'-methylethynyl-d4T (**114**)	O	C≡CCl	> 63	63 ± 21
7	4'-chloroethynyl-d4T (**115**)	O	C≡CMe	4.0 ± 1.6	> 100
8	4'-cyanol-d4T (**123**)	O	C≡N	7.0 ± 2.6	> 100
9	carbocayclic 4'-ethynyl-d4T (**135**)	CH_2	C≡CH	> 100	> 100
10	difluoromethylene- 4'-ethynyl-d4T (**145**)	CF_2	C≡CH	> 100	> 100

[a] Effective concentration required to achieve 50% protection from HIV.
[b] Cytotoxic concentration required to inhibit MT-2 cells by 50%.
[c] The highest concentration tested.

Table 6: Anti-HIV-1 (IIIB strain) activity and cytotoxicity of 4'-carbon-substituted stavudine analogues in MT-4 cells [63]

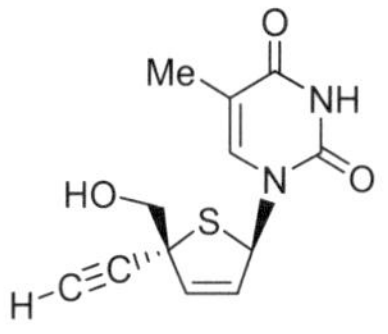

(−)-**158**: X = S, R = C≡CH
(+)-**158**: X = S, R = C≡CH

Entry	Compound	X	R	EC_{50} (μM)[a]	CC_{50} (μM)[b]
1	d4T (**104**)	O	H	0.51	100
2	4'-ethynyl-d4T (**103**)	O	C≡CH	0.060	>100
3	(−)-4'-thio- 4'-ethynyl-d4T ((−)-**158**)	S	C≡CH	0.37	>100
4	(+)-4'-thio- 4'-ethynyl-d4T ((+)-**158**)	S	C≡CH	> 20	>100

[a] Inhibitory concentration required to achieve 50% protection of MT-4 cells against the cytopathic effect of HIV-1 III_B.
[b] Cytotoxic concentration required to reduce the viability of mock-infected MT-4 cells by 50%.

In conclusion, one would readily expect that suitable 4′-substituents should possess an sp-hybridized carbon atom like ethynyl and cyano group, and its size should be as small as possible because methyl-**114** and chloroethynyl nucleosides **115** decreased the activity.

Development of Improved Synthetic Method for 4′-Ed4T

For evaluating 4′-Ed4T **103** in preclinical and clinical studies, alternative synthetic methods suitable for its large scaled preparation were needed, because the route shown in Scheme **27** is unfavorable due to the inaccessibility of a highly concentrated acetone solution of DMDO. These facts led us to develop easy, cheap and large scale synthetic methods. To this end, three promising synthetic routes have been developed.

Nucleophilic Substitution Method Utilizing 4′-Benzoyloxythymidine Derivative [73]

We envisioned that nucleophilic ethynylation of nucleoside derivatives having leaving group at the 4′-position would constitute the most straightforward route to 4′-Ed4T (**103**). Therefore, we first thought that regioselective vicinal diacetoxylation reaction of 4′,5′-unsaturated d4T **159** by reacting with $Pb(OAc)_4$. Thus, when **159** was reacted with $Pb(OAc)_4$ (1.5 equiv), two products **160** and **161** were detected by TLC analysis (Scheme **39**). Although silica gel column chromatography allowed the isolation and structural confirmation of these products (**160**, *ca.* 35%; **161**, 50%), the 4′-acetoxy derivative **160** appeared to be too unstable for further reaction, liberating **161** during evaporation of the solvent or even on standing at rt. This fact led us to examine diacyloxylation of 4′,5′-unsaturated derivative (**162**).

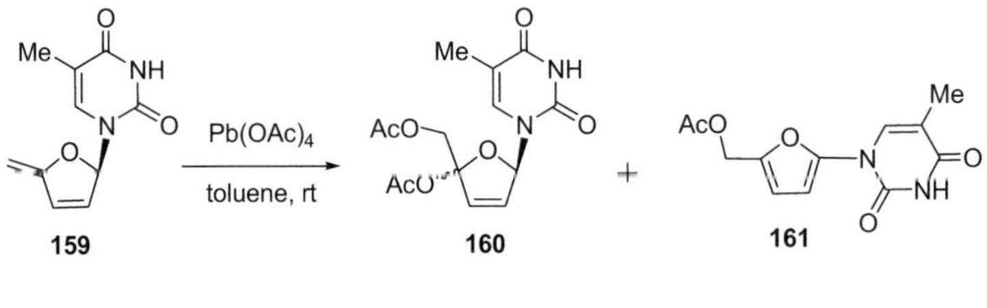

Scheme 39: Diacetoxylation of 4',5'-unsaturated d4T derivative **159** [73].

When **162** was reacted with $Pb(OAc)_4$ under the above reaction conditions, a mixture of the diastereomers of 4′-acetoxy derivative **163** was obtained (Scheme **40**), but the yield was only 28%. The main product in this reaction was the aldehyde **164** (60%). It is conceivable that acidic reaction media encourages protonation to the 4′-acetoxy group of **163**, which accelerates attack of nucleophile to its carbonyl group. Based on this assumption, the diacetoxylation was reexamined by adding bases. After several attempts (imidazole and collidine), the presence of *i*-Pr_2NEt (1.5 equiv) was found to prevent the formation of **164** completely, but the yield of **163** (32%) was not improved.

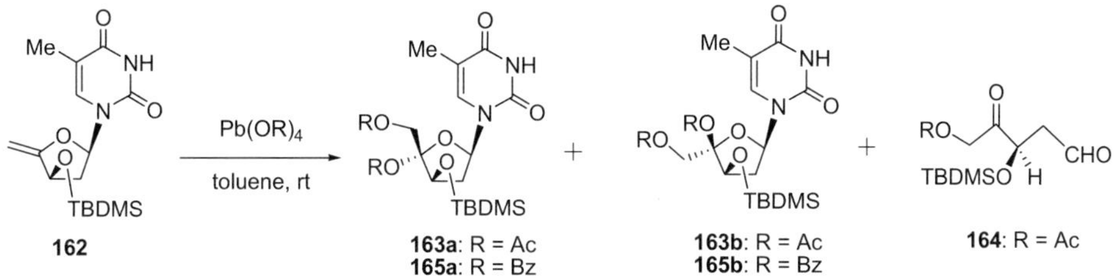

Scheme 40: Diacyloxylation of 4',5'-unsaturated thymine nucleosides **162** [73].

It has been reported that although $Pb(OAc)_4$ did not work for vicinal diacetoxylation of styrene, use of lead tetracarboxylate prepared from higher carboxylic acids gave styrene glycol dicarboxylates. When **162** was reacted with $Pb(OBz)_4$, prepared from $Pb(OAc)_4$ and benzoic acid, in the presence of *i*-Pr_2NEt in toluene at rt, the 4′-benzoyloxy derivative **165** could be obtained in 71% yield (**165a/165b** = 1/0.8) without forming the aldehyde. The stereochemistry of **165a** and **165b** was confirmed by their NOE experiments: **165a**, H-5′b/H-6 (3.4%) and H-5′a/H-6 (1.4%); **165b**, H-5′b/H-3′ (0.7%).

Next, 4′-benzoyloxy derivative **165** was reacted with Me_3Al as a model experiment. As shown in Scheme **41**, in this reaction, three isomeric products were formed. The minor product was the expected 4′-methyl derivative **167** (15%) and the other two products were found to be spiro-nucleosides. HPLC separation of the mixture followed by NOE experiment led us to propose the depicted 4′-configuration for the both diastereomers.

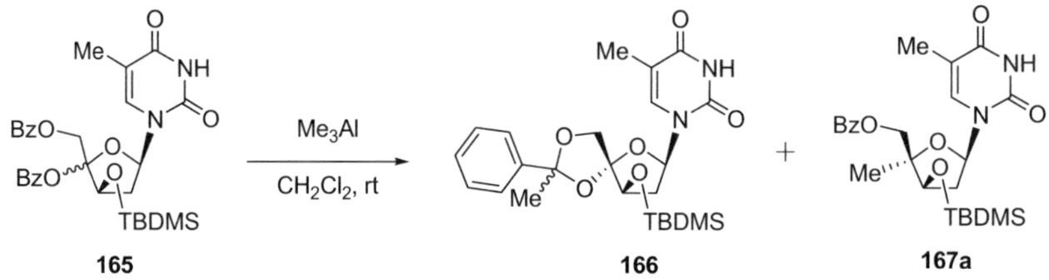

Scheme 41: Reaction of **165** with Me_3Al [73].

On the other hand, when **165** was reacted with $MeAlCl_2$ (4.0 equiv) in CH_2Cl_2 for 2 h at 0 °C (Scheme **42**), the 4′-methyl derivative was not detected, but instead two isomeric 4′-chlorinated products (**168a**, 53%; **168b**, 14%) were obtained. Independent treatment of the isolated **168a** or **168b** with $MeAlCl_2$ in CH_2Cl_2 again resulted in a mixture of both compounds, showing that they are interconvertible in the presence of $MeAlCl_2$. It was found that further treatment of the above reaction mixture containing **168** with Me_3Al (6.0 equiv, at rt for 23 h) gave the 4′-methyl derivatives (**167a**, 14%; **167b**, 19%) in one-pot manner. Although the yield of **167** was not high, formation of the spiro derivative **166** was suppressed to a trace amount.

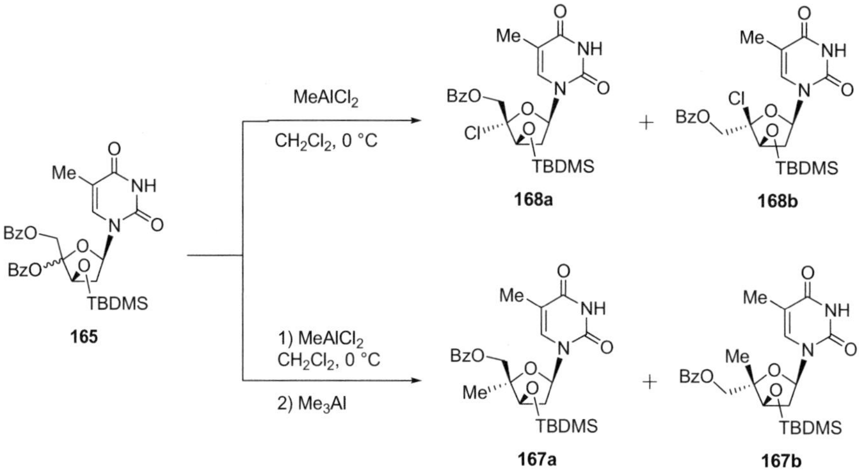

Scheme 42: Reaction of **165** with $MeAlCl_2$ or $MeAlCl_2/Me_3Al$ [73].

Next, ethynylation at the 4′-position of **165** was explored. One-pot treatment of **165** with $MeAlCl_2$ followed by $(HC{\equiv}C)_3Al$ did not allow the introduction of an ethynyl group. However, reaction of $Me_3SiC{\equiv}CAl(Et)Cl$ furnished the desired 4′-ethynyl derivative **169** as a single isomer in 51% yield. During this ethnylation reaction of **165**, the ethynylaluminum reagent was found to be capable of chlorinating **165**, and that the 4′-ethynylation gradually took place. Thus, when **165** was reacted with 8.0 equiv of $Me_3SiC{\equiv}CAl(Et)Cl$ in CH_2Cl_2 at rt overnight (Scheme **43**), **169** was formed as a single stereoisomer in 62% yield. This ethynylation can be performed in several ten grams scale. When the reaction of $Me_3SiC{\equiv}CAl(Et)Cl$ with the two isomers was independently carried out, both **168a** and **168b** gave **169** exclusively in 71% and 50% isolated yields, respectively.

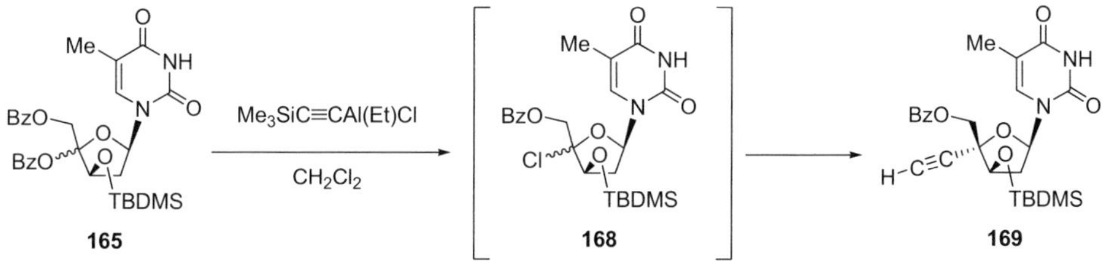

Scheme 43: Reaction of **165** with $Me_3SiC{\equiv}CAl(Et)Cl$ [73].

At present time, the clear explanation for the reason why **168** gave the desired 4′-α-ethynyl derivative **169** exclusively, while it gave two isomeric 4′-methyl derivatives (**167a** and **167b**, Scheme **42**) upon reacting with Me_3Al, is not available. However, the 3′-β-*O*-TBDMS group had played an important role in the above ethynylation, because the 4′-benzoyloxy derivative **170** with the opposite 3′-configuration gave the 4′-β-ethynylated product **171** exclusively, in 31% yield (Scheme **44**).

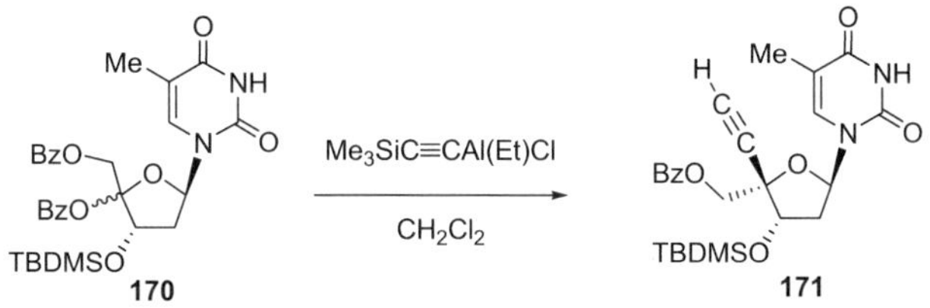

Scheme 44: Reaction of **170** with $Me_3SiC{\equiv}CAl(Et)Cl$ [73].

Finally, the above-prepared **169** was transformed into 4′-Ed4T **103** by reaction sequence shown in Scheme **45**. Thus, desilylation of **169** with Bu_4NF gave the 3′-hydroxyl derivative **172** in 97% yield. Then, **172** was subjected to sulfonylation by reacting $(CF_3SO_2)O$ in the presence of pyridine in THF. The resulting 3′-*O*-triflate **173** was not isolated, instead extracted with $CHCl_3$, and the crude reaction mixture was treated with DBN/CH_3CN to lead to the formation of the protected 4′-Ed4T. Removal of the 5′-*O*-benzoyl group of the protected 4′-Ed4T was carried out in a one-pot manner by adding MeOH to the elimination reaction mixture. Utilizing this protocol, 4′-Ed4T **103** could be obtained in 69% yield from **172**.

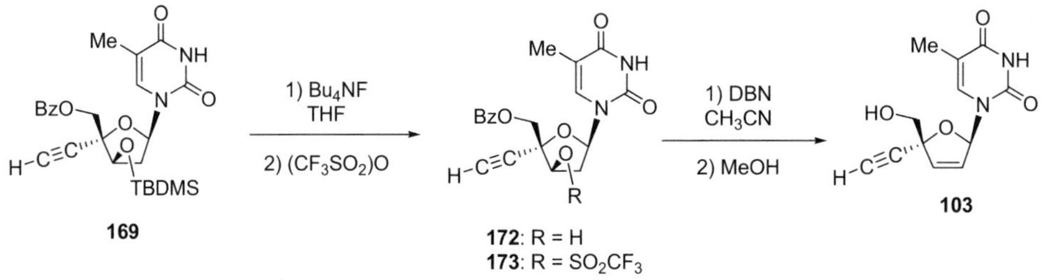

Scheme 45. Synthesis of 4'-Ed4T **103** [73].

<u>Furfuryl Alcohol Method</u> [74]

Furfuryl alcohol was treated with *N*-bromosuccinimide (NBS) in the presence of NaOAc and $NaHCO_3$ in THF at 0 °C to give the pentopyranose derivative (**174**) as a racemic mixture (Scheme **46**). The hemiacetal **174** was converted to the corresponding acetate **175**. The (±)-acetate **175** was subjected to optical resolution by means of lipase-catalyzed hydrolysis and the (−)-acetate ((−)-**176**) could be obtained in high optical purity. When (−)-**176** was next reacted with lithium trimethylsilylacetylide, prepared from trimethylsilylacetylene and *n*-butyl lithium, the respective propargyl alcohol **177** was obtained. Compound **177** was transformed into the diol **178** by reacting with lipase PS in a mixture of CH_3CN, *n*-hexane and 2-propanol at 40 °C. The diol **178** is presented in equilibrium with 4-trimethylsilylethynyl-2′,3′-dideoxy-2′,3′-didehydroribose **179**. The ribose derivative **179** was reacted with Ac_2O/pyridine/DMAP in THF to give the di- *O*-acetate **180**. Next, the di-*O*-acetate **180** was glycosidated with silylated thymine, prepared from thymine and *N*,*O*-bis-trimethylsilylacetamide (BSA), in the presence of TMSOTf to furnish the protected 4′-Ed4T **181** as an anomeric mixture. Finally, deprotection of **181** with 1 M NaOH and the recrystallization of the resulting anomeric mixture provided 4′-Ed4T **103**.

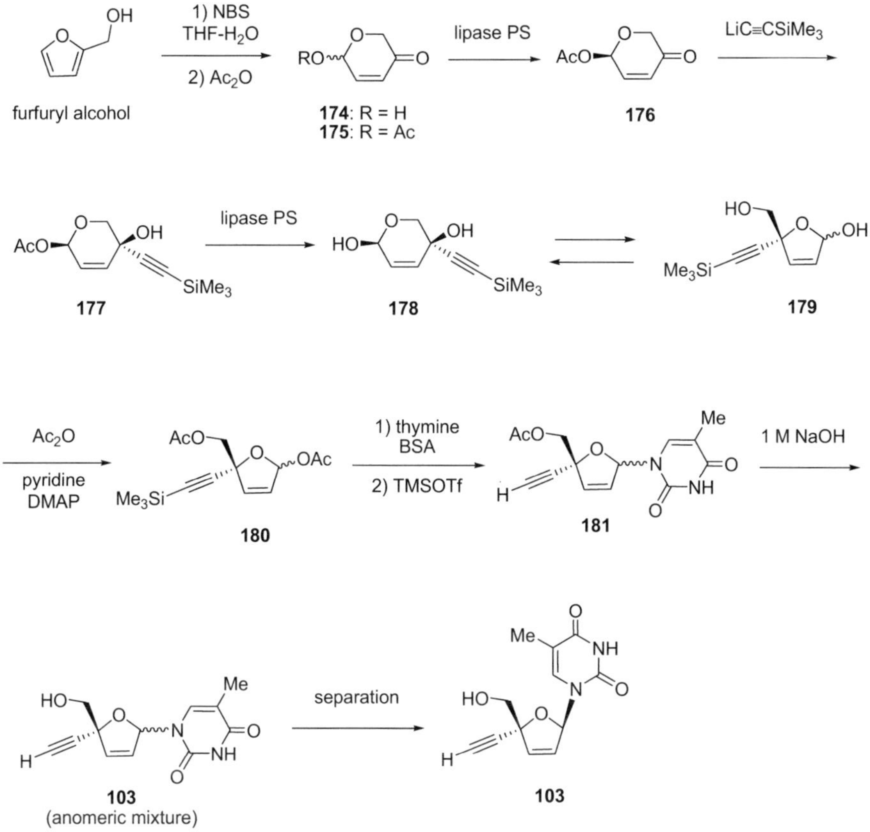

Scheme 46: Synthesis of 4'-Ed4T **103** from furfuryl alcohol [74].

Levoglucosenone Method [74]

When levoglucosenone was reacted with lithium trimethylsilylacetylide (LiC≡CSiMe$_3$) at-30 °C, nucleophilic 1,2-addition from the concave face of the α,β-unsaturated moiety of the starting material proceeded to give propargyl alcohol **182** stereoselectively (Scheme **47**). Acetolysis of the cyclic acetal moiety of **182** was carried out by reacting with Ac_2O in the presence of conc.H_2SO_4 to furnish the tri-*O*-acetate **183**. Regioselective removal of the acetyl group of the anomeric position was performed by treatment of **183** with hydrazine hydrate to give the hemiacetal **184**. Hydride reduction of **184** and silylation of the primary hydroxyl group of the resulting diol **185** gave the mono-alcohol **186**. The di-*O*-acetate **186** was transformed to the triol **187** and subsequent oxidative cleavage of the glycol moiety of **187** gave aldehyde **188**. The aldehyde **188** is in equilibrium with 4-ethynyl-2,3-

didehydro-2,3-dideoxyribose **189**. Compound **189** was acetylate and the resulting glycosyl donor **190** was reacted with silylated thymine in the presence of TMSOTf in CH_2Cl_2 to furnish the glycoside **191**. Finally, 4′-Ed4T **103** could be obtained through desilylation with Bu_4NF in a mixture of ether and hexane.

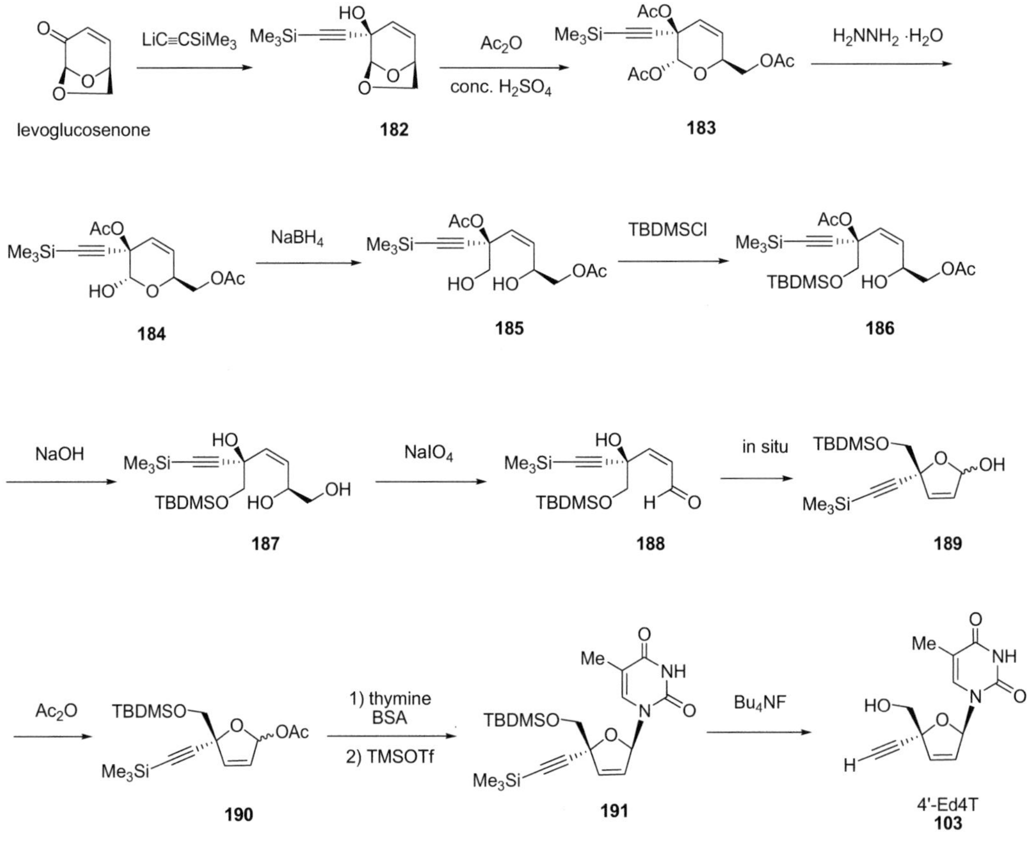

Scheme 47: Synthesis of 4'-Ed4T **103** from levoglucosenone [74].

Antiviral Activity of 4′-Ed4T

When the anti-HIV-1 activity of 4′-ethynylstavudine (4′-Ed4T) was evaluated in MT-4 cells and peripheral blood mononuclear cells (PBMCs) and compared to that of stavudine (d4T) and lamivudine (3TC), 4′-Ed4T was found to be more active than d4T and 3TC (Table **7**). The 50% effective concentration (EC_{50}) of 4′-Ed4T was 0.070 μM in MT-4 cells infected with HIV-1 III_B strain. This value was approximately 4.4-fold lower than that of the parental compound d4T. In addition, 4′-Ed4T also proved highly active against both X4 HIV-1 (III_B) and R5 HIV-1

(Ba-L) in PBMCs. The EC_{50}s were 0.0019 and 0.0076 μM against the III_B and Ba-L strains, respectively. Again, these values were 10-and 6.2-fold lower than those of d4T. On the other hand, 4′-Ed4T appeared to be less cytotoxic than d4T. These results indicate that 4′-Ed4T is a more potent and selective inhibitor of HIV-1 replication in cell cultures than d4T.

Table 7: Anti-HIV-1 activity of 4′-Ed4T, d4T, and 3TC in MT-4 cell cultures[a] [62]

Compound	Virus	Cell	EC_{50}[b] (μM)	CC_{50}[c] (μM)
4′-Ed4T	III_B	MT-4	0.070 ± 0.041	> 100
		PBMC	0.0019 ± 0.0002	56 ± 3
	Ba-L	PBMC	0.0076 ± 0.0013	
d4T	III_B	MT-4	0.31 ± 0.07	79 ± 19
		PBMC	0.019 ± 0.004	28 ± 7
	Ba-L	PBMC	0.047 ± 0.027	
3TC	III_B	MT-4	0.60 ± 0.03	> 100

[a] Data are taken from the reference 1.
[b] 50% effective concentration.
[c] 50% cytotoxic concentration.

The anti-HIV-1 activity of 4′-Ed4T was also evaluated for various reverse transcriptase (RT) inhibitor-resistant mutants. It was found that the activity was affected by the nucleoside RT inhibitor-associated mutations (NAMs) and the M184V mutation of HIV-1 RT [62]. The reduction of activity was several-fold, depending on the absence or presence of additional amino acid mutations. 4′-Ed4T retained potent antiviral activity against the mutants harboring the Q151M and K65R mutations, which confer resistance to most nucleoside RT inhibitors (NTRIs) and tenofovir disoproxil fumarate (TDF), respectively. As expected, the K103N mutation, which confers a high level resistance to non-nucleoside RT inhibitors (NNRTIs), did not affect the activity of 4′-Ed4T. However, the K103N mutation appeared to compensate the effect of the M184V mutation on the resistance to 4′-Ed4T [62].

A variety of Gag/protease/RT-recombinant viruses were generated from clinical samples harboring selected sets of the NRTI-resistant mutations, such as NAMs, M41L/L210W/T215Y (TAM41), D67N/K70R/T215F/K219Q (TAM67), K65R, L74V, and Q151M in the absence or presence of K103N and M184V [75]. These viruses were examined for their susceptibility to 4′-Ed4T, TDF, abacavir (ABC), d4T, zidovudine (AZT), and 3TC. In this system, the anti-HIV-1 activity of 4′-Ed4T was modestly reduced in the viruses carrying NAMs, TAM41, and TAM67 together with the K103N and M184V mutations (Fig. **9A** and **9B**). Similar results were obtained for TDF. In contrast, some of the recombinant viruses showed a high level of resistance to ABC, d4T, AZT, or 3TC. Interestingly, viruses carrying the Q151M mutation were found to be hypersensitive to 4′-Ed4T (Fig. **9A**). This nature of 4′-

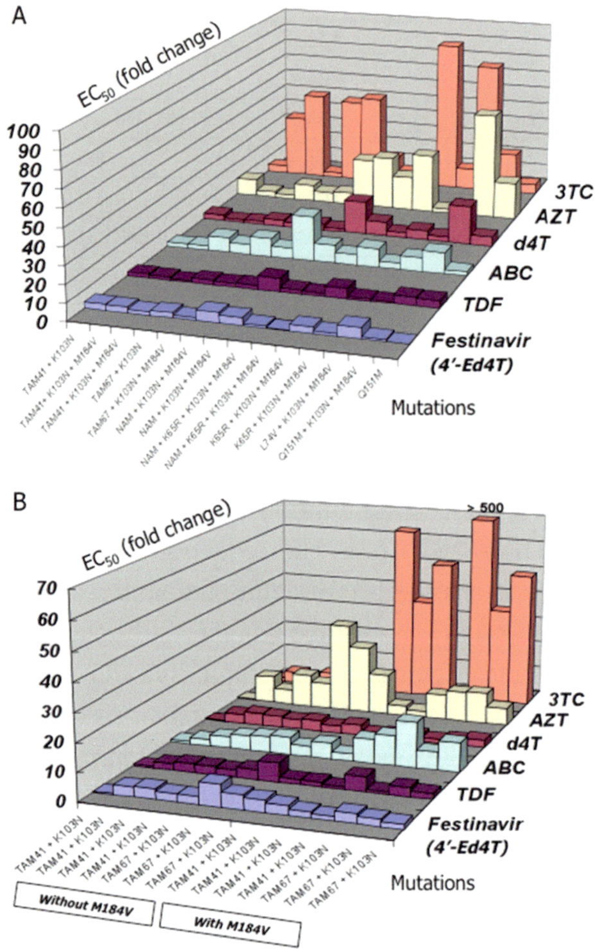

Figure 9: Anti-HIV-1 activity of NRTIs including 4′-Ed4T against various RT mutants. Gag/protease/RT-recombinant viruses were generated from clinical samples harboring various NRTI-and NNRTI-resistant mutations and examined for their susceptibility to the indicated compounds. The antiviral activity of each compound against the mutants are expressed as fold-change in its EC_{50}s compared to the EC_{50} to the wild-type virus [76].

Ed4T was also observed in our previous study [75]. Thus, the resistance profile of 4′-Ed4T is quite unique and different from those of other NRTIs. Furthermore, when the anti-HIV-1 activity of 4′-Ed4T was examined in combination with other NRTIs and NNRTIs, 4′-Ed4T displayed strong synergistic interaction with efavirenz and moderate one with ABC, TDF, and NVP [76 and unpublished data].

To obtain resistant viruses *in vitro*, serial passages of HIV-1 (III_B)-infected MT-4 cells in the presence of escalating concentrations of 4′-Ed4T and 3TC were conducted. 3TC induced a virus harboring the M184V mutation on day 29 ($3TC_{29D}$). This mutant was completely resistant to 3TC (Table **8**). However, 4′-Ed4T proved only 2-fold less active against $3TC_{29D}$ compared to the wild-type. The virus approximately 10-fold resistant to 4′-Ed4T ($Ed4T_{81D}$) was obtained on day 81 after incubation of the infected cells. The RT sequence analysis revealed that $Ed4T_{81D}$ carried the three mutations P119S, T165A, and M184V [62]. However, the resistant virus did not have any amino acid mutations in the thumb, connection, and RNaseH domains of RT [76]. The purine nucleoside analog 4′-ethynyl-2-fluoro-2′-deoxyadenine (4′-EFdA) has been reported as a highly potent and selective inhibitor of HIV-1 replication [77]. In fact, 4′-EFdA was more active against HIV-1 than 4′-Ed4T in our assay (Table **8**). However, $Ed4T_{81D}$ was also less (approximately 25-fold) susceptible to 4′-EFdA, probably due to the structural similarity (the ethynyl group at the 4′-position) between 4′-Ed4T and 4′-EFdA.

Table 8: Anti-HIV-1 activity of 4′-Ed4T, 4′-EFdA, and 3TC against resistant strains in MT-4 cells [62]

Strain	**EC_{50}[a] (μM)**		
	4'-Ed4T	**4'-EFdA**	**3TC**
III_B (wild type)	0.22 ± 0.13	0.0011 ± 0.0003	2.0 ± 0.8
III_B ($3TC_{29D}$)	0.41 ± 0.08	0.014 ± 0.004	> 20
III_B ($Ed4T_{81D}$)	2.3 ± 1.4	0.028 ± 0.012	> 20
CC_{50}[b] (μM)	> 20	8.4 ± 0.9	> 20

[a] 50% effective concentration.
[b] 50% cytotoxic concentration.

Biology, Pharmacology and Clinical Studies of 4′-Ethynylstavudine

Since the discovery of the anti-HIV activity of zidovudine (AZT) in the 1980s [78, 79], the US Food and Drug Administration (US FDA) has approved over 30 antiretroviral agents for the treatment of HIV. However, the search for anti-HIV agents continues unabated due to limitations of current antiretroviral therapy (ART): (1) varying potencies and inability to eradicate the virus; (2) drug-induced toxicities; (3) evolution of drug resistant HIV strains on treatment; and (4) pill burden and frequent dosing schedules. Therefore, an ideal antiretroviral agent should have the following attributes: (1) potency; (2) favorable or negligible toxicity profile; (3) high genetic barrier to development of resistance; (4) no cross resistance to other agents; and (5) potential to be co-formulated with other agents into a fixed-dose combination (FDC) regimen. 4′-Ed4T promises to be an ideal nucleoside analog with higher potency and therapeutic index, longer half-life of active metabolites in cells, without much impact on mitochondrial DNA (mt-DNA) concentration in cell culture, effective against multidrug resistant (MDR) HIV, and difficulty in selecting for HIV resistant viruses probably due to the interaction of the compound with HIV reverse transcriptase (RT) [61, 80]. Here, we describe the pre-clinical and clinical studies of 4′-Ed4T.

Preclinical Studies of 4′-Ethynlstavudine

Potency: Among 4′-substituted compounds synthesized, [80] 4′-Ed4T was potent than stavudine (d4T), the parent compound. The potency of 4′-Ed4T may be explained by: (1) its binding characteristics to HIV RT; (2) intracellular accumulation of the active metabolites; and (3) persistent of activity when drug was removed from cell culture. In steady-state enzymatic analyses, 4′-Ed4T triphosphate (4′-Ed4TTP) inhibited the DNA polymerase activity of RT more efficiently than d4T triphosphate (d4TTP), and the inhibition was more effective with RNA template than with DNA template [16]. 4′-Ed4TTP had much lower *K*i value in the inhibition of RT compared to the *K*i value of d4TTP. Moreover, 4′-Ed4TMP was incorporated by RT with DNA/RNA substrate 3-fold less than incorporation of d4TMP. Thus the binding of 4′-Ed4TTP to RT-P/T complex is an important factor than incorporation of 4′-Ed4TTP. Pre-steady-state kinetic studies and computer modeling showed that the 4′-ethynyl group of 4′-Ed4TTP may dock and bind to a hydrophobic pocket in the RT active site. This might explain why 4′-Ed4TTP is a better RT inhibitor than d4TTP. The hydrophobic pocket plays a critical role in HIV RT activity (Table **9**) [80]. The hydrophobic pocket is formed by the side chains of A114, Y115, M184, F160 and D185 [81]. When these residues were mutated to A114M, A114L, Y115Q, F160A, F160L, and M184F,

RT activity was completely lost, except for M184V and M184A mutants [80, 81]. The mutant M184V could affect the binding of incoming dNTP as a result of a gap or groove created between the polymerase and the DNA of the nascent base pair leading to 3 to 5-fold resistance to 4′-Ed4T.

Table 9: Pre-staedy-state kinetic parameters for dTMR, d4TMP, and 4′-Ed4TMP incorporation by wt RT and the M184V mutant with DNA/DNA and DNA/RNA P/Ts [80]

P/T	Sequence
DNA/RNA 23-/36-mer	5′-TCAGGTCCCTGTTCGTTCGGGCGCCAC-3′ 3′-CGAAAGUCCAGGGACAAGCCCGCGGUGACGAUCUCU-5′
DNA/DNA 23-/36-mer	5′-TCAGGTCCCTGTTCGGGCGCCAC-3’ 3′-CGAAAGTCCAGGGACAAGCCCGCGGTGACGATCTCT-5′

P/T	Enzyme	dTTP		
		Kd **(μM) (mean ± SD)**	***k*pol (S^{-1}) (mean ± SD)**	***k*pol/*Kd* ($\mu M^{-1}S^{-1}$)**
DNA/DNA	wt RT	15. 4 ± 2.9	22.6 ± 1.3	1.47
	M184V	73.2 ± 8.0	22.4 ± 0.9	0.31
DNA/RNA	wt RT	67.1 ± 10.2	65.0 ± 3.9	0.97
	M184V	143.9 ± 25.0	41.7 ± 3.5	0.29

P/T	Enzyme	d4TTP			Selectivity[a]
		Kd **(μM) (mean ± SD)**	***k*pol (S^{-1}) (mean ± SD)**	***k*pol/*Kd* ($\mu M^{-1}S^{-1}$)**	
DNA/DNA	wt RT	48.0 ± 4.8	16.0 ± 0.5	0.33	4.5
	M184V	605 ± 285	29.8 ± 10.4	0.05	6.2
DNA/RNA	wt RT	40.8 ± 9.2	18.4 ± 1.4	0.45	2.2
	M184V	232.3 ± 50.0	29.6 ± 3.6	0.13	2.2

[a] Selectivity is calculated by dividing the efficiency of dTTP (*k*pot/*Kd*) by the efficiency of d4TTP or 4'-Ed4TTP.

P/T	Enzyme	4’-Ed4TTP			Selectivity[a]
		Kd **(μM) (mean ± SD)**	***k*pol (S^{-1}) (mean ± SD)**	***k*pol/*Kd* ($\mu M^{-1}S^{-1}$)**	
DNA/DNA	wt RT	15.8 ± 2.4	12.1 ± 0.5	0.77	1.9
	M184V	168.1 ± 25.6	18.9 ± 1.1	0.11	2.8
DNA/RNA	wt RT	11.4 ± 2.7	11.7 ± 30.8	1	0.97
	M184V	43.4 ± 13.9	9.7 ± 0.8	0.22	1.3

[a] Selectivity is calculated by dividing the efficiency of dTTP (*k*pot/*Kd*) by the efficiency of d4TTP or 4'-Ed4TTP.

The peak concentrations in cells of the metabolites occurred at 2 h for AZT and at 12 h for both 4′-Ed4T and stavudine. Interestingly, the rate of phosphorylation of 4′-Ed4T was slower than d4T, but faster than AZT. 4′-Ed4T intracellular triphosphate metabolites concentration was higher than that of AZT at 24 h in culture [82]. 4′-Ed4T monophosphate was the major metabolite, which contributed most to the accumulation of the triphosphate over a 12 hour period. This was consistent with TMP kinase activity on 4′-Ed4T, the rate limiting-step, observed previously [83]. Most importantly, 4′-Ed4TTP, the active metabolite, had a longer half-life ($t_{1/2}$ 8.0 to 9.7 h) than diphosphate ($t_{1/2}$, 2.4 to 5.1 h) and monophosphate ($t_{1/2}$, 1.4 to 2.4 h) after the drug was removed from cell culture [17]. The persistence of intracellular 4′-Ed4TTP translated to a more durable anti-HIV-1 activity. The comparative rank order of the inhibitors to protect cells from HIV infection after 48 h of removal of drug from cell culture was 4′-Ed4T > LFD4C > didanosine (DDI) > d4T > lamivudine (3TC) > AZT > emtricitabine (FTC) > nevirapine (NVP) [84]. That is, 4′-Ed4T could protect uninfected cells against HIV replication longer than AZT, d4T, and most of currently used HIV drugs. In a viral rebound studies, viral rebound occurred after removal of all the inhibitors from culture. After 48 h of removal of inhibitor from cell culture, the rank order of concentration of inhibitor required to keep viral rebound at 50% was DDI < 4′-Ed4T < LFD4C < FTC < d4T < 3TC < NVP < AZT [85]. The durability of antiviral activity of 4′-Ed4T in culture may be due to: (1) the relative stability of the triphosphate and that the monophosphate (which is less likely effluxed from the cells [84]) may continue to form 4′-Ed4TTP; (2) inefficient removal of incorporated 4′-Ed4T from terminal viral DNA by Exos; and (3) inability of 4′-Ed4TTP metabolites to be transported out of the cell [86] as compared to the metabolites of AZ [86].

Toxicity: During the era of AZT monotherapy, some patients developed skeletal muscle myopathies [87]. Histological examination of their muscle biopsies revealed mitochondrial pathologies [88, 89]. These patients had decreased amounts of mitochondrial DNA (mtDNA), RNA, and proteins in their muscles [90]. *In vitro* studies demonstrated that NRTIs inhibit polymerase gamma (Pol-γ), the enzyme responsible for replication of mtDNA, leading to depletion of mtDNA content and subsequent mitochondrial dysfunction [91-94]. *In vitro* studies are used to predict the effect of various inhibitors on mitochondria. For instance, the *in vitro* hierarchy of inhibition of pol-γ by NRTIs is ddC > ddI > d4T ≥ AZT > 3TC = ABC = TDF [95]. Interestingly, the IC_{50} for inhibition of pol γ and pol β by 4′-Ed4TTP was at least 100-fold greater than that for d4TTP (Table **10**) [16]. This may explain why 4′-Ed4T caused much less cellular toxicity and mitochondrial DNA depletion than d4T in cell culture studies [15]. The underlying molecular mechanism of less inhibition of 4′-Ed4TTP to pol γ and pol β than d4TTP could be due to subtle differences in the interaction of the 4′-position of these two compounds at the active site of at pol γ and pol β. In long-term cultures of human proximal tubule epithelium, skeletal muscle, or differentiated adipocytes, 4′-Ed4T had minimal effect on cytotoxicity or mtDNA content compared to the effect of d4T, adefovir, and ABC [18]. Moreover, in rats and cynomolgus monkeys, high dosed of 4′-Ed4T showed no evidence of renal or bone toxicity [19]. Thus, the safety profile of 4′-Ed4T is better than that of Tenofovir. High doses of tenofovir resulted in renal and bone toxicity in these animal models [20-25].

Table 10: Action of 4′-Ed4TTP on major human DNA polymerases [16]

DNA polymarase	IC_{50} (μM)[a,b]			
	4'-ED4TTP	D4TTP	ddTTP	Aphidicolin
α	>100	>100	ND[c]	5
β	>100	1		ND[c]
γ	~100	1		ND[c]
δ		40		ND[c]
ε	>100	>100	ND	5

[a] The ID_{50} values represent means from at least three independent experiments with standard deviation less than 20%.
[b] When 0.3 mM dTTP was used in the assay.
[c] ND, not determined.

Potential for fixed-dose combination formulation: The sine qua non of HIV treatment since 1996 is combination of highly active antiretroviral drugs. When these drugs are used in combination, lower doses may achieve desired antiviral effect with less toxicity. In pre-clinical studies, 4′-Ed4T had synergy with 3TC and LFd4C against HIV and was additive in combination with ddI or AZT [15]. Therefore, 4′-Ed4T could be given in combination with several approved antiretroviral drugs in the clinic. 4′-Ed4T is a thymidine analog in the same class as AZT and d4T. However, the phosphorylation of 4′-Ed4T by TK-1 may not explain its potency over d4T. Since its antiviral effect could be neutralized by dThd but not by dCyd, 4′-Ed4T (like d4T) acts as a dThd analog; however, the antiviral mechanism of action of 4′-Ed4T could still be quite different from that of d4T. D4T was efficiently phosphorylated to the triphosphate metabolite than 4′-Ed4T. Could 4′-Ed4TMP be one of the active metabolite in addition to 4′-Ed4TTP? Furthermore, 4′-Ed4T is not a substrate for thymidylate phosphorlyase and may explain its pharmacokinetic advantages over d4T [15].

Resistance: In an initial selection for 4′-Ed4T drug resistance study by Nitanda *et al.* [62] presented above, on day 26 M184V mutation was observed followed by additional mutations (P119S and T165A) on day 81. The M184V and triple (M184V/P119S/T165A) mutants were reported to confer 3-5-fold and 130-fold resistance to 4′-Ed4T, respectively. This was intriguing as the P119S and/or T165A have not been observed in HIV-1-infected treatment-experienced individuals. The clinical significance of these mutations was unknown. Further resistance studies had been carried out. The P119S, T165A, and M184V mutations were introduced into an NL4-3 background to assess the role of each of these mutations. Compared with wild type virus, single RT mutations (P119S or T165A) did not show resistance to 4′-Ed4T, however, the M184V and P119S/T165A/M184V strains conferred 3-and 5-fold resistance, respectively [17]. The P119S/M184V and T165A/M184V variants showed about 4-fold resistance to 4′-Ed4T. The differences in the growth kinetics of the variants were less than 3-fold. The P119S/M184V and T165A/M184V mutations were inhibited with 8 to 13-fold efficiency by 4′-Ed4TTP than wild type RT [16]. These findings led to reexamination of the viral strains from the original drug resistance selection [62]. Re-assessment of the original P119S/T165A/M184V mutant strain with 130-fold resistance, revealed only 3-5-fold resistance to 4′-Ed4T instead of the 130-fold resistance previously observed (Baba *et al.*, unpublished results). Could the previously observed high resistance be due to additional mutations in the RT and/or other genes, or that this virus is either difficult to recover from storage due to a poor replication capacity? Based on recent studies and the structural modeling of interaction of HIV RT-primer complex and 4′-Ed4TTP, a virus with such a high degree of resistance will be difficult to select for under 4′-Ed4T therapy [17].

Mutations selected for during *in vitro* passage may not necessarily represent the mutation pathway that will evolve during clinical use, therefore, true resistance to 4′-Ed4T is yet to be demonstrated in clinical studies. In a cross-resistance profile study of 4′-Ed4T, virus containing a K65R mutation showed a 0.4-fold change in 50% effective concentration (EC_{50}) *versus* the wild type, while viruses with the Q151M complex mutations (without M184V) showed changes in EC_{50} *versus* wild type of 0.23-to 0.48-fold [27]. L74V-containing virus was sensitive to 4′-Ed4T, while an M184V mutant virus had a 2-to 3-fold decrease in susceptibility. Susceptibility to 4′-Ed4T decreased with increasing numbers of thymidine analog mutation pattern 1 (TAM-1) pathway mutations, while the number of mutations in the TAM-2 pathway did not affect the susceptibility to any extent The T69 insertion complex caused a 22-fold decrease in susceptibility to 4′-Ed4T. Common non-NRTI (NNRTI) mutations were susceptibility to 4′-Ed4T. 4′-Ed4T has also been shown to be active against drug-resistant clinical isolates and different HIV-1 subtypes [96]. Thus evolution of clinically relevant resistance to 4′-Ed4T may be difficult even in the presence of a baseline M184V mutant virus, a pre-requisite for selecting for highly 4′-Ed4T resistant virus in *in vitro* studies.

Clinical Studies of 4′-Ed4T

A Phase Ia single-blind, placebo-controlled, sequential dose escalation study in healthy male volunteers was conducted to evaluate the safety, tolerability, and pharmacokinetics of 4′-Ed4T [96]. Sixty-three of 64 subjects completed the study. Subjects were randomized into 8 treatment groups (10, 30, 100, 300, 600, and 900 mg in fed state, and 100 and 300 mg in fasting state), each with eight subjects (6 received 4′-Ed4T treatment dosage and 2 received placebo). 4′-Ed4T was safe; the most common AE reported was fatigue (2 in treatment group and 1 in placebo group). All AEs reported were mild to moderate and did not appear to be related to the study drug. No laboratory, vital signs or physical examination, and EKG changes were observed.

There was a linear dose-exposure relationship of mean plasma concentrations of 4′-Ed4T for all the dose ranges studied. The area under the curve (AUC) increased in a dose-dependent manner. The median T_{max} values of 4′-Ed4T in the fed state ranged from 1 to 2 hours. The metabolism of 4′-Ed4T displayed first-order kinetics. The median $T_{1/2}$ ranged from 2 to 4 hours. Fed or fasting state did not affect the C_{max} or AUC_{0-24} of 4′-Ed4T. For all the dose ranges, >50 of 4′-Ed4T was excreted unchanged in the urine. These results are promising for further development of 4′-Ed4T for HIV therapy. To date, the missing piece is whether resistance to 4′-Ed4T will develop in the clinic. Ongoing and future clinical trials will inform on this.

In a Phase IIa clinical trial, a total of 32 treatment-experienced subjects, who were off ART three months before study enrollment, were randomized (3:1) to receive different doses of 4′-Ed4T (*e.g.*, 100, 200, 300, and 600 mg) or placebo once daily for 10 days. Each of the 4 treatment groups had 6 and 2 subjects receiving study drug and placebo, respectively. 4′-Ed4T was well tolerated and the adverse events were not dose-dependent and most of them were mild; the investigators concluded that the events were unlikely related to study treatment. Consistent with the findings in Phase Ia trial, 4′-Ed4T reached C_{max} in approximately 1-2 hours for all the doses studied. Moreover, the 4′-Ed4T there was a linear dose-exposure relationship for all the dose ranges studied. Thus, the plasma C_{max} and AUC were proportional to the dose ranges. Also, the plasma AUC correlated with the antiviral activity. Median decrease in plasma HIV-1 RNA at day 11 from baseline was 0.97, 1.15, 1.28, and 1.15 log10 copies/mL for 100, 200, 300, and 600 mg dose ranges, respectively. The pattern of decrease in plasma HIV-1 RNA from baseline is similar to that observed with tenofovir Phase II trial [97]. However, the dosing schedule in the tenofovir trial was different; subjects received assigned dose of tenofovir for one day and then had a 7-day period of washout followed by daily tenofovir dose for 28 consecutive days. Moreover, about 60% of the subjects in the tenofovir study were treatment-experienced compared to 100% treatment-experienced subjects in the 4′-Ed4T study. Although there were variations in increase in CD4+ T cell from baseline, the median CD4+ T cell increase observed at days 11 and 24 was 71.0-178.50 cells/μL for all dosing ranges except that of 600 mg at day 24 (-20.00 to 145.50 cells/ μL) [106]. At baseline, only one subject harbored T21T/S mutation in the HIV RT gene. This subject received 600 mg daily dose and at days 11 and 17 the mutation had disappeared. Two subjects who received 300 mg daily dose had K70K/R and K219K/R, respectively, on day 17, which were not present in earlier time points. Of note, all three subjects with pre-existing or acquired NRTI mutations responded well to 10 days of 4′-Ed4T. The HIV-1 RNA decline at day 11 from baseline for T215T/S, K70K/R, or K219K/R was 1.91, 1.42, or 1.58 $\log_{10}$ copies/mL. The investigators concluded that 100 mg daily dose of 4′-Ed4T was expedient based on the safety profile, favorable pharmacokinetics, potent antiviral activity and CD4+ T cell gain in a 10 day period. Phase IIb study in treatment-naïve HIV-1-infected individuals is in progress [98].

ACKNOWLEDGEMENTS

Financial supports from the Japan Society for the Promotion of Science (KAKENHI No.24590144 to K. Haraguchi) are gratefully acknowledged. Also, this work was supported by Public Health Service grant AI-38204 from NIAID to Y.C.C. Y.C.C. is a fellow of the National Foundation for Cancer Research. E.P was supported by grant K08AI074404 from NIAID.

The authors are also grateful to Miss Y. Odanaka and Mrs. M. Matsubayashi (Center for Instrumental Analysis, Showa University) for technical assistance with NMR, MS, and elemental analyses.

CONFLICT OF INTEREST

The authors confirm that this chapter contents have no conflict of interest.

REFERENCES

[1] European AIDS Clinical Society. Guidelines version 6.1. Available from: http://www.europeanaidsclinicalsociety.org/images/stories/EACS-Pdf/EACSGuidelines-v6.1-English.pdf; 2012 Accessed 01.04.13.

[2] Panel on Antiretroviral Guidelines for Adults and Adolescents. Guidelines for the use of antiretroviral agents in HIV-1-infected adults and adolescents 2012 update. Available from: http:// aidsinfo.nih.gov/contentfiles/lvguidelines/adultandadolescentgl.pdf; 2012 Accessed 05.18.12.

[3] World Health Organization. Antiretroviral therapy for HIV infection in adults and adolescents: recommendations for a public health approach 2010 revision. Available from:<http:// whqlibdoc.who.int/publications/2010/9789241599764_eng.pdf>; 2010 Accessed 08.02.12.

[4] Cherry CL, Skolasky RL, Lal L, *et al.* Antiretroviral use and other risks for HIV-associated neuropathies in an international cohort. Neurology 2006; 66(6):867-73.

[5] Moore RD, Wong WM, Keruly JC, *et al.* Incidence of neuropathy in HIV-infected patients on monotherapy *versus* those on combination therapy with didanosine, stavudine and hydroxyurea. AIDS 2000; 14(3):273-78.

[6] Hendrickson SL, Kingsley LA, Ruiz-Pesini E, *et al.* Mitochondrial DNA haplogroups influence lipoatrophy after highly active antiretroviral therapy. J Acquir Immune Defic Syndr 2009; 51(2): 111-16.

[7] Haubrich RH, Riddler SA, DiRienzo AG, *et al.* Metabolic outcomes in a randomized trial of nucleoside, nonnucleoside and protease inhibitor-sparing regimens for initial HIV treatment. AIDS 2009; 23(9): 1109-18.

[8] Lactic Acidosis International Study Group. Risk factors for lactic acidosis and severe hyperlactataemia in HIV-1-infected adults exposed to antiretroviral therapy. AIDS 2007; 21(18): 2455-64.

[9] Moreno A, Quereda C, Moreno L, *et al.* High rate of didanosine related mitochondrial toxicity in HIV/HCV-coinfected patients receiving ribavirin. Antivir Ther 2004; 9(1): 133-38.

[10] Reisler RB, Murphy RL, Redfield RR, *et al.* Incidence of pancreatitis in HIV-1-infected individuals enrolled in 20 adult AIDS clinical trials group studies: lessons learned. J Acquir Immune Defic Syndr 2005; 39(2): 159-66.

[11] Bedimo R, Maalouf NM, Zhang S, *et al.* Osteoporotic fracture risk associated with cumulative exposure to tenofovir and other antiretroviral agents. AIDS 2012; 26(7): 825-31.

[12] Scherzer R, Estrella M, Li Y, *et al.* Association of tenofovir exposure with kidney disease risk in HIV infection. AIDS 2012; 26(7): 867-75.

[13] Strategies for Management of Anti-Retroviral Therapy/INSIGHT, DAD Study Groups. Use of nucleoside reverse transcriptase inhibitors and risk of myocardial infarction in HIV-infected patients. AIDS 2008; 22(14): F17-F24.

[14] Sabin CA, Worm SW, Weber R, *et al.* Use of nucleoside reverse transcriptase inhibitors and risk of myocardial infarction in HIVinfected patients enrolled in the D:A:D study: a multi-cohort collaboration. Lancet 2008; 371(9622): 1417-26.

[15] Dutschman GE, Grill SP, Gullen EA, *et al.* Novel 4′-substituted stavudine analog with improved anti-human immunodeficiency virus activity and decreased cytotoxicity. Antimicrob Agents Chemother 2004; 48(5): 1640-46.

[16] Yang G, Dutschman GE, Wang CJ, *et al.* Highly selective action of triphosphate metabolite of 4′-ethynyl D4T: a novel anti-HIV compound against HIV-1 RT. Antiviral Res 2007; 73(3): 185-91.

[17] Yang G, Paintsil E, Dutschman GE, *et al.* Impact of novel human immunodeficiency virus type 1 reverse transcriptase mutations P119S and T165A on 4′-ethynylthymidine analog resistance profile. Antimicrob Agents Chemother 2009; 53(11): 4640-46.

[18] Wang F, Flint OP. BMS-986001, an HIV nucleoside reverse transcriptase inhibitor, does not degrade mitochondrial DNA in longterm primary cultures of cells isolated from human kidney, muscle and adipose tissue. Antimicrob Agents Chemother 2013; 57(12): 6205-12.

[19] Guha M, Pilcher G, Moehlenkamp J, *et al.* Absence of renal and bone toxicity in non-clinical studies of BMS-986001, a nucleoside reverse transcriptase inhibitor (NRTI) of human immunodeficiency virus (HIV). In: 19th International AIDS Conference. Washington, USA; July 22, 2012. Abstract TUPE041.

[20] Castillo AB, Tarantal AF, Watnik MR, *et al.* Tenofovir treatment at 30 mg/kg/day can inhibit cortical bone mineralization in growing rhesus monkeys (Macaca mulatta). J Orthop Res 2002; 20(6): 1185-89.

[21] Kohler JJ, Hosseini SH. Subcellular renal proximal tubular mitochondrial toxicity with tenofovir treatment. Methods Mol Biol 2011; 755: 267-77.

[22] Lebrecht D, Venhoff AC, Kirschner J, *et al.* Mitochondrial tubulopathy in tenofovir disoproxil fumarate-treated rats. J Acquir Immune Defic Syndr 2009; 51(3): 258-63.

[23] Tarantal AF, Marthas ML, Shaw JP, *et al.* Administration of 9-[2-(*R*)-(phosphonomethoxy)propyl]adenine (PMPA) to gravid and infant rhesus macaques (Macaca mulatta): safety and efficacy studies. J Acquir Immune Defic Syndr Hum Retrovirol 1999; 20(4): 323-33.

[24] Van Rompay KK, Brignolo LL, Meyer DJ, *et al.* Biological effects of short-term or prolonged administration of 9-[2-(phosphonomethoxy) propyl]adenine (tenofovir) to newborn and infant rhesus macaques. Antimicrob Agents Chemother 2004; 48(5): 1469-87.

[25] Van Rompay KK, Durand-Gasselin L, Brignolo LL, *et al.* Chronic administration of tenofovir to rhesus macaques from infancy through adulthood and pregnancy: summary of pharmacokinetics and biological and virological effects. Antimicrob Agents Chemother 2008; 52(9): 3144-60.

[26] Bristol-Myers Squibb. Data on file. J Clin Pharm unpublished data, 2011.

[27] Li Z, Terry B, Olds W, *et al. In vitro* cross-resistance profile of nucleoside reverse transcriptase inhibitor (NRTI) BMS-986001 against known NRTI resistance mutations. Antimicrob Agents Chemother 2013; 57(11): 5500-08.

[28] Matsuda A. Recent development of anti-HIV nucleosides. J Synth Org Chem, Jpn 1990; 48(10): 907-20.

[29] Huryn DM, Okabe M. AIDS-driven nucleoside chemistry. Chem Rev 1992; 92(8): 1745-68.

[30] Nucleosides and Nucleotides as Antitumor and Antiviral Agents; Chu, C. K., Baker, D. C., Eds.; Plenum Press: New York, 1993.

[31] Ichikawa E, Kato K. Sugar-modified nucleosides in past 10 years, a review. Current Medicinal Chemistry 2001; 8(4): 385-423.

[32] De Clercq E. The design of drugs for HIV and HCV. Nature Review 2007; 6: 1001-18.

[33] Modified Nucleosides in Biochemistry, Biotechnology and Medicine; Herdewijn, P., Eds: Wiley-VCH Verlag GmbH & Co. KGaA; Weinheim, 2008.

[34] Chemical Synthesis of Nucleoside Analogues; Merino, P., Eds: John Wiley & Sons; Hoboken, New Jersey, 2013.

[35] McCarthy JR Jr, Robins RK, Robins MJ. Purine nucleosdes. XXII. Synthesis of angustmycin A (decoynine) and related unsaturated nucleosides. J Am Chem Soc 1968; 90(17): 4993-99.

[36] Pierra C, Amador A, Benzaria S, *et al.* Synthesis and pharmacokinetics of valopicitabine (NM283), an efficient prodrug of the potent anti-HCV agent 2′-C-methylcytidine. J Med Chem 2006; 49(35): 6614-20.

[37] Hattori H, Tanaka M, Fukushima M, *et al.* Nucleosides and Nucleotides. 158. 1-(3-*C*-Ethynyl-β-D-*ribo*-pentofuranosyl)cytosine, 1-(3-*C*-ethynyl-β-D-*ribo*-pentofuranosyl)uracil, and their nucleobase analogues as new potential multifunctional antitumor nucleosides with a broad spectrum of activity. J Med Chem 1996; 39(25): 5005-11.

[38] O-Yang C, Wu HY, Fraser-Smith EB, Walker KAM. Synthesis of 4′-cyanothymidine and analogs as potent inhibitors of HIV. Tetrahedron Lett 1992; 33(1): 37-40.

[39] Itoh Y, Haraguchi K, Tanaka H, *et al.* Divergent and stereocontrolled approach to the synthesis of uracil nucleosides branched at the anomeric position. J Org Chem 1995; 60(3): 656-62.

[40] Kodama T, Shuto S, Ichikawa S, *et al.* A highly stereoselective samarium diiodide-promoted aldol reaction with 1′-phenylseleno-2′-keto nucleosides. synthesis of 1′-α-branched uridine derivative. J Org Chem 2002; 67(22): 7706-15.

[41] Haraguchi K, Itoh Y, Matsumoto K, *et al.* Stereoselective synthesis of 1′-*C*-branched arabinofuranosyl nucleosides *via* anomeric radicals generated by 1,2-acyloxy migration. J Org Chem 2003; 68(5): 2006-09.

[42] Kumamoto H, Murasaki M, Haraguchi K, *et al.* Nucleophilic addition of benzenethiol to 1′,2′-unsaturated nucleosides: 1′-*C*-phenylthio-2′-deoxynucleosides as anomeric radical precursors. J Org Chem 2002; 67(17): 6124-30.

[43] Kodama T, Shuto S, Nomura M, *et al.* An efficient method for the preparation of 1′α-branched-chain sugar pyrimidine ribonucleosides from uridine: the first conversion of a natural nucleoside into 1′-substituted ribonucleosides. Chem Eur J 2001; 7(12): 2332-40.

[44] Sugimoto I, Shuto S, Mori S, *et al.* Nucleosides and nucleotides. 183. synthesis of 4′α-branched thymidines as a new type of antiviral agent. Bioorg Med Chem Lett.1999; 9(3): 385-88.

[45] Sugimoto I, Shuto S, Matsuda A. A one-pot method for the stereoselective introduction of a vinyl group *via* an atom-transfer radical-cyclization reaction with a diphenylvinylsilyl group as a temporary connecting tether. synthesis of 4′α-C-vinylthymidine, a potent antiviral nucleoside. J Org. Chem.1999; 64(19): 7153-57.

[46] Jung ME, Toyohara A. Preparation of thymidines by substitution of the thymidinr 5′-ester. J Org Chem 2001; 64(8): 2624-35.

[47] Smith JG. Synthetically useful reactions of epoxides. Synthesis 1984; 629-56.

[48] Ashwell M, Jones AS, Walker RT. The synthesis of some branched-chain-sugar nucleoside analogues. Nucleic Acids Res 1987; 15(5): 2157-66.

[49] Adam W, Balas J, Hadjarapoglou L. A convenient preparation of acetone solution of dimethyldioxirane., Chem Ber 1991; 124(10): 77.

[50] Curci R, Fiorentiono M, Troisi L, *et al.* Epoxidation of alkenes by dioxirane intermediates generated in the reaction of potassium caroate with ketones. J Org Chem 1980; 45(23): 4758-60.

[51] Murray RW, Jeyaman R. Dioxiranes: synthesis and reaction of methyldioxiranes., J Org Chem 1985; 50(16): 2847-53.

[52] Haraguchi K, Kubota Y, Tanaka H. Ring opening of nucleoside 1’,2’-epoxides with organoaluminum reagents: stereoselective entry to ribonucleosides branched at the anomeric position. J Org Chem 2004; 69(6): 1831-36.

[53] Haraguchi K, Konno K, Yamada K, *et al.* Electrophilic glycosidation employing 3,5-*O*-(di-*tert*-butylsilylene)-*erythro*-furanoid glycal leads to exclusive formation of the β-anomer: synthesis of 2′-deoxynucleosides and its 1′-branched analogues. Tetrahedron 2010; 66(25): 4587-4600.

[54] Kubota Y, Haraguchi K, Kunikata M, *et al.* Anti *versus* syn opening of epoxides derived from 9-(3-deoxy-β-D-*glycero*-pento-3-enofuranosyl)adenine with Me_3Al: factors controlling the stereoselectivity. J Org Chem 2006; 71(3): 1099-03.

[55] Maag H, Rydzewski RM, McRoberts MJ, *et al.* Synthesis and anti-HIV activity of 4′-azido- and 4′-methoxynucleosides. J Med Chem 1992; 35(8): 1440-51.

[56] Nomura M, Shuto S, Tanaka M, *et al.* Synthesis and biological activities of 4′-α-branched-chain sugar pyrimidine nucleosides J Med Chem 1999; 42(15): 2901-08.

[57] Ohrui H, Kohgo S, Kitano K, *et al.* Synthesis of 4′-*C*-ethynyl β-D-arabino-and 4′-*C*-ethynyl-2′-deoxy-β-D-ribo-pentofuranosylpyrimidines and-purines and evaluation of their anti-HIV activity. J Med Chem 2000; 43(23); 4516-25.

[58] Kodama E, Kohgo S, Kitano K, *et al.* 4′-Ethynyl nucleoside analogs: potent inhibitors of multidrug-resistant human immunodeficiency virus varinats *in vitro*. Antimicrob Agents Chemother 2001; 45(5): 1539-46.

[59] Leland DL, Kotick MP. Studies on 4-*C*-(hydroxymethyl)pentofuranose. Synthesis of 9-[4-*C*-hydroxymethyl]-α-L-*threo*-pentofuranosyl]adenine. Carbohydr Res 1974; 38; C9-C-11.

[60] Haraguchi K, Takeda S, Tanaka H. Ring opening of 4′,5′-epoxynucleosides: a novel stereoselective entry to 4′-*C*-branched nucleosides. Org Lett 2003; 5(9): 1399-02.

[61] Haraguchi K, Takeda S, Tanaka H, *et al.* Synthesis of a highly active new anti-HIV agent 2′,3′-didehydro-3′-deoxy-4′-ethynylthymidine. Bioorg Med Chem Lett 2003; 13(19): 3775-77.

[62] Nitanda T, Wang X, Kumamoto H, *et al.* Anti-human immunodeficiency virus type 1 activity and resistance profile of 2′,3′-didehydro-3′-deoxy-4′-ethynylthymidine *in vitro*. Antimicrob Agents Chemother 2005; 49(8): 3355-60.

[63] Tanaka H, Haraguchi K, Kumamoto H, *et al.* 4′-Ethynylstavudine (4′-Ed4T) has potent anti-HIV-1 activity with reduced toxicity and shows a unique activity profile againsy drug-resistant mutant. Antiviral Chemistry & Chemotherapy 2005; 16(4): 217-21.

[64] Haraguchi K, Itoh Y, Takeda S, *et al.* Synthesis and anti-HIV activity of 4′-cyano-2′,3′-didehydro-3′-deoxythymidine. Nucleosdes Nucletides Nucleic Acids 2004; 23(4): 647-54.

[65] Kumamoto H, Haraguchi K, Tanaka H, *et al.* Synthesis of (±)-4′-ehtynyl-and 4′-cyano carbocyclic analogues of stavudine (d4T). Nucleosides Nucleotides Nucleic Acids 2005; 24(2): 73-83.
[66] Kumamoto H, Haraguchi K, Ida M, *et al.* Synthesis of (±)-4′-ehtynyl-5′,5′-difluoro-2′,3′-dehydro-3′-deoxy-carbocyclic thymidine: a difluoromethylidene analogue of promising anti-HIV agent Ed4T. Tetrahedron 2009; 65(36): 7630-36.
[67] Kumamoto H, Nakai T, Haraguchi K, *et al.* Synthesis and anti-HIV-1 activity of 4′-branched (±)-4′-thiostavudines. J Med Chem 2006; 49(26): 7861-67.
[68] Kato K, Suzuki H, Tanaka H, *et al.* Stereoselective synthesis of 4′-α-alkylcarbovir derivatives based on an asymmetric synthesis or chemoenzymatic procedure. Chem Pharm Bull 1999; 47(9): 1256-64.
[69] Haraguchi K, Takahashi H, Shiina N, *et al.* Stereoselective synthesis of the β-anomer of 4′-thionucleosides based on electrophilic glycosidation to 4-thiofuranoid glycals. J Org Chem 2002; 67(17): 5919-27.
[70] Haraguchi K, Takahashi H, Tanaka H. Stereoselective entry to 1′-C-branched 4′-thionulcosides from 4-thiofuranoid glycals: synthesis of 4′-thioangustmycin C. Tetrahedron Lett 2002; 43(32): 5657-60.
[71] Haraguchi K, Shiina N, Yoshimura Y, *et al.* Novel stereoselective entry to 2′-β-carbon-substituted 2′-deoxy-4′-thionucleosides from 4-thiofuranoid glycals. Org Lett 2004; 6(16); 2645-48.
[72] Haraguchi K, Takahashi H, Tanaka H, *et al.* Synthesis and antiviral activities of 1′-carbon-substituted 4′-thiothymidines. Bioorg Med Chem 2004; 12(20): 5309-16.
[73] Haraguchi K, Sumino M, Tanaka H. Nucleophilic substitution at the 4′-position of nucleosides: new access to a promising anti-HIV agent 2′,3′-didehydro-3′-deoxy-4′-ethynylthymidine. J Org Chem 2006; 71(12): 4433-38 and references cited therein.
[74] JP WO02009/084655 A1 2009.7.9.
[75] Weber J, Weberova J, Vazquez AC, *et al.* Drug susceptibility profile of OBP-601, a novel NRTI, using a comprehensive panel of NRTI and/or NNRTI resistant viruses. 15th Conference on Retroviruses and Opportunistic Infections, Boston, MA. 2008; Abstract #726b.
[76] Haraguchi K, Taleda S, Kubota Y, *et al.* From the chemistry of epoxy-sugar nucleosides to the discovery of anti-HIV agent 4′-ethynylstavudine – festinavir. Curr Pharm Des 2013; 19(10): 1880–97.
[77] Nakata H, Amano M, Koh Y, *et al.* Activity against human immunodeficiency virus type 1, intracellular metabolism, and effects on human DNA polymerases of 4′-ethynyl-2-fluoro-2′-deoxyadenosine. Antimicrob. Agents Chemother 2007; 51(10): 2701–08.
[78] Mitsuya H, Broder S. Inhibition of the *in vitro* infectivity and cytopathic effect of human T-lymphotrophic virus type III/lymphadenopathy-associated virus (HTLV-III/LAV) by 2',3'-dideoxynucleosides. Proc Natl Acad Sci U S A. 1986; 83(6): 1911-15.
[79] Mitsuya H, Weinhold KJ, Furman PA, *et al.* 3'-Azido-3'-deoxythymidine (BW A509U): an antiviral agent that inhibits the infectivity and cytopathic effect of human T-lymphotropic virus type III/lymphadenopathy-associated virus *in vitro*. Proc Natl Acad Sci U S A. 1985; 82(20):7096-100.
[80] Yang G, Wang J, Cheng Y, *et al.* Mechanism of inhibition of human immunodeficiency virus type 1 reverse transcriptase by a stavudine analogue, 4'-ethynyl stavudine triphosphate. Antimicrob Agents Chemother 2008; 52(6): 2035-42.
[81] Longley MJ, Ropp PA, Lim SE, *et al.* Characterization of the native and recombinant catalytic subunit of human DNA polymerase gamma: identification of residues critical for exonuclease activity and dideoxynucleotide sensitivity. Biochemistry 1998; 37(29): 10529-39.

[82] Paintsil E, Dutschman GE, Hu R, *et al.* Intracellular metabolism and persistence of the anti-human immunodeficiency virus activity of 2',3'-didehydro-3'-deoxy-4'-ethynylthymidine, a novel thymidine analog. Antimicrob Agents Chemother 2007; 51(11): 3870-79.
[83] Hsu CH, Hu R, Dutschman GE, *et al.* Comparison of the phosphorylation of 4'-ethynyl 2',3'-dihydro-3'-deoxythymidine with that of other anti-human immunodeficiency virus thymidine analogs. Antimicrob Agents Chemother 2007; 51(5): 1687-93.
[84] Wang X, Tanaka H, Baba M, *et al.* Retention of metabolites of 2',3′-didehydro-3′-deoxy-4′-ethynylthymidine, a novel anti-human immunodeficiency virus type 1 thymidine analog, in cells. Antimicrob Agents Chemother 2009; 53(8): 3317-24.
[85] Paintsil E, Grill SP, Dutschman GE, *et al.* Comparative study of the persistence of anti-HIV activity of deoxynucleoside HIV reverse transcriptase inhibitors after removal from culture. AIDS Res Ther 2009; 6: 5.
[86] Zimmerman TP, Mahony WB, Prus KL. 3'-azido-3'-deoxythymidine. An unusual nucleoside analogue that permeates the membrane of human erythrocytes and lymphocytes by nonfacilitated diffusion. J Biol Chem 1987; 262(12): 5748-54.
[87] Gertner E, Thurn JR, Williams DN, *et al.* Zidovudine-associated myopathy. Am J Med 1989; 86(6 Pt 2): 814-18.
[88] Dalakas MC, Illa I, Pezeshkpour GH, *et al.* Mitochondrial myopathy caused by long-term zidovudine therapy. N Engl J Med 1990; 322(16): 1098-105.
[89] Dalakas MC, Semino-Mora C, Leon-Monzon M. Mitochondrial alterations with mitochondrial DNA depletion in the nerves of AIDS patients with peripheral neuropathy induced by 2'3'-dideoxycytidine (ddC). Laboratory investigation; a journal of technical methods and pathology 2001; 81(11): 1537-44.
[90] Dagan T, Sable C, Bray J, *et al.* Mitochondrial dysfunction and antiretroviral nucleoside analog toxicities: what is the evidence? *Mitochondrion.* 2002;1(5):397-412.
[91] Lewis W, Dalakas MC. Mitochondrial toxicity of antiviral drugs. Nat Med 1995; 1(5): 417-22.
[92] Chen CH, Cheng YC. Delayed cytotoxicity and selective loss of mitochondrial DNA in cells treated with the anti-human immunodeficiency virus compound 2',3'-dideoxycytidine. J Biol Chem 1989; 264(20): 11934-37.
[93] Chen CH, Vazquez-Padua M, Cheng YC. Effect of anti-human immunodeficiency virus nucleoside analogs on mitochondrial DNA and its implication for delayed toxicity. Mol Pharmacol 1991; 39(5): 625-28.
[94] Brinkman K, Smeitink JA, Romijn JA, *et al.* Mitochondrial toxicity induced by nucleoside-analogue reverse-transcriptase inhibitors is a key factor in the pathogenesis of antiretroviral-therapy-related lipodystrophy. Lancet 1999; 354(9184): 1112-15.
[95] Lim SE, Copeland WC. Differential incorporation and removal of antiviral deoxynucleotides by human DNA polymerase gamma. J Biol Chem 2001; 276(26): 23616-23.
[96] Urata Y, Paintsil E, Cheng YC, *et al.* Randomized, placebo-controlled single-ascending-dose study to evaluate the safety, tolerability and pharmacokinetics of the HIV nucleoside reverse transcriptase inhibitor, BMS-986001, in healthy subjects. J Clin Pharmacol 2013; 54(6): 657-64.
[97] Barditch-Crovo P, Deeks SG, Collier A, *et al.* Phase i/ii trial of the pharmacokinetics, safety, and antiretroviral activity of tenofovir disoproxil fumarate in human immunodeficiency virus-infected adults. Antimicrob Agents Chemother 2001; 45(10): 2733-39.
[98] Cotte L, Dellamonica P, Raffi F, *et al.* Randomized placebo controlled study of the safety, tolerability, antiviral activity, and pharmacokinetics of 10-day monotherapy with BMS-986001, a novel HIV NRTI, in treatment-experienced HIV-1-infected subjects. Clinical Science 2013; 63(3): 346-54.

CHAPTER 6

HIV Integrase – Biology and Inhibitor Design

Victoria Hann and Mark Ashton*

Department of Pharmacy, Health and Wellbeing, University of Sunderland, Sunderland, Tyne and Wear, UK

Abstract: In recent years, HIV integrase has emerged as an important target for the development of new HIV inhibitors. Following the synthesis of viral DNA by reverse transcriptase, integrase performs two functions; 3'-processing and strand transfer/ integration. The catalysis of both functions by the enzyme relies on the presence of magnesium ions (Mg^{2+}) in the active site. All three of the current FDA approved integrase inhibitors operate as strand transfer inhibitors and have chelation of the Mg^{2+} ion as an integral part of their respective pharmacophores. Interesting new developments in the field involve the targeting of one or more of the range of cellular cofactors involved in the integration process and inhibitors with a novel mode of action known as allosteric inhibitors.

Keywords: Allosteric, chelation, dolutegravir, elvitegravir, integrase, LEDGF/p75, PIC, 3'-processing, strand transfer, raltegravir, retrovirus.

INTRODUCTION

Historical Perspective and Development of the Field

The two decades post 1960 saw a significant revolution in the field of virology with discoveries involving both reverse transcription and the integration of proviral DNA into the genome's of infected cells. Initially, the suggestion by Howard Temin of a flow of genetic information in retroviruses contrary to the widely accepted Central Dogma of molecular biology was difficult the scientific community to accept. His hypothesis, in which an RNA virus was able to stably alter the host's genome by incorporating its genetic material into the cell's DNA was revolutionary. The independent discovery of an RNA-dependent DNA polymerase (RT) by Baltimore [1] and Temin and Mizutani [2] helped to prove

***Corresponding author Mark Ashton:** Department of Pharmacy, Health and Wellbeing, University of Sunderland, UK; Tel: +44 (191) 5153503; E-mail. mark.ashton@sunderland.ac.uk

Temin's provirus hypothesis but also help to open up the development of molecular biology.

Subsequent to the work on identifying and characterising RTs, various groups worked on identifying the enzyme responsible for the integration of the provirus into the host genome. This work involved different viruses, and provided important support to the provirus hypothesis [3-5]. The identification of HIV-1 integrase (IN) quickly followed those initial studies [6, 7].

HIV-1 Integrase

The retrovirus HIV-1 has limited genetic makeup (~10Kb) though it has to carryout multiple and distinct functions in order to complete the multiple steps in its replicative cycle, as a result of this the virus takes advantage of cellular proteins and pathways. Integrase (IN) is one of only 3 enzymes encoded by all retroviral genomes. The other two are proteases and reverse transcriptase, each of which plays an essential role in virus replication. Integration is a critical step in the retroviral replication cycle as it ensures a stable association between the viral DNA and the host cell genome. The primary role of the enzyme IN is to catalyse the insertion of the proviral DNA into the genome of the infected cells. IN belongs to the functionally diverse superfamily of DDE nucleotidyltransferases [8], these share a common mechanism of metal ion-dependent (Mg^{2+} in the case of HIV-1 IN) phosphodiesterase bond cleaving and joining.

To initiate replication in a host cell the virus must first adhere to the plasma membrane of the host cell. This begins with the binding of the viral envelop glycoprotein gp120 to the CD4 cell surface receptor. This initiates a conformational change in gp120, which enables gp120 to bind to the CXCR4 or CXCR5 chemokine co-receptor. Binding to the co-receptor triggers a conformational change in the viral envelop glycoprotein gp41, which is responsible for inducing fusion of the viral envelop with the cell membrane.

Once the viral core enters the cytoplasm, it is uncoated exposing a nucleoprotein complex known as the reverse transcription complex (RTC), the viral RNA is reverse transcribed within the RTC [9, 10]. The p66/p51reverse transcriptase heterodimer converts the genome viral RNA in to linear, blunt ended, double stranded complimentary DNA (cDNA) containing a copy of the viral long term repeat (LTR) at both ends.

Following reverse transcription the proviral DNA is primed for integration by the enzyme IN. IN carries out two fundamental activities required for integration of retroviral DNA into the host cells chromosomal DNA. The first of which is 3'-processing and this involves the removal of two nucleotides from each 3' end of the viral DNA. IN specifically recognises the conserved 5'-CA in the HIV LTR and processes the viral DNA ends adjacent to the conserved 5'-CA sequence, liberating the pGT_{OH} dinucleotide from each 3'end, generating reactive 3'-hydroxyls at both ends of the viral DNA [11].

The multistep integration process begins with the formation of the stable synaptic complex (SSC) or intasome, in which a tetramer of IN bridges the pair of newly transcribed viral DNA ends. 3'-Processing of the viral DNA converts the SSC into a cleaved donor complex (CDC). After 3'-processing the replication intermediate gains the ability to catalyse DNA strand transfer, 3' processing marks the transition from RTC to preintegration complex (PIC). The intasome is the structure within the PIC that catalyses integration. The PIC is a nucleoprotein complex in which the viral DNA is associated with both viral and cellular proteins [12-15]. *Via* the microtubule the PIC is translocated to the nucleus. How the PIC is transported through the nuclear membrane is still unclear but the prevailing hypothesis is that it probably does so *via* the nuclear pore complex [16, 17]. Once in the nucleus the cellular protein LEDGF/p75 tethers the PIC to favoured chromatin acceptor sites. Engagment of the CDC with the target DNA converts the CDC into the target capture complex (TCC).

The second activity is to catalyse the integration reaction; the covalent insertion of viral DNA into the host cells genome, which is known as strand transfer. IN DNA strand transfer activity utilizes the 3' hydroxyl groups at the end of the viral DNA to attack a pair of phosphodiester bonds in the target DNA. At the site of insertion the target DNA strands are separated by 5 nucleotides with a 5' protruding stagger. The 3' ends of the processed viral DNA are joined to the 5' ends of the target DNA, the 5' ends of the viral DNA and the 3' ends of the target DNA which are unpaired remain unjoined. The integration of viral 3' DNA ends into the target DNA converts the TCC into a strand transfer complex (STC).

IN is responsible for the catalysis of 3’ processing and DNA strand transfer steps of integration however cellular proteins complete the integration process. Completion of integration involves removal of the two unpaired nucleotides at the 5’ ends of the viral DNA, gap repair of the single strand connections between viral DNA and target DNA followed by the ligation of the 5’ ends of the viral DNA to the target DNA. Gap repair yields a 5-base pair (bp) duplication of target DNA, the sequence of which is defined by the staggered cut in the target DNA.

Upon completion of integration the provirus remains in the host cell and is stably maintained and replicated along with cellular DNA through cycles of cell division. A small percentage of the preintergrated cDNA in the nucleus is converted into a dead end by product circles containing one or two LTRs.

Integrase is Mechanistically and Structurally Similar to Transposases Enzymes

The mechanisms by which retroviruses integrate a DNA copy of their genome into the host’s cellular DNA resembles that of transposons [18]. Transposons are mobile DNA elements that are able to move from one location on the genome to another. There are many different types and they can be divided in to two classes; class 1 retrotransposons require reverse transcription whereas class 2 DNA transposons do not. All class 2 DNA transposons encode the protein transposase, which is required for the cutting and joining of DNA. Transposases are divided into several families depending on their mechanism of transposition. IN shares many structural and functional features with the DDE family of transposases [19]. DDE transposases are named after their characteristic motif of three acidic residues (two aspartic acids (D) and one glutamic acid (E), which coordinate a divalent metal ion required for catalysis. They also contain a common structural motif, an RNase H-like fold which brings the 3 catalytic residues into close proximity [18, 20].

Two steps are common to all transposition reactions catalysed by DDE transposases. The first of which is hydrolysis of phosphodiester bonds at the inverted terminal repeats of the transposon DNA which generates free 3’-OH groups. The second is the joining of the two 3’ ends of the transposon DNA to the target DNA (DNA strand transfer), which is catalysed by the same divalent cation bound active site [21]. The way in which different DDE transposases generate a DNA substrate for strand transfer varies [22]. The site of insertion of the target DNA strands are off set with a 5' protruding stagger. Cellular DNA polymerases carry out gap repair of the single strand connection between the transposed DNA and the target DNA, resulting in a short duplication of the target DNA at the site of insertion, which is a hallmark feature of DNA transposition.

As with retroviral integration, DNA transposition is also carried out within the context of a protein-DNA complex know as a transpososome (synaptic complex). This complex contains at least two transposases enzymes bound to the transposon DNA ends [23-25]. HIV IN is believed to form a tetrameric assembly within its synaptic complex

Integrase Structure

IN is a 288 amino acid protein (32KDa) encoded at the 3'-end of the HIV *pol* gene. It is made up of three clearly independent domains, shared by all retroviral IN proteins. They are comprised of the N terminal domain (NTD), catalytic core domain (CCD), and the C terminal domain (CTD), each of which plays an essential role in enzymatic activity. The three domains are connected by flexible linkers, which are all capable of homodimerisation.

Structural studies of most retroviral IN proteins have been hampered by the poor solubility and stability of the protein, as well as the flexibility of the linkers between the domains. The entire full length HIV-1 IN protein has proved difficult to crystallize and to date the full length enzyme structure has remained elusive. However, X-ray crystallography and/or nuclear magnetic resonance (NMR) structures of the three domains of HIV-1 IN have been resolved individually or as two domain constructs [26].

N-terminal Domain (Amino Acids 1-49)

The NTD structure was resolved by NMR. It adopts a helix-turn-helix fold formation utilising conserved His12, His16, Cys-40 and Cys-43 residues (HHCC motif, analogous to the zinc finger), to effectively bind a single Zn^{2+} ion, which has been shown to be involved in IN multimerisation and enzyme catalytic activity [27, 28]. The NTD has also been shown to specifically bind the viral DNA during integration.

Catalytic core Domain (Amino Acids 50-212)

The CCD structure was resolved by X-ray crystallography [8]. Structural studies of the CCD revealed that HIV-1 IN belongs to a large superfamily of polynucleotydyl transferases [8]. The CCD comprises the enzyme's active site, which contains a highly conserved traid of acidic residues, D64, D116 and E152 (DDE motif) [29, 30] and mutations of these residues abolish catalytic activity. The CCD adopts an RNase H fold which harbours the DDE motif that is common to all retroviral IN proteins [31]. The D64 and D116 residues that comprise the DDE motif coordinates the binding of a pair of Mg^{2+} ions which are required for the catalysis of 3' processing and DNA strand transfer reactions (43). Although the isolated CCD is capable of 3' processing, the full length protein is required for DNA strand transfer to proceed. The CCD interacts with both viral DNA and target DNA during integration, it also forms the major contacts for IN multimerisation.

C-terminal Domain (Amino Acids 213-288)

The CTD structure was resolved by NMR, and is the least conserved of all three domains. It folds in to a 5-strand beta barrel, the +ve charged regions on its surface adopts a Src homology 3 (SH3) fold [32, 33]. It is believed to bind both specifically and non-specifically to DNA, although the non-specific binding is thought to mainly be involved in the stability of the IN complex. The CTD also contributes to IN multimerisation.

It is now widely accepted that IN functions as a multimeric complex. Two-domain IN constructs, site-directed mutagenesis and cross-linking of IN-DNA complexes have provided most of our understanding of the structural organisation of the HIV IN tetramer and how it complexes with viral DNA. However they only shed light on the possible structure, the full length structure is required to fully reflect the actual structural architecture of HIV-1 IN and how it complexes with viral DNA, as IN domains are linked by flexible linkers and therefore their spatial interpretation may differ. Complementation studies, in which individually inactive proteins were combined to form active IN complexes, were the first to demonstrate that IN functions as a tetramer. The major breakthrough in our understanding of the multimeric state of IN was provided by the structure of prototype foamy virus (PFV) IN complexed with DNA. This breakthrough has also shown that some of the predicted HIV-1 IN-DNA complex models are incorrect [34].

Catalytic Activities of Integrase

IN carries out a number of catalytic functions which are critical for the viral replication cycle, namely 3' processing and DNA strand transfer reaction. These two reactions occur *in vivo* in a sequential manner, they are spatially and temporally separated and energetically independent. Mutagenesis studies of retroviral INs demonstrated that 3' processing and DNA strand transfer are effected in parallel, demonstrating that the two reactions share a common active site. Biochemical studies have established that 3' processing and DNA strand transfer are catalysed by a single step mechanism which does not involve a covalent intermediate between IN and DNA. Both reactions are S_N^2-type nucleophilic substitution reactions [35], assisted by a divalent metal ion (Mg^{2+} or Mn^{2+}) which activates the attacking nucleophile and destabilises the scissile phosphodiester bonds [36-38].

3'-Processing is a highly specific reaction which involves the removal of two nucleotides from each 3' end of the viral DNA. IN specifically recognises the conserved 5'-CA in the HIV LTR. Mutations in this sequence completely abolishes catalytic activity, however the integrity of the flanking sequences is much less important. A water molecule is commonly used as the nucleophile source for the 3' processing reaction. IN processes the viral DNA ends adjacent to the conserved 5'-CA sequence, cleaving off the terminal pGT_{OH} dinucleotide from each 3'end, generating reactive 3'-hydroxyls at both ends of the viral DNA. The resulting CA_{OH} 3'-hydoxyl groups then serve as the nucleophiles for the second reaction, DNA strand transfer. IN uses the 3'-hydroxyl groups to attack a pair of phosphodiester bonds, generating a staggered cut in the chromosomal DNA, the site of attack is separated by 5 nucleotides on each DNA strand. The 3' ends of the processed viral DNA are covalently joined to the 5' ends of the target DNA, in which the 5' ends of the viral DNA and the 3' ends of the target DNA, which are unpaired, are unjoined. The single strand gaps created by integration are repaired by cellular proteins, which involves the removal the 2 unpaired nucleotides at the 5' ends of the viral DNA, filling in the single strand gaps, and ligation of the 5' ends of viral DNA to target DNA. This yields a 5 base pair duplication of target DNA a long side the integrated viral DNA.

IN alone can catalyse concerted integration *in vitro* [39-42], although it has been shown that IN activity can be stimulated by the presence of some viral and cellular proteins, suggesting IN may not work alone *in vivo*. The ability of IN to perform concerted integration requires tetramer formation [11, 43-46]. Although it is somewhat unclear as to whether a tetramer or just a dimer of IN is required for 3'-processing [47]. *In vitro* a dimer is sufficient however mutations which prevent teramerisation have been shown to impair 3' processing [43, 48].

IN has been demonstrated to carry out a third catalytic reaction, disintegration. However there is no evidence that this reaction occurs *in vivo.* Disintegration is the apparent reverse reaction of DNA strand transfer. In the presence of a divalent metal ion and DNA that is structurally similar to the product of the strand transfer reaction IN can catalyse the reversal of strand transfer reaction to free the viral DNA from the target DNA [49]. Unlike 3'- processing and strand transfer which require the full length IN, only the CCD is required for the disintegration reaction [50, 51].

The Reaction Mechanism

HIV IN, like all other members of the retroviral IN superfamily [20], requires divalent metal ions in order to execute its two functions, namely, 3'-processing and strand transfer. The nature of the divalent metal ion in HIV IN is thought to be Mg^{2+} *in vivo* [52], although Mn^{2+} enhances enzyme activity *in vitro* [53]. Studies with IN enzymes from other viruses have shown activity to be maintained with a range of divalent metal ions [54].

The metal ions, or cofactors, are key to the functioning of the enzyme [37] and are contained within the catalytic core domain (CCD) [8, 55]. The CCD, which is highly conserved amongst retroviral IN enzymes [56] is composed of residues 51-212 which contain the essential D,D(35)E motif. The carboxylate anions of the amino acid residues, two aspartates (D64 and D116) and one glutamate (E152) residue help to provide the correct coordination geometry for the Mg^{2+} ions; six ligands in an octahedral geometry.

Although there is no crystal structure for the complete HIV-1 IN enzyme and available data for the core domain [57, 58] indicates a single divalent metal binding site, work with the prototype foamy virus (PFV) [46, 59] strongly supports the two metal model of enzyme catalysis [60, 61]. This model relies on the cooperation of the two divalent metal cations to promote the necessary transesterification reactions. In the 3'-processing reaction, Mg^{2+} ion A acts as a Lewis acid [62] to increase the basicity of a water molecule, thereby initiating attack at the scissile phosphate leading to cleavage of the terminal dinucleotides from the 3' end of the viral DNA. The ST reaction is dependent on Mg^{2+} ion B and involves IN joining the 3' ends of the viral DNA to the host DNA.

Both transesterification reactions occur in a stereospecific manner with respect to the phosphate [63] involving an S_N2-like mechanism; Mg^{2+} ion B is pivotal in helping to facilitate this second transesterification reaction by stabilizing the trigonal bipyramidal transition state and the 3' oxyanion leaving group.

Integrase-DNA Nucleoprotein Complexes

Upon infection of the host cell, viral DNA is synthesized in the cytoplasm of the cell by reverse transcription. The reverse transcribed viral cDNA then forms part of the nucleoprotein complex, known as the PIC. The structure and organisation of PICs is poorly defined due to their low abundance in extracts from infected cells. The general consensus is that HIV-1 PICs are composed of a tetramer of IN tightly bound to two viral DNA ends (known as an intasome) along with other viral proteins, including nucleocapsid, reverse transcriptase, matrix and Viral protein R (Vpr). Several host cellular proteins have also been identified as components of the PIC, including barrier to autointegration protein (BAF), high mobility group chromosomal protein A1 (HMGA1), LEDGF/p75 as well as others.

The structure of the intasome within the viral nucleoprotein complex changes throughout the different stages of integration. Binding of IN to the viral LTR generates a SSC, 3' processing of the viral DNA converts the SSC into a CDC, binding of the CDC to target DNA converts the CDC to a TCC. Completion of strand transfer generates a STC.

The intasome is the basic recombination unit required for integration *in vitro*. Intasomes are very stable structures which remain tightly bound even when challenged with high ionic strength, they can be assembled *in vitro* with purified IN and synthetic oligonucleotides that mimic viral DNA. These complexes have been used extensively to study 3' processing and DNA strand transfer reactions and these biochemical studies have answered many of the questions regarding the mechanisms of the integration pathway, however, to date no high resolution crystal structure of the HIV-1 intasome is available. Although the recent development of a highly soluble hyperactive IN may facilitate structural studies of the HIV-1 intasome [64].

The X-ray crystal structure of the functional PFV SSC and STC intasomes was an enormous breakthrough in our understanding of the entire retroviral integration pathway, providing a great deal of insight into the details of intasome assembly and integration reaction mechanisms [46, 59, 65]. This major advance was facilitated by the biophysical properties of the PFV IN enzyme. Unlike HIV-1 IN, PFV IN is remarkably soluble and is able to assemble functional intasomes with short oligonucleotide DNA substrates and is highly efficient at concerted integration *in vitro* [56].

As expected from partial structures, the intasome is composed of a tetramer of IN, which comprises of a dimer of a dimer, with each dimer containing an inner and outer subunit. Only one of the monomers within each dimer pair is bound to a single viral DNA end. The pair of IN dimers, both attached to single viral DNA ends come together to form the intasome. All three domains of the inner monomer form contacts with the viral DNA and each other. Each viral DNA end interacts with both inner IN subunits. As predicted from previous studies of 1 and 2 domain constructs, the inner monomers harbour the active site; DDE required for catalysis and the NTD of each monomer engages with the CCD from the opposing IN monomer with its bound DNA in *trans,* which aids to stabilise the tetramer. Only the CCD of the outer monomer is resolved, both the NTD and CTD subunits are disordered in the crystals and their functions are currently unknown. The outer subunits do not interact with the viral DNA or each other leading to the idea that they may play a supporting role. As repeatedly observed in the 1 and 2 domain IN structures the CCD-CCD dimer interface is observed, however this CCD-CCD interface is between the inner DNA bound CCD of IN and the outer CCD of IN, confirming that there is only one active site per IN dimer.

Both PFV pre-catalytic TCC and post-catalytic STC intasomes have been co-crystallised [59]. These structures identified that target DNA binds along the groove between the symmetrical IN dimers, the target DNA binds in a highly kinked conformation with a dramatic expansion of the major groove and a compression of the minor groove, which allows the intasomes active site access to the scissile phosphodiester bonds within the target DNA. The majority of contacts between the PFV intasome and the target DNA are mediated through hydrogen bonds to the phosphodiester backbone. As expected from the lack of target DNA sequence specificity the target DNA base contacts with IN are few. Although the TCC and STC appear to be identical in their structural organisation, there are subtle differences in their conformation. Within the TCC the scissile phosphodiester is positioned within the active site, whereas the phosphodiester joining viral DNA and the target DNA sits outside of the active site. Studies of the TCC, Mg^{2+} bound structure are consistent with a two metal ion mechanism of action previously described.

Although the overall HIV-1 IN and PFV IN amino acid sequence identity is relatively low and the length of the interdomain linkers varies [30, 47]. They share a high degree of amino acid sequence identity within their active site [56]. The ability of IN strand transfer inhibitors (INSTI's) to actively bind to both PFV IN and HIV-1 IN suggests their structural organisation is similar. Given that they are functionally and structurally similar it would be highly unlikely that the HIV-1 IN intasome structural organisation would drastically differ from that of PFV.

To date three groups have modelled HIV-1 IN based on the PFV IN intasome structure. Two of these are structural based models produced by superimposing the HIV-1 IN domain structures onto the full length PFV IN. A recent study has used a different approach, using sequence alignment with PFV IN they have produced a homology based model of HIV-1 IN [66]. The two different model based approaches slightly differ from one another, although overall HIV-1 IN's predicted structural organisation is extremely similar to that of PFV IN. However until the full length HIV IN-DNA bound structure is determined, these two models provide the best insight into the structural architecture of HIV-1 IN.

Target DNA Site Selection

Retroviruses must covalently integrate DNA copies of their genome into host cell chromosomes in order to replicate. Although DNA target site selection is primarily not sequence specific, which is logical as this would disadvantage the virus. Chromosomal integration site selection is not a random process. This is not really surprising given the location of viral genome integration has significant consequences for both the virus and host cell. A poor choice of integration site can have profound effect on the transcriptional efficiency of the viral DNA, for example, integration into silent regions of the genome will lead to poor transcription of the viral DNA and therefore poor replication. This also applies to host cells as viral integration can also markedly effect gene expression leading to entire gene inactivation or enhanced gene expression, which in turn could lead to tumorigenesis if the host gene is an oncogene.

Several factors influence integration site selection, including local chromatin features and primary DNA sequences. Retroviral IN exhibit a preference for weak conserved palindromic sequences, The preferred HIV-1 intergration site is (-3) TDG↓GTWACCHA (the arrow indicates the position of the scissile phosphodiester bond and the underlined section marks the 5bp target site duplication) [67]. Distortion of target DNA, with outwardly facing major grooves strongly promotes integration [59]. Chromatin bound proteins can either facilitate integration by bending the DNA or inhibit integration by sterically blocking IN binding.

Integration target site selection differs amongst retroviruses, HIV-1 favours insertion into the bodies of active genes located within gene dense regions of the chromosome, whereas MLV preferentially integrates into transcription start sites and CpG islands [68]. ASIV has no significant pattern of integration, although they demonstrate a week preference for transcription units [69]. The distinct integration patterns observed for the different retroviruses suggest that their chromatin interactions are all unique and individual to each retrovirus. There are currently three models to explain the integration target site selection of the different retroviruses; Chromatin accessibility model, Cell Cycle model and the Tethering model. The structure of chromatin has been shown to play a role in target site selection, with integration sites favouring bent target DNA such as outward facing major grooves of the nucleosomal DNA. The Cell Cycle model postulates that although HIV-1 is able to infect both dividing and non-dividing cells, it may be similar to MLV in that there may be a preference for cells to enter mitosis in order for the virus to enter the nucleus, *i.e.,* changes to the chromosomal DNA during the cell cycle may influence target site selection. The Tethering model suggests an interaction of viruses with chromosomal bound cellular proteins which acts to tether them to favoured integration target sites.

There is now an overwhelming body of convincing evidence supporting the role of LEDGF/p75 in the tethering of HIV-1 IN to favoured chromatin acceptor sites. HIV-1 integration target site selection into active transcription units is aided by its binding to the cellular protein LEDGF/p75 [70, 71]. LEDGF/p75 was first identified as a HIV-1 IN binding partner in affinity screens [72, 73]. It has been shown to only bind to lentivirus IN proteins [74-76]. Knockdown of LEDGF/p75 leads to relocalisation of IN into the cytoplasm. The preference of HIV-1 to intergrate into active transcription units is also reduced in LEDGF/p75 knockout cells [77]. Disruption of the LEDGF/p75-HIV-1 IN interaction leads to a decrease in HIV-1 replication but has no effect on IN catalytic activity.

IN INHIBITORS [78-80]

Introduction

IN is the last of the three viral enzymes to be exploited as a target for the development of anti-HIV drugs [81-83]. The enzyme represents an important target since there is no human equivalent and work in this area is now starting to deliver new valuable agents against HIV.

All of the three Food and Drug Administration (FDA) approved IN inhibitors, raltegravir [84], elvitegravir [85, 86], and dolutegravir [87] are members of the strand transfer (ST) class of IN inhibitors; raltegravir and elvitegravir are first generation ST inhibitors and dolutegravir is a second generation [88] inhibitor.

With the continued development of new models for various aspects of IN function [89-91] based on the new discoveries in the structural biology of INs, agents that target all aspects of HIV IN's function will hopefully be added to this important class of inhibitors.

Strand Transfer Inhibitors (STI)

Although a large number of the details are missing from the inhibitor-binding model, certain features are clear. Only the ST reaction is inhibited by the STIs and they only bind to the enzyme when it's complexed with DNA [92, 93]; the bases of the LTR unit of the viral DNA are important for both STI binding and catalytic efficiency [41, 94, 95]

Work with the IN enzymes from various viruses [11, 44, 93, 96, 97] has provided information on the mechanism by which STI operate. By employing the synaptic complex (SC; viral DNA and an IN tetramer formed by the association two IN dimers) [97] as an *in vitro* model of the PIC, valuable insight in to the ST inhibition has been gained. Following association of the viral DNA with the IN tetramer, the SC binds to the target DNA to form a strand transfer complex (STC) which joins the viral DNA with the target DNA.

The STI appear to operate as interfacial inhibitors [98, 99] and by binding with the SC they adjust its configuration which precludes the binding of the target DNA [11, 46, 93, 100-102]. The currently accepted model of STI involves the binding of the STI to the Mg^{2+} ions in the active site of IN, which blocks DNA access [103].

Metal Chelation

β-Diketoacids and Derivatives

Initial work in this area was based on simple β-diketo acids and has been reviewed previously [104-106]. Two early β-diketo acid development candidates, L-708,906 and L-731,988 (no 1) were identified from a screen of a sample collection and were some of the first inhibitors of the ST reaction identified [107].

A key part of the pharmacophore is the 'β-diketo' moiety which has been shown to be important for metal chelation. The pharmacophore is effectively composed of two domains; a hydrophobic domain made up of either an aryl or heteroaryl unit and a hydrophilic domain constituted from the β-diketo carboxylic acid (or bioisostere) [108, 109]. A subsequent study extended the SAR for the pharmacophore by exploring the effect of substituents in the aryl ring and their effect on binding efficiency [110] (Fig. **1**).

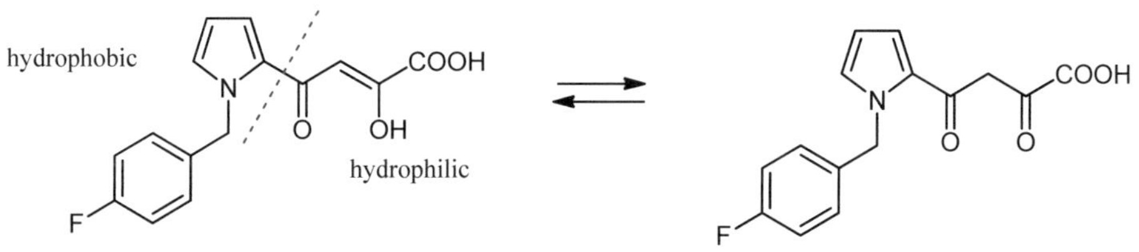

(1), L-731,988 (H_2L^2)
enol form

(1), L-731,988 (H_2L^2)
keto form

Figure 1: Keto-enol forms of the ST inhibitor L-731,988. Also indicated are the two domains of the pharmacophore, the hydrophobic and hydrophilic.

Even simple β-dicarbonyl (1,3-dicarbonyl) compounds exhibit keto-enol tautomerism [111] and form varying amounts of a stable enol; studies with the various β-diketo IN development candidates have shown that it is the enol form of the drug that binds to the Mg^{2+} ions. The enol form gives rise to a planar, conjugated system that provides a fixed geometry conducive to metal chelation and X-ray studies have revealed that the bond angles and bond lengths satisfy the coordination requirements of Mg^{2+} ions [53, 112]. These studies also served as the basis for the development of a model for the binding of the Mg^{2+} ions by the 'keto-enol' form of the β-diketoacid unit [54].

The model proposed that the β-diketo acid acts as a bidentate ligand (the β-keto-enol acid could also serve as a tridentate ligand) with the hard Lewis basic oxygen centres coordinating with the hard Lewis acid magnesium ions. Additional valuable structural data for the binding model came from a comparison of X-ray data for the β-diketo ST inhibitor, 5-CITEP (2) Fig. **2**) [112] and the calculated bond distances of the Mg^{2+} ions in the X-ray structure of avian sarcoma virus (ASV) integrase [54]. Further support for the binding model was obtained from

IN mutants selected by β-diketo ST inhibitors which were found to have mutations around the DDE motif of the active site [107, 113, 114] and the absence of β-diketoacid binding without Mg^{2+} or Mn^{2+} ions [53, 92, 110].

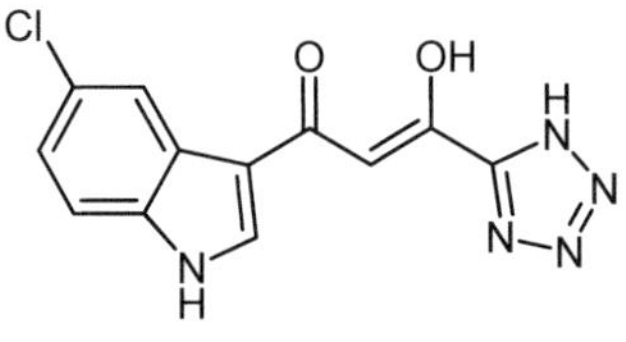

(2), 5-ClTEP

Figure 2: 1-(5-chloroindol-3-yl)-3-hydroxy-3-(2H-tetrazol-5-yl)propenone (2, 5-ClTEP).

A comprehensive theoretical study [115] of four ST inhibitors and various experimental studies have also supported the 'enol' form of the β-diketo acids [116-118] as the 'binding' form. Studies have also been undertaken to try to establish the nature of the metal-ligand complexes generated by the various ST inhibitors [119]. Ligand (Fig. **1**, (1), H_2L^2) was shown to mainly form a complex with Mg^{2+} ions that had the stoichiometry Mg_2L_2 [117] at physiological pH.

Using the initial SAR studies and the binding model for metal chelation, the pharmacophore of the original substituted β-diketo acids was explored and more appropriate drug-like candidates advanced. A key part of the hydrophilic portion of the original pharmacophore was the carboxylic acid. Various diaryl diketone derivatives were investigated and it was observed that replacement of the carboxylic acid with a range of nitrogen containing heterocycles with a Lewis basic centre, essentially maintained activity [120-122]. The inclusion of nitrogen containing heterocyclic substituents in the central aryl ring also produced inhibitors with good potency (Fig. **3**).

It had been previously noted that an important feature of the β-diketo acid pharmacophore was the planar keto-enol unit which was conjugated to the aryl group. With this in mind, groups GlaxoSmithKline (GSK), Shionogi & Co. and Merck explored alternative planar chelating templates to replace the β-diketo unit and reported compounds employing both the quinoline and 1,6-naphthyridine motifs [123].

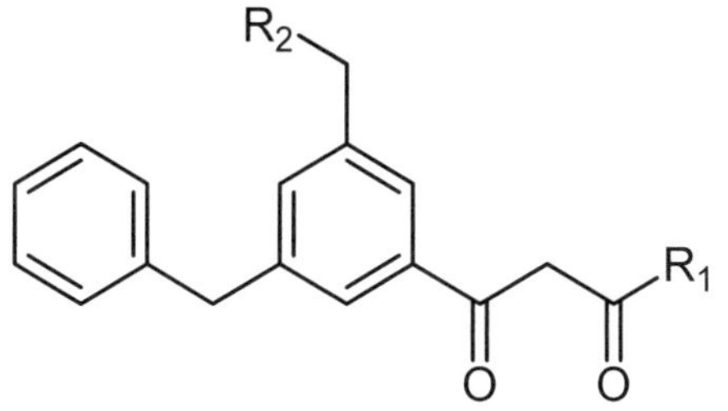

R_1 and R_2 = range of nitrogen containing heterocycles as per references

Figure 3: R1 and R2 represent a range of nitrogen containing heterocycles.

The 8-hydroxyquinoline system is well known to be a good ligand for metal chelation [124] and early analogues did exhibit ST inhibitory properties but were shown to be toxic in cell based assays, hence development was discontinued. The 1,6-naphthyridine unit offered certain advantages over the 8-hydroxyquinoline system and was explored further in a series of analogues.

Compound (No. 3), a substituted 8-hydroxy-1,6-naphthyridine and compound (No. 4; L-870,810) were both potent inhibitors of ST and HIV replication. In addition, L-870,810 had very good pharmacokinetic properties and reached phase II in development [125, 126] before development was terminated due to issues with toxicity. Other naphthyridine skeletons have also been explored [127-131] (Fig. **4**).

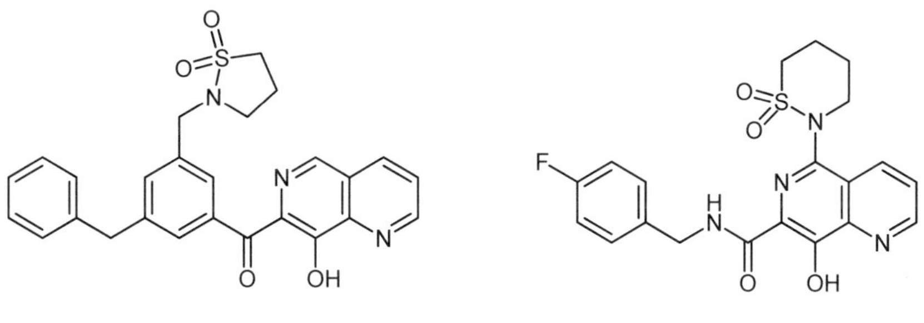

(3) (4), L-870,810

Figure 4: Naphthyridine based IN ST inhibitors.

Running in parallel to the '8-hydroxyquinoline and 1,6-naphthyridine' program, a group at Merck was looking to develop inhibitors against Hepatitis C (HCV) polymerase and had also identified small molecule metal chelating ligands; a simple β-diketo acid, meconic acid and a dihydroxypyrimidine derivative were all shown to inhibit the target enzyme *via* metal chelation [132, 133]. Extensive comparative SAR [134] studies of the 1,6-naphthyridine and dihydroxypyrimidine systems revealed that a key feature of both series was the coplanar metal binding motif that presented two Lewis basic centres (either the oxygen of a carbonyl group, or the nitrogen of a heterocyclic ring) and a hydroxyl group sandwiched between the Lewis basic centres.

Pyrimidine Containing and Related ST Inhibitors

ST inhibitors employing the pyrimidone (and related derivatives) system have been studied extensively and have been reviewed [135].

Raltegravir

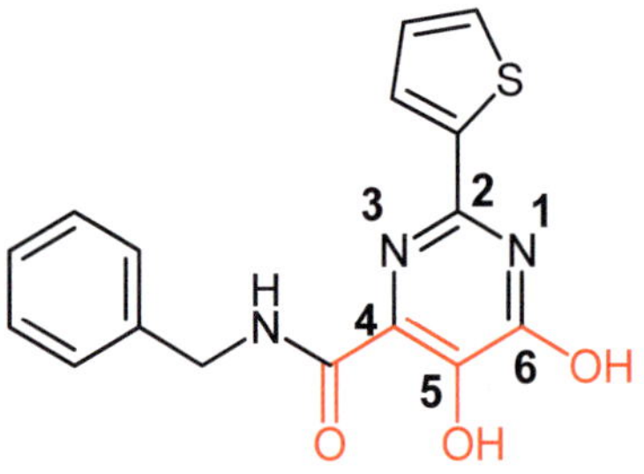

(5)

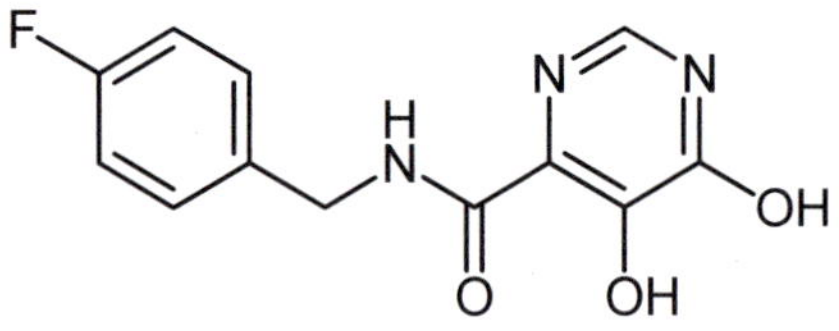

(6)

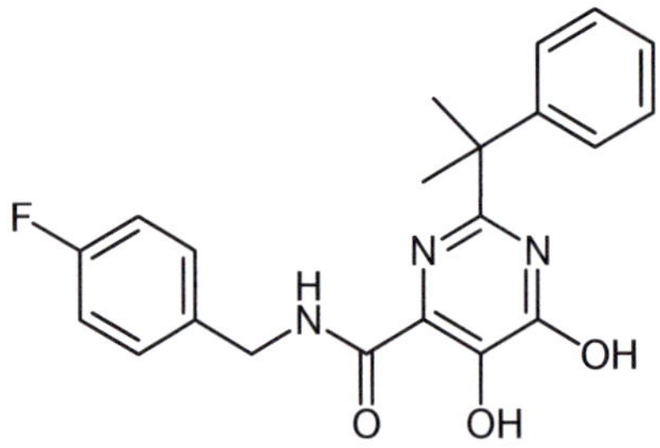

(7)

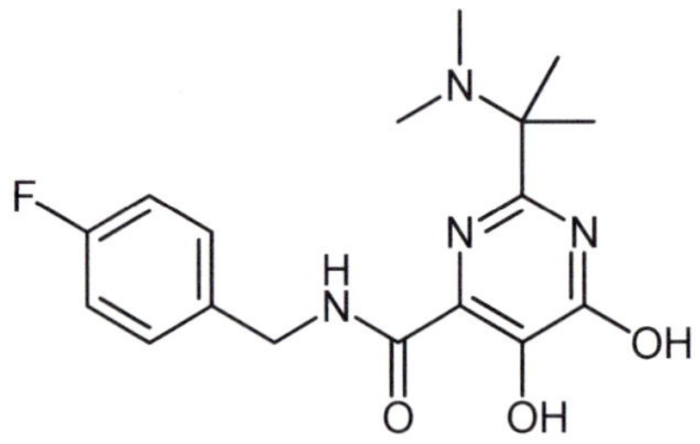

(8)

Figure 5: Early development candidates from the raltegravir programme; metal binding motif shown in red.

Compound (5) [136] emerged from a development program at Merck as a suitable lead candidate for further development as a ST inhibitor of IN. Initial SAR studies to evaluate the impact of the 'benzylamide' portion of the pharmacophore highlighted the 4-fluorobenzyl and the 3,5-dichlorobenzyl derivatives as having good ST inhibitory activity in an *in vitro* IN assay, but both poor cell permeability and plasma protein binding precluded further development. Removal of the thiophene ring from the 2-position (6) of the pyrimidine ring maintained ST activity (*in vitro*; IC_{50} = 60nM) [136, 137] and hence suggested that since substituents in the 2-position were not intimately involved in binding to the active site, substituents could be introduced in to that position to improve the physiochemical properties of analogues of (5).

A benzyl group in the 2-position produced a derivative with good *in vitro* potency and compound (7) with a dimethylbenzyl group in the 2-position had a number of very favourable characteristics, but unfortunately was highly bound to serum protein. Replacement of the phenyl group of (7) with two methyl groups (8) produced a very promising development candidate, but due to problems with toxicity, its development had to be halted (Fig. **5**) [136, 137].

Further analogues with various basic groups in the 2-position of the pyrimidine ring showed varying degrees of activity but were not developed further for a range of issues, however, they did serve as a successful starting point for the development of substituted pyrimidinones, culminating in (9) [138].

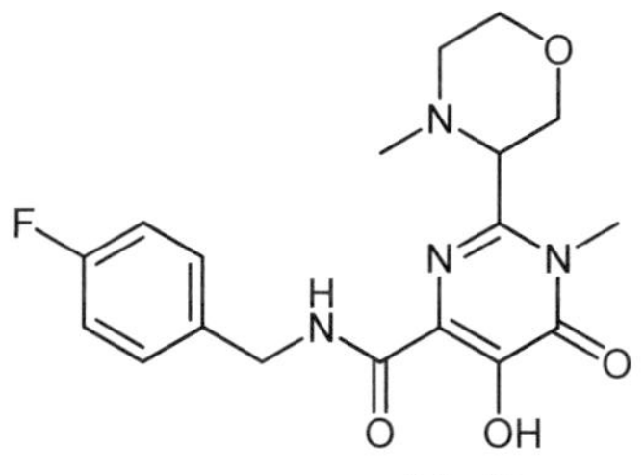

(+)- (9)

Figure 6: Raltegravir development candidate.

Compound (9) (Fig. **6**) had very favourable physiochemical properties coupled with good antiretroviral activity and excellent pharmacokinetic characteristics, however, due to a positive Ames test development was stopped. Returning to compound (8), the Merck development team looked to again adjust the C-2 substituent to improve the 'drug-like' qualities while maintaining the metal chelating and hydrophobic portions of the pharmacophore. The pyrimidine ring was exchanged for a pyrimidinone ring (N-methylpyrimidinone) and a range of substituents were introduced in to the 2-position; the inclusion of N, N-dimethyl oxalamide gave a compound with excellent potency in the ST assay (IC_{50} = 10 nM). The compound also benefitted from other favourable properties, including, low levels of plasma protein binding, good bioavailability and an absence of geneotoxicity [139]. However, the compound was considerably less active against IN containing either of two mutations, F121Y and N155S [140-142] and was not developed. Further optimisation of the C-2 substituent produced compound (Fig. **7**, (10) raltegravir) [139, 143].

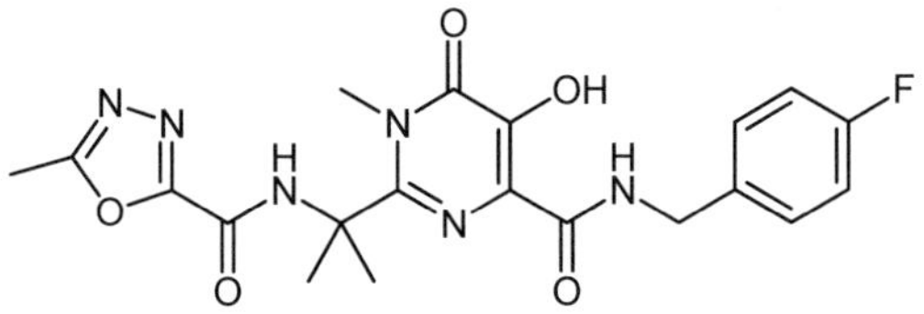

(10)

Figure 7: Raltegravir.

Following the successful launch of raltegravir, further SAR studies for the pyrimidone and pyrimidine scaffolds have been reported in the literature, including a recent study with a series of 5-hydroxy-6-oxo-1,6-dihydropyrimidine-4-carboxamide analogues that suggested that the compounds may be useful in evading one of the main raltegravir resistance pathways (Y143R/C) [144].

Modifications at the 1-position [145], the 2-position [146-148], 3-position [149], 6-position [150], and the 7 and 9-positions [151] have all been explored. An interesting use of the pyrimidine-2,4-dione scaffold included the development of a dual inhibitor against HIV-1 RT and IN [152].

Seo *et al.* disclosed a new pyridinone based scaffold that demonstrated good inhibition of the ST reaction, IC_{50} 6 nM, however, due to cell permeability, a prodrug was evaluated which showed good anti-HIV activity in cell culture (EC_{50} 9 ± 4 nM, CC_{50} 135 ± 7 μM, therapeutic index = 15,000) [153, 154]

Elvitegravir and Two Ring Systems

The original β-diketo acid based IN inhibitors made use of the coplanar 'enol' form of the β-diketo acid motif to facilitate metal chelation *via* what is likely to be tridentate coordination and subsequent inhibitors maintained the triad of Lewis basic centres for metal chelation. The development group at JT Inc. [155] initially looked at a simple substituted quinolone, 4-quinolone-3-carboxylic acid (Fig. **8**; No 11;IC_{50} = 1600nM, EC_{50} = 30000 nM)

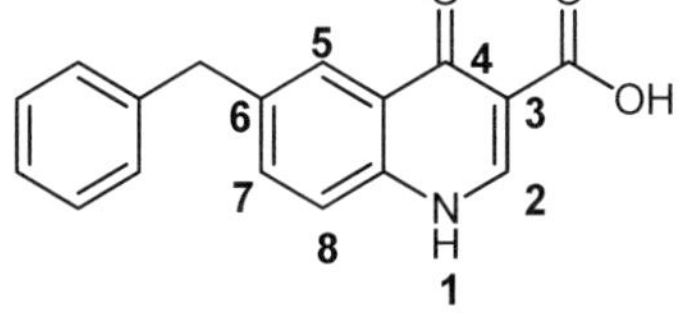

(11)

Figure 8: Initial development lead.

The metal coordination was from the carbonyl group in the 4-position and the carboxylic acid in the 3-position *via* a hard Lewis acid-base interaction. By analogy with the raltegravir development, the aryl group (hydrophobic portion of the pharmacophore) was found to be important for efficient binding to the active site [110, 156]. SAR studies suggested that the incorporation of halogen substituents in to the aryl ring would lead to significant improvements in binding, with 2-fluoro and 3-chloro substituents being optimal (Fig. **9**; No (12) and (13)).

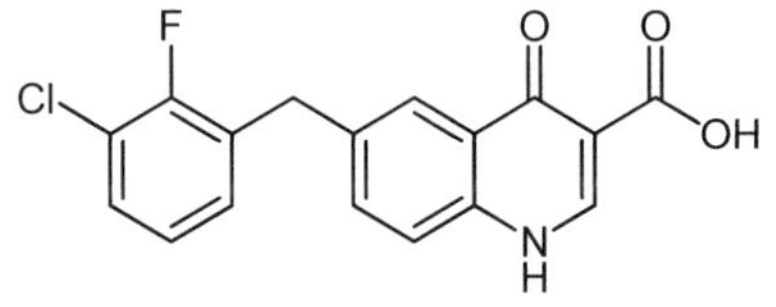

(12)

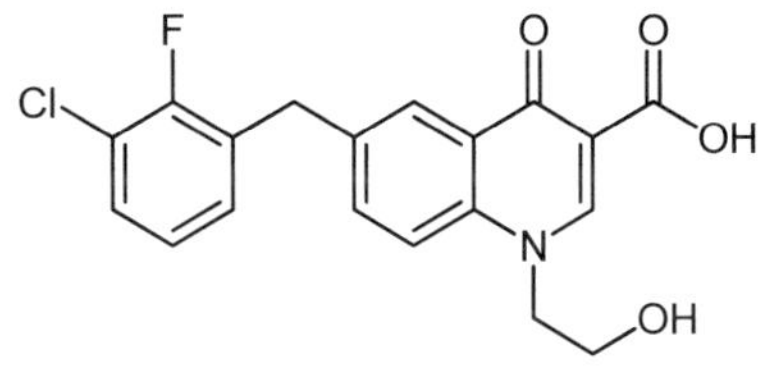

(13)

Figure 9: The inclusion of the halogens greatly improved the inhibition of ST activity.

The hydroxyethyl group was shown to be the optimal substituent for the 1-position and examination of the 7-position identified a methoxy group as the best substituent for that position; the two substituents gave compound (No.14) (Fig. **10**) which showed good activity, IC_{50} = 9.1nM and EC_{50} = 17.1nM.

Final SAR driven modifications eventually led to elvitegravir (Fig. **10**; No 14).

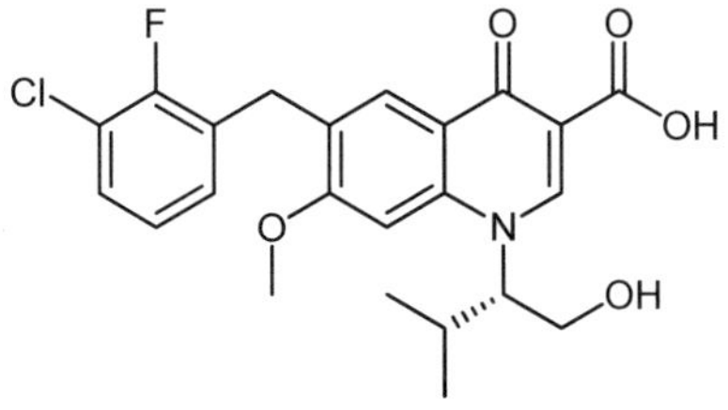

(14)

Figure 10: Elvitegravir.

Elvitegravir is not used as a single agent IN inhibitor due to its metabolism by the CYP3A isoform of cytochrome P450 and is instead used as a combination therapy [157]; the once-daily co-formulation of elvitegravir, cobicistat [158] (a CYP3A inhibitor/pharmacokinetic enhancer), emtricitabine and tenofovir disoproxil fumarate is marketed as Quad® [86].

Compounds characterised by structures like (Fig. **11**, (15-16) in which R=H or OH were originally reported to have low micromolar inhibitory potency against HIV-1 IN (ST IC_{50} = 2.4μM) [159]. Further modification of the scaffold by the introduction of a range of substituents in the 4-position was undertaken to try to find compounds with good antiviral potency against the common resistance mutations; Y143R, N155H, G140S/Q148H, R263K and G118R [160]. The majority of the new analogues, (17) exhibited single-digit nanomolar antiviral activity against the wild type IN and one of the compounds tested compared favourably to dolutegravir against a panel of IN mutants.

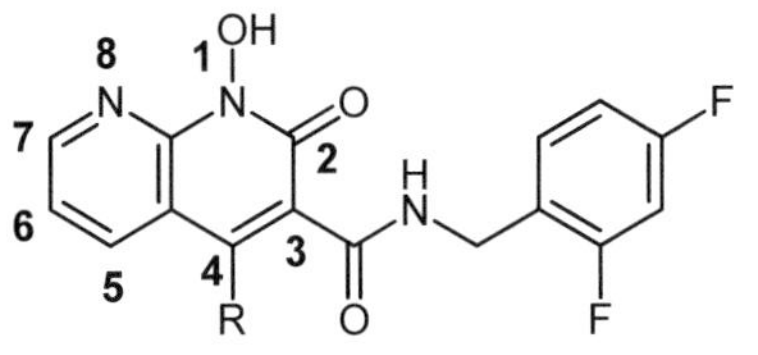

(15), R = H
(16), R = OH
(17), R = NR^1R^2
R^1,R^2 = aryl, alkyl or H

Figure 11: 1-hydroxynaphthyridine series.

The bicyclic, second generation integrase inhibitor, (Fig. **18**, (27) MK-0536) has been reported to exhibit an improved pharmacokinetic profile compared to the first generation inhibitors and maintain activity against enzymes carrying the three main raltegravir resistance mutations [161].

Tricyclic Based Scaffolds

Doultegravir

An excellent review of the development of doultegravir has been published recently by Johns *et al.* [162]. Doultegravir is the first second generation STI to be approved by the FDA and it offers significant advantages over the first generation IN inhibitors, in particular, an excellent resistance profile maintaining activity against viruses expressing all of the common resistance mutations that are observed with raltegravir and elvitegravir [163]. Twenty years of activity in the STI field has established a reasonably good model of inhibitory activity for the various structurally diverse classes of STI and a key feature for all STIs are, a planar metal chelating motif (bidentate or tridentate complexation) and a hydrophobic domain.

The development of doultegravir started with a SAR study with a series of naphthyridine and naphthyridinone derivatives to explore the hydrophobic portion of the motif, particularly, the 'reach of the hydrophobic arm' It was found that by extending the distance of the hydrophobic 'aryl' unit further from the metal chelating core of the scaffold, compounds with a higher degree of potency were obtained [164, 165], possibly by facilitating a better interaction with the hydrophobic portion of one of the bases from the viral DNA [166].

In common with all other STIs, the metal-binding portion of the pharmacophore needed a series of Lewis basic centres for complexation with the Mg^{2+} ion(s) [167]. Initially, the doultegravir team examined the carbamoylpyridone (Fig. **12**; (18) with three oxygen centres (Lewis bases) [168] and the 4-fluoro substituted benzyl ring for hydrophobic binding. The compound, which had reasonable physiochemical and pharmacokinetic properties, proved to be a good starting point for development.

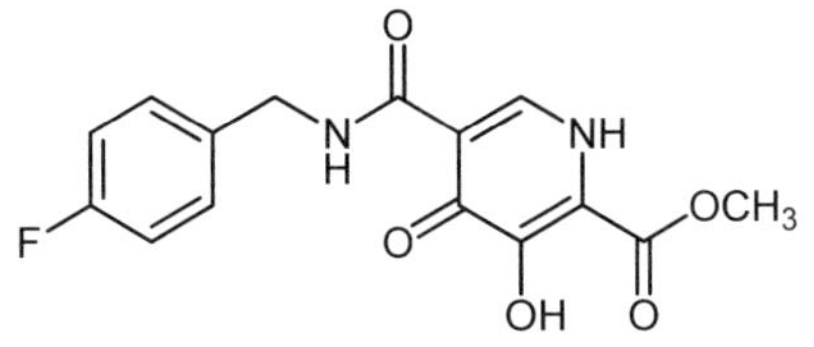

(18)

Figure 12: Initial lead in dolutegravir programme.

The replacement of the C-2 ester with an amide failed to produce the desired outcome due to disruption of the planarity of the metal chelating motif, however, the introduction of a cyclic amide (effectively construction of a pyrimidone ring), yielding the three compounds in Fig. **13**. [162] did produce active compounds, and all three of the bicyclic carbamoylpyridones were more potent than (18) against the wild-type virus, but unfortunately with 16/17 potency was not maintained with the Q148K mutant (a common mutation seen with raltegravir) [169].

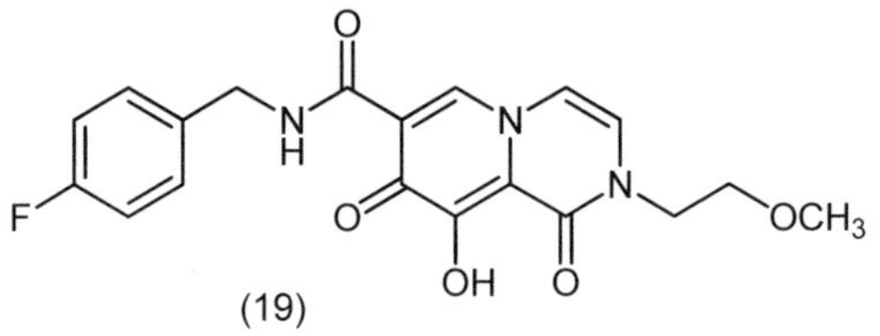

(19)

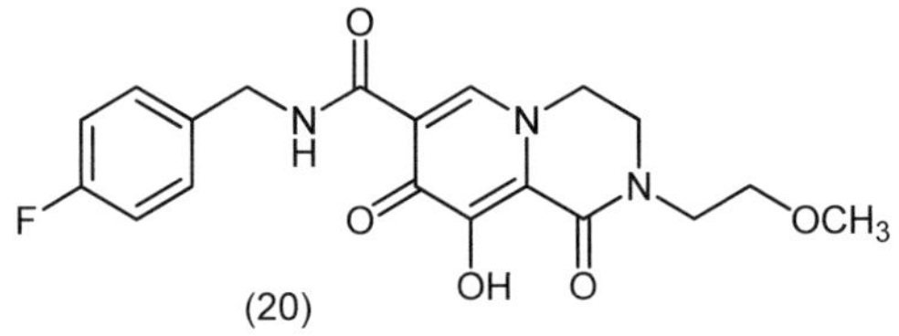

(20)

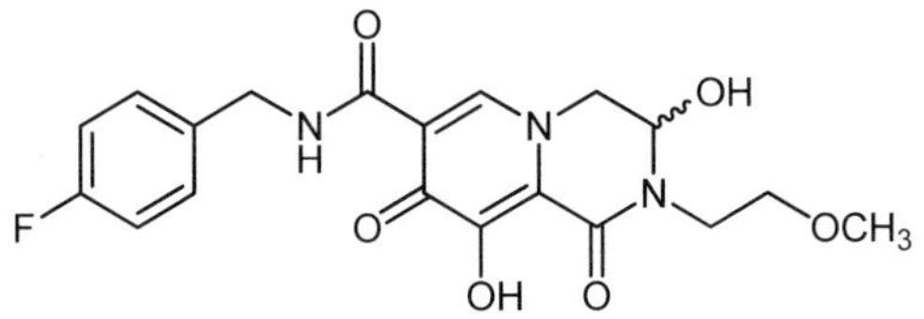

(21)

Figure 13: Carbomylpyridinone development candidates.

The low oral bioavailability of compound (21) was addressed by the formation of a ring leading to compound (Fig. **14**, (22)).

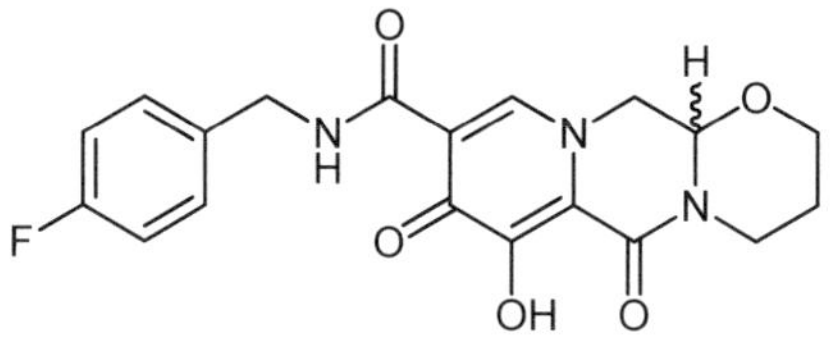

(22)

Figure 14: Construction of the third ring to improve the bioavailability.

The tricyclic carbamoylpyridone (22) was a potent antiviral agent when assayed [170], having an IC_{50} = 2nM. Additional work with the R and S enantiomers of (22) showed that although the R and S enantiomers were virtually equipotent antiviral agents, the S enantiomer was highly protein bound [162]. A further SAR study looking at the third saturated ring was undertaken and produced a series of compounds with good physiochemical properties, good pharmacokinetic and pharmacodynamic properties and ultimately led to doultegravir (Fig. **15**, (23)).

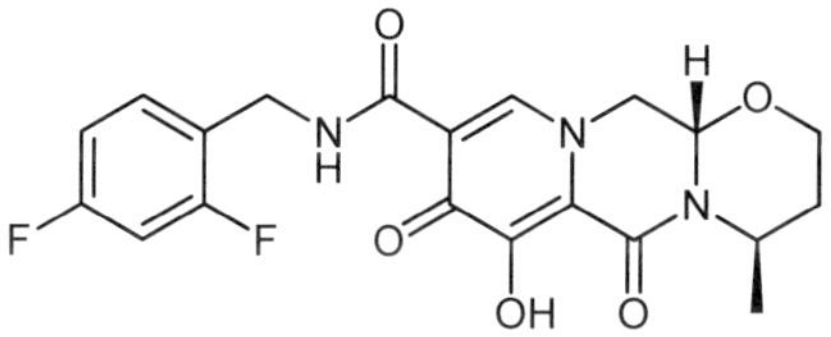

(23), dolutegravir

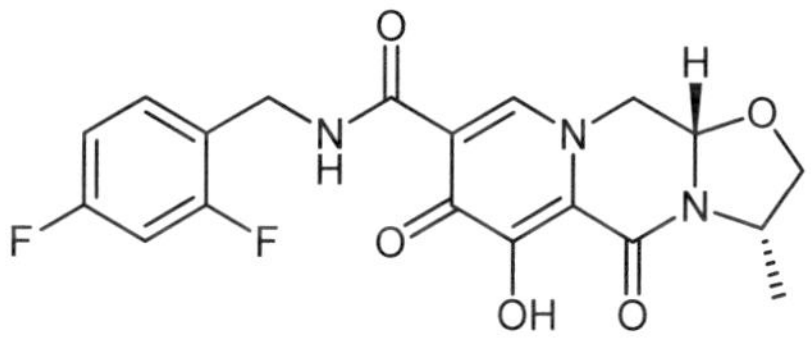

(24), S/GSK1265744

Figure 15: Second generation ST IN inhibitors.

Doultegravir is licensed for once-a-day dosing without a boosting agent [87, 162, 163, 171]. A particularly attractive feature of S/GSK1265744 Fig. **15**, (No. 24) is the potential it offers as a long-acting antiviral agent that could help to address the adherence challenge [172, 173]. Currently a Phase IIa trial by ViiV Healthcare is looking to evaluate the use of S/GSK1265744 as a long acting injectable formulation [174].

An early development compound with a tricyclic ring system as a scaffold was introduced by a team at Gilead. By employing an internally developed computational model of IN [175] and using the published inhibitor L-870,810 the team identified the tricyclic ring system (Fig. **16**, (25)). The tricyclic ring system provided a good framework for both metal chelation, *i.e.,* a planar arrangement of Lewis basic centres, and the hydrophobic *para*-fluorbenyl unit for hydrophobic interactions.

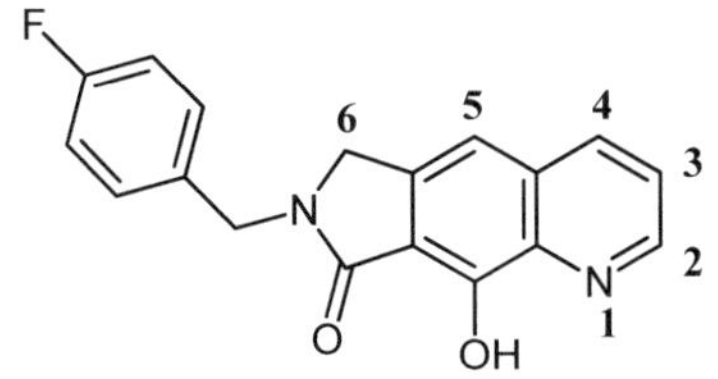

(25)

Figure 16: Early tricyclic ring scaffold.

SAR studies explored the various positions of compound (25) in order to improve both the potency and pharmaceutical characteristics. The C-5 and C-6 positions were examined and a range of different heterocycles compared to the pyridine system which ultimately led to GS-9160 (Fig. **17**, (26); IC_{50} = 28nM for ST).

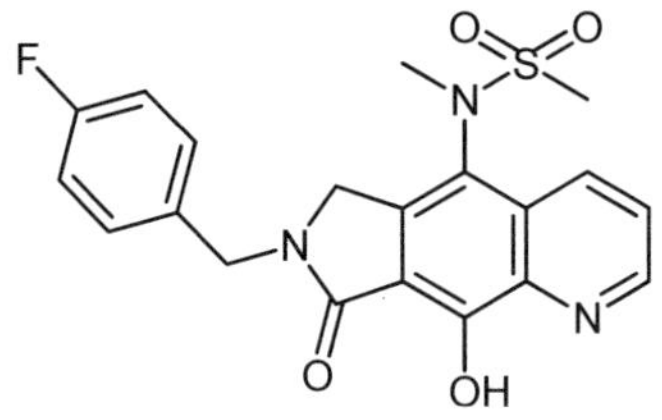

(26), GS-9160

Figure 17: GS-9160.

The second generation inhibitor, (Fig. **18**, (28) MK-2048) has been demonstrated to have activity against viruses that are resistant to raltegravir and elvitegravir, although resistance mutations have been observed [176]. A recent publication describes a patent from Merck that outlines additional second generation STIs with improved resistance profiles and pharmacokinetics [177].

Other Scaffolds

A series of dihydro-1H-isoindole derivatives, of which XZ-259 is archetypal (Fig. **19**; (29)) have been reported to be IN inhibitors operating by chelation of the

Mg^{2+} ions in the active site with concomitant displacement of the nucleobase (terminal adenosine) of the viral DNA which is consistent with the ST inhibitor model [178-180]. XZ-259 showed very good potency in antiviral assays both against wild-type and ralvitegravir strains.

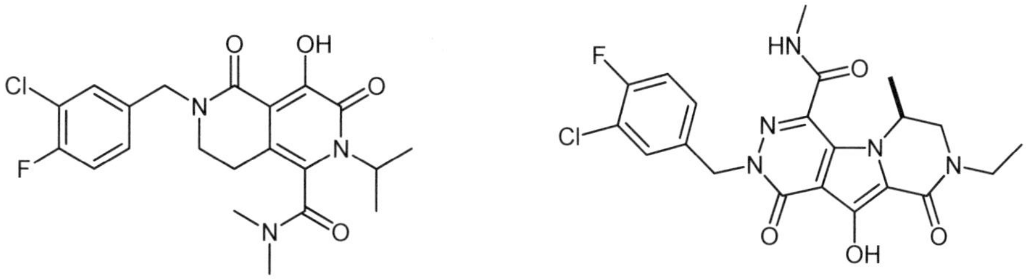

(27), MK-0536 (28), MK-2048

Figure 18: Second generation ST IN inhibitors reported by Merck.

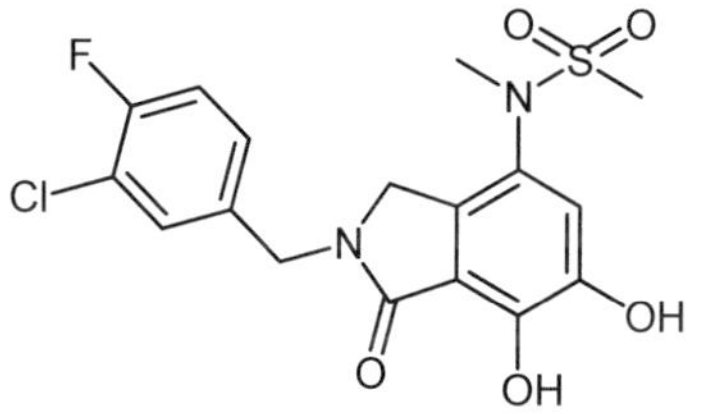

(29), XZ-259

Figure 19: Dihydro-1H-isoindole scaffold.

Screening of an internal library of chemical entities by scientists at Pfizer led to the identification of two classes of heterocyclic compounds that displayed activity in a scintillation proximity assay (SPA) [US Patent 7,135,482 – 2006]. The azaindole carboxylic acids (Fig. **20**; (30)) and β-carboline carboxylic acids (31) gave IC_{50} values in the range of 08.4-7.5 μM [181].

Both scaffolds were modified by the introduction of a hydroxamic acid (32) and (33) in place of the original carboxylic acid, a change that improved potency in enzymatic assays; 40-fold increase with azaindole hydroxamic acid (Ar = 2,4-difluorobenzene) and a more modest improvement with β-carboline; IC_{50} = 3.8 μM for acid (30) verses IC_{50} = 0.23 μM (Ar = 4-fluorobenzene) for hydroxamic acid (32). The β-carboline series suffered from cytotoxicity in the low micromolar range.

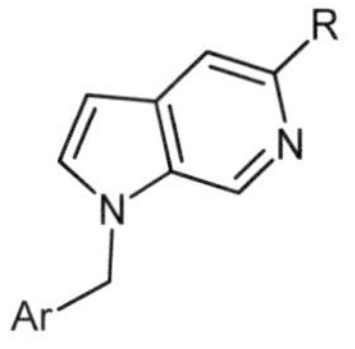

(30), R = CO_2H
(32), R = CONHOH

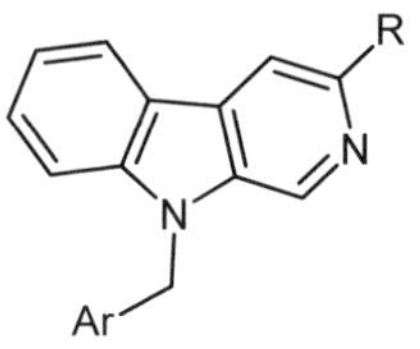

(31), R = CO_2H
(33), R = CONHOH

Figure 20: Azaindole and β-carboline scaffolds.

The quinolone 3-carboxylic acid scaffold which was originally disclosed by a group from Japan Tobacco was explored computationally using an algorithm that allowed the generation of a common feature pharmacophore model [182]. The original search returned 56 possible hits which were purchased and evaluated with several compounds showing activity; $IC_{50} < 100$ μM [183].

A series of salicylic acid derivatives were identified by Botta *et al.* using a virtual screening protocol reported previously [184-186]. The series, exemplified by (Fig. **21**, (34)) showed both inhibitory potency against IN and antiviral activity in cellular assays.

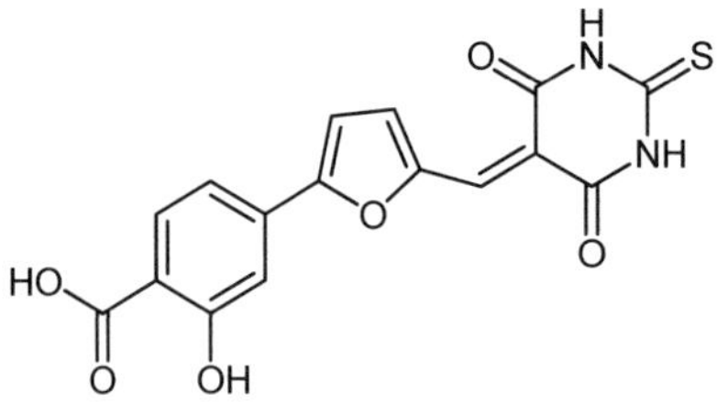

(34)

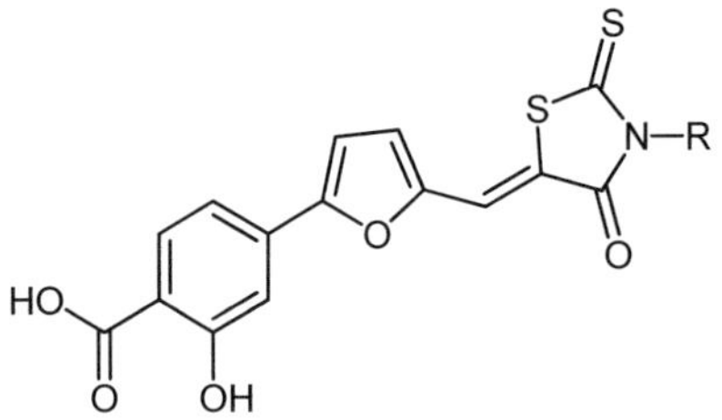

(35)

Figure 21: Scaffolds based on salicylic acid.

SAR studies allowed the pharmacophore to be explored and it was reported that the acid group was paramount for activity; hydroxyl groups in the aryl ring improved potency; the 3-position of the furan ring did not tolerate the introduction of substituents with activity being diminished in each case; the thiobarbituric acid could be exchanged for a range of heterocycles without affecting activity. Further work [187] reported the replacement of the thiobarbituric acid heterocycle with either a benzyl unit, or rhodanine (Fig. **21**, (35)) derivatives. The benzyl derivatives invariably resulted in compounds that were inactive (one derivative was active at very low levels), whilst the substituted rhodanine derivatives were active in IN inhibition assays.

Styrylquinoline IN Inhibitors

Styrylquinoline inhibitors are readily accessible compounds involving a simple condensation reaction (acid or base catalysed) between a substituted methyl (4, 2, or 3) quinoline and the appropriate substituted aldehyde [123]. The compounds have been reviewed previously [188], including a detailed Structure Activity Relationship of a small series of styrylquinoline inhibitors [189]. The mechanism of action of the styrylquinoline IN inhibitors is not known with certainty, but the inhibitors do generate resistance mutations in the *pol* gene, and appear to inhibit both the 3'-processing reaction and ST, possibly by interfering with LTR IN binding [190-192]. The compounds do also form complexes with a range of metal ions [193].

Some of the most active members of this family discovered to date are represented by the multi-hydroxy substituted derivatives (Fig. **22**) [194, 195]. The key features of the pharmacophore are a polar group at C-7 (typically a carboxylic acid which is ionized at physiological pH), a hydroxyl group at C-8, the quinoline nitrogen (basic centre) and a high degree of overall hydrophobicity (Table **1**).

A particularly interesting feature of the styrylquinoline class of compounds, is their activity against strains of virus that are resistant to a number of current anti-HIV drugs [191].

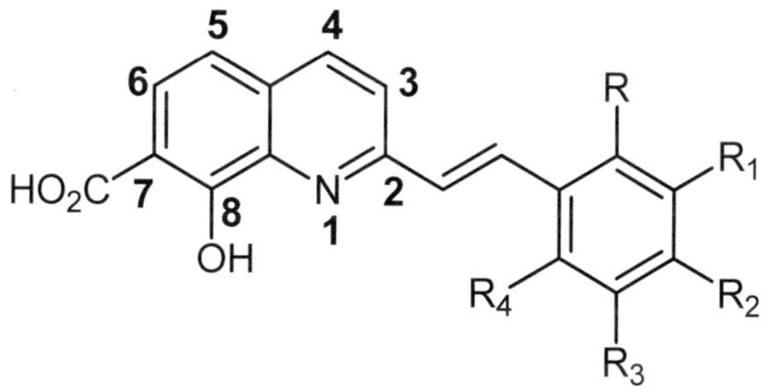

Figure 22: The styrylquinoline scaffold.

Table 1: Biological activities of selected substituted styrylquinoline compounds; data taken from Ref. [145, 146]

Compound	Substituents	*In vitro* IN inhibition		Antiviral Activity and Cytotoxicity	
		3' Processing (IC_{50}, μM)	ST (IC_{50}, μM)	(IC_{50}, μM)	(TC_{50}, μM)
I	$R,R_2,R_4 = H$ $R_1, R_3 = OH$	3.2	3.2	>100	>100
II	$R_1,R_3,R_4 = H$ $R, R_2 = OH$	3.7	2.8	80	>100
III	$R,R_4 = H$ $R_1,R_2 = OH$ $R_3 = OCH_3$	0.7	2.8	1-5	250

Inhibition of IN by Peptide Molecules

Early work in this area established that peptides could inhibit the activities of HIV-1 IN [196].

A group at Merck & Co. (Fig. **23**) isolated a range of small peptides from a series of fungi; a cyclic peptide (WIN66306) from *Aspergillus flavipus* [197] and two linear peptides from *Dendrochiump sp.* [198]. The linear peptides, integramide A (36) and integramide B (37) were most active with both compounds showing inhibition of both the 3'-processing reaction and the strand transfer reaction. Inhibition for 3'-processing was integramide A (IC_{50} = 17 μM) and integramide B (IC_{50} = 10 μM), and inhibition of the strand transfer reaction for both A and B was (IC_{50} = 60 μM), however due to issues with cellular toxicity the development of both compounds was halted.

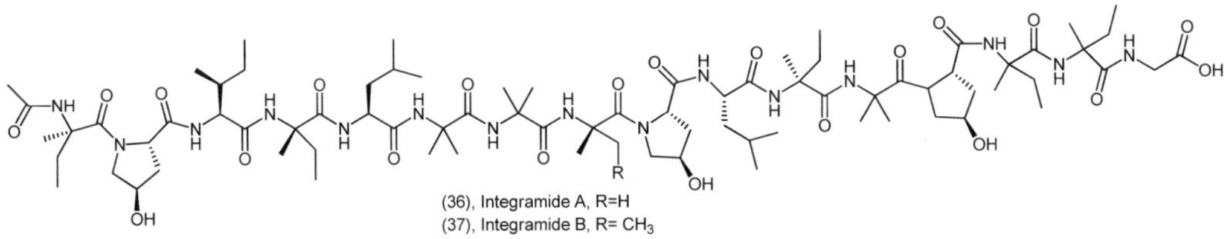

Figure 23: Integramide A and B.

Many components of the PIC interact with each other in a regulatory capacity, exemplified by the effect that RTand IN have on one another [199-201]. Vpr, which is also a component of the PIC, interacts with IN *via* its C-terminal domain inhibiting its activity [202]. Screening of a peptide library derived from the HIV-1 gene products identified a number of small peptides that inhibited the ST reaction of IN *in vitro* and some Vpr-derived peptides showed inhibitor activity against 3'-processing [203].

A series of modified crystalline libraries provided inhibitors that could inhibit all three reactions catalysed by IN at the nanomolar range [204].

The group of Neamati has been quite active in the development of peptides targeting IN function and two approaches have been pursued by the group. Two sets of peptides derived from the HIV-1 HXB2 Pol genome were tested against IN [205, 206]. In a follow up paper [207], one of the original lead peptides was modified with a hydrocarbon staple [208]. The stapled peptides not only showed antiviral activity, but were also internalized by cells.

Inhibition of IN by blocking protein-protein interactions has been reviewed by Friedler *et al.* [209] and much of the current focus of effort in this area is centred on the crucial interaction between IN and LEDGF/p75. It is likely that due to the nature of the interaction between IN and LEDGF/p75, agents like peptides, that can act over a relatively large portion of the protein's surface will be effective at disrupting the interplay between IN and LEDGF/p75 [210-213].

Deadman *et al.* reported a series of linear and cyclic peptides derived from the LEDGF/p75 protein. The peptides, which all synthesised by solid phase chemistry, fitted the LEDGF/p75 pocket and were useful in identifying previously undescribed bonding interactions [214].

A group at KU Leuven have previously demonstrated small cyclic peptides could bind to the LEDGF/p75 protein and interfere with its binding to IN [215]. A follow-up study identified the nature of the interaction between one of the peptides, LP21 and LEDGF/p75 [216].

Nucleotide-Based Inhibitors of IN

This area has previously been reviewed [217] and although there has been some promising early work [218], there are no examples of late stage development candidates from this category.

Natural Product Derived IN Inhibitors [219, 220]

Many natural products and natural product derivatives have been reported to show inhibitory activity against HIV-1 IN, mainly through inhibition of the ST reaction.

Fukiic acid [221] which is structurally similar to chicoric acid [222] was evaluated for antiviral activity [223] and was shown to be able to effectively inhibit reactions catalysed by IN, but to be inactive against viral replication in a MT-4 assay. Unfortunately, fukiic acid was shown to be 5-fold more toxic than chicoric acid.

Caffeoylglycolic acid derivatives of chicoric acid, so called 'halfmer' of chicoric acid were synthesised and evaluated for antiviral activity [224]. The compounds showed activity that was comparable to L-chicoric acid. Caffeoyl-anilides, formed by merging the caffeoyl and anilide moieties were evaluated as potential inhibitors of both IN and CCR5 docking [225].

Lamellarin α 20-sulfate [226], a marine natural product was demonstrated to be active against both the PIC and purified IN.

Additional examples include, cytosporic acid [227], integric acid [228], daphane diterpenes [229] and labdane analogues [230].

Miscellaneous in Inhibitors

Screening of the National Cancer Institute drug data-base in the USA identified a number of structural classes of molecule that showed inhibitory activity against HIV-1. Two distinct classes of molecule were identified as inhibitors of IN.

The tropolone derivatives identified from the screening programme all inhibited the ST reaction with α-hydroxytropolone (NSC 18806) being one of the most active inhibitors with an IC_{50} 4.8 ± 2.5 μM [231]. Hydroxytropolones were also shown to inhibit HIV-1 RT [232].

Screening of the database also identified a number of tetracyclines that possessed inhibitory activity against IN [233].

Phenanthrene-β-diketo acid derivatives [234, 235] have previously been demonstrated to have modest activity against the ST step and in some cases, also 3'-processing.

A range of ionic liquids [236] were evaluated in gel based assays for both 3'-processing and ST inhibition [237]. The authors reported that some of the ammonium and imidazolinium-based ionic liquids did inhibit the ST reaction and a few ionic liquids actually inhibiting both reactions although no mechanism for the activity was proposed.

A series of synthetic polyamides, bisdistamycins and lexitropsins were shown to selectively bind the conserved AT sequences in the LTR with a general correlation between oligomeric form and potency, for example, the monomers were relatively inactive at micromolar concentrations, whereas the dimeric forms were generally more potent [238].

Integrase Co-Factors

Although IN is both necessary and sufficient to carry out the catalytic steps of DNA integration *in vitro* numerous proteins have been observed to interact with IN and potentially play a functionally relevant role in the integration process, including targeting PICs to particular chromatin regions, nuclear import of PICs across the nuclear membrane and inhibition of autointegration [239-242]. These proteins are known as IN co-factors. A majority of these proteins where identified using high through put screening, yeast 2 hybrid (Y2H) screening, co-immunopurification (co-IP) and full length genome RNAi screens. However, thorough validation is required to confirm their status as a true co-factor. A number of methods are used for this including siRNA knockdown followed by western blotting and quantitative RT PCR, along with co-localization studies. To date a number of IN co-factors have been identified and validated, although many still required full validation.

LEDGF/p75

LEDGF/p75 is by far the most extensively studied IN co-factor. It is a 74kD protein ubiquitously expressed, chromatin associated protein. It was initially discovered as a human transcriptional co-activator [243]. However the exact cellular functions of LEDGF/p75 are incompletely understood. LEDGF/p75 interacts with several other cellular proteins including, menin mixed-lineage leukemia (MML) a histone methyltransferase complex involved in transcriptional regulation [244], the transposase pogZ [245], menin a nuclear tumour suppressor protein which links LEDGF/p75 with MLL, JP02 a C-myc binding protein [246, 247] and cdc7-activator of S-phase kinase (ASK) which is required for DNA replication during S-phase of the cell cycle.

LEDGF/p75 has been suggested to play a role in transcriptional regulation; over expression of LEDGF/p75 was found to increase transcription of a number of stress related genes [248-255], regulation is mediated by binding of LEDGF/p75 to heat shock and stress related elements in the promoters [249-252, 255]; cell survival, the addition of recombinant LEGDF/p75 or overexpression of LEDGF/p75 has been shown to promote cell survival in a variety of cell types. This protection is most likely attributed to LEDGF/p75 transcriptional activation of stress response genes [248]. LEDGF/p75 has also been reported as a substrate for caspase 3 and 7 during apoptosis, cleavage of LEDGF/p75 by these caspases results in 2 protein fragments which lack any prosurvival activity [256]; autoimmunity, the autoantigen properties of LEDGF/p75 was first identified by antibodies which recognised a ~70kD protein (LEDGF/p75) present in the nucleus of cells from patients with several chronic inflammatory diseases [257].

LEDGF/p75 belongs to the hepatoma derived growth factor (HDGF) related protein (HRP) family, based on sequence similarities [258]. It is 530 amino acids in length and comprised of two small folded domains. The N-terminal region contains a Pro-Trp-Trp-Pro (PWWP) domain (amino acids 1-92), a functional nuclear localisation sequence (NLS) (amino acids 148-156) and 2 AT-hook like motifs, together they are responsible for the tight association of LEDGF/p75 with chromatin [259, 260]. The C-terminal region contains the highly conserved IN binding domain (IBD), which is essential for IN binding (amino acids 347-429) [261-264]. The IBD has also been reported to be involved in the interactions of LEDGF/p75 with its previously mentioned binding partners, pogZ, JP02, menin and MLL. The LEDGF/p75 gene encodes a splice variant, p52 which shares the same N-terminal 325 amino acids but have different C-terminal regions. p52's C-terminal region is considerably smaller, 8 amino acids in length compared to 205 amino acids for p75 and therefore lacks the IBD and is unable to bind HIV-1 IN.

The structure of the IBD has been determined by NMR and is composed of a bundle of 4 long α helices [265]. Mutagenesis studies have revealed 3 amino acids

(Ile365, Asp366 and Phe406) at one end of the α helical bundle are essential for HIV-1 IN-LEDGF/p75 binding [265]. The IBD interacts with HIV-1IN through its CCD. IBD-CCD 2 domain constructs have demonstrated that the side loop of IBD containing residues Ile365 and Asp366 are inserted into the CCD dimer interface of one IN in the dimer and the other side loop containing residues Phe406 and Val408 are packed against the hydrophobic patch on the other IN in the dimer. The overall structure is a pair of IBDs bound to two equivalent positions on the IN CCD dimer. The NTD of HIV IN has also been shown to be involved in LEDGF/p75 binding. The positively charged residues on one side of the IBD interact with three Glu acidic residues of the NTD. This interaction is proposed to stabilise high affinity binding observed between LEDGF and HIV-1 IN. LEDGF binding has also been suggested to stabilise an IN tetramer by binding the NTD and CCD from the two different dimers, as demonstrated by disruption of the HIV-1 IN NTD-CCD abolishes tetramerisation and significantly reduces catalytic activity.

LEDGF/p75 was originally identified by co-IP as a HIV-1 IN binding partner. The nuclear distribution of IN has been shown to perfectly match that of LEDGF/p75. LEDGF/p75 binds to lentiviral IN but is unable to bind to IN from other retroviral genera [74, 76, 266]. *In vitro* assays have shown LEDGF/p75 significantly enhances HIV-1 IN DNA strand transfer activity. It was initially debatable as to whether LEDGF/p75 promoted efficient HIV-1 integration in cells as several studies produced conflicting results, however later findings have demonstrated that small residual amounts of LEDGF/p75 in the cell is sufficient to carry out almost wild type level of HIV-1 replication. Following on from these observations multiple groups have gone on to produce solid evidence in support of the role of LEDGF/p75 in HIV-1 integration target site selection. Y2H screening and site directed mutagenesis studies demonstrated that HIV-1 harbouring a single mutation disrupts HIV-1 IN-LEDGF/p75 interactions resulting in defective viral replication without any significant effect on catalytic activity. It was also reported to abolish chromosomal tethering, however it had no effect on nuclear import of HIV-1 IN. In support of LEDGF/p75s role in integration target site selection, analysis of integration in LEDGF/p75 knock down cells, which maintained normal levels of infection, integration was shown to be less frequent in transcription units and more frequent in GC-rich DNA. Several studies have used overexpression IBD constructs, which lack the PWWP and AT hooks required for LEDGF/p75 chromatin binding to demonstrate LEDGFs role in integration, additionally replacing the N-terminal portion of LEDGF/p75 with that from other chromatin binding proteins redirects integration target site selection. In further support of LEDGF/p75s role in tethering HIV-1 IN to active transcription units during integration, mapping of LEDGF/p75 chromatin binding profile has shown it preferentially binds to active transcription units.

All this taken together provides overwhelming evidence that LEDGF/p75 plays and important part in HIV-1 integration target site selection.

Integrase Interacting Protein (INI1)

INI1 is a homolog of yeast SNF5, and the core subunit of the ATP-dependant SW1/SNF chromatin remodelling complex [267]. INI1 is a 385 amino acid long protein which comprises of 3 highly conserved regions, repeat 1 and 2, a coiled-coiled domain termed a homology region 3 (HR3) at the C-terminal [268]. Repeat 1 and 2 are involved in protein-protein interactions and are required for INI1 multimerisation [269], repeat 1 has also been shown to be necessary and sufficient for IN binding [268]. INI1 also binds DNA non-specifically, Das *et al.* [269] have identified the INI1 proposed DNA binding domain, and demonstrated that it's involved in concentration dependant multimerisation of INI1.

INI1 was the first protein shown to interact with IN [270], INI1-IN interaction is through the CCD of IN. INI1 is believed to play a role in many stages of the HIV-1 replication including integration, viral transcription and viral assembly [271, 272]. The pre-integration role of INI1 involves its binding of IN. *In vitro* studies have shown that INI1 is able to both stimulate and inhibit IN activity [271-273], dependant on the concentration of IN [270], however these two opposing activities probably occur at different time points in the viral replication cycle.

Multimerisation of INI1 is believed to be requred for IN binding and can be attributed to its inhibition of integration [269], binding of INI1to IN is believed to form a high molecular weight complex which is inactive [269]. A recent study has clarified the INI1 mediated inhibition of IN, a study of the structure and function relationship of a complex of full length IN, full length LEDGF/p75 with INI1 IN binding domain and viral DNA, have shown they bind together in a 4/2/2/2 formation. Functional assays show INI1 IN binding domain inhibits 3' processing however it does not interrupt viral DNA binding. This is explained by the complex binding structure, in which INI1 IN binding domain sits in the target DNA binding site, resulting in inhibition of integration. These results suggest INI1 maintains IN in a stable inactive conformation, preventing any non-specific interactions and stabilising the IN tetramer whilst it travels to its target integration site [274]. Interestingly, studies by Das *et al.* suggest that DNA binding to INI1 may be necessary to stimulate IN activity [269]. Furthermore, *in vitro* studies demonstrate that the direct interaction between IN and the SW1/SNF complex promotes remodelling of the nucleosome which is required for efficient viral DNA integration.

Post-integration INI1 functions may facilitate proviral transcription by enhancing Tat function [275-279]. INI-1 and SW1/SNF are directly involved in Tat dependant activation of transcription at the HIV LTR, overexpression of INI1increases Tat-induced LTR transactivation. Overexpression of the INI IN binding site has been shown to inhibit HIV-1 assembly by specifically binding to the viral gag-pol protein [271].

Barrier to Autointegration (BAF)

BAF is required for many cellular functions including chromatin organisation, gene regulation and nuclear envelop assembly. BAF is a component of the lamina, it transiently interacts with histones, lamins and LEM (lamina-associated polypeptide emerin MAMN1)-domain proteins, including the nuclear protein emerin [280], suggesting it also plays an important role in nuclear assembly. It is a highly conserved 89 amino acid protein, which forms a dimer that connects two strands of double stranded DNA [281]. Each monomer contains 2 helix-hairpin-helix (HHH) motifs, believed to be the DNA binding surface. HHH binding to DNA is entirely non-specific, amide groups on the protein backbone bind to DNA phosphates [281, 282]. BAFs cellular distribution varies depending on the cell cycle stage.

BAF was originally discovered as a component of the retroviral PIC [283]. In further support for a role of BAF in HIV-1 replication, the addition of BAF to salt stripped PICs restored their integration activity as well as the native structure of the synaptic complex. BAF is proposed to compact viral DNA making it inaccessible to self-destructing autointegration (integration into itself) [283]. Further support for a role of BAF in viral replication came from the finding that BAF also interacts with LAP2α an inner nuclear membrane LEM protein [284]. Lap2α was identified as a component of the MLV PIC [284], furthermore knockdown of LAP2α significantly inhibited viral replication [285]. Whether this effect is a direct effect of LAP2α or an indirect effect mediated through LAP2α-BAF-viral DNA complex remains to be established. A recent study suggests HIV-1 interacts with a different inner nuclear membrane LEM protein during infection, siRNA knockdown of emerin in both dividing and non-dividing cells has demonstrated that BAF is required for the association of viral DNA with emerin and for the ability of emerin to support normal HIV-1 infectivity [280]. However further studies have contested the role of emerin in HIV-1 infectivity as knockdown of BAF or emerin had no effect on HIV-1 infectivity in HeLaP4 cells or mouse fibroblasts [286].

Transportin SR2 (TRN-SR2, Tnop3, Transportin-3)

TRN-SR2 belongs to the importin-β superfamily of karyopherins [287]. It was first identified as nuclear import factor for serine/arginine rich (SR) proteins, which are essential mRNA splice factors. TRN-SR2 recognises SR proteins *via* their NLS which is comprised of sequences rich in Arg/Ser, known as an RS domain. Phosphorylation of the SR proteins is believed to initiate the RanGTP-dependant nuclear import by TRN-SR2 [287-289]. TRN-SR2 directly binds its cargo in the cytoplasm and transports it to the nucleus *via* an interaction with nuclear pore proteins [288]. TRN-SR2 is also able to import other proteins which do not belong to the SR protein family [290, 291].

TRN-SR2 is a 975 amino acid protein, encoded for by the TNPO3 gene and comprised of α-helical repeats, it is structurally similar to importin 13 [292]. The N-terminal region is believed to directly bind Ran GTP and shares a high degree of amino acid sequence identity with importin 13 [293], the C-terminal region is thought to be the binding region for its cargo proteins [292, 294].

TRN-SR2 was initially identified as a co-factor for early stage HIV replication by genome wide siRNA screening [295]. Its specific interaction with HIV-1 IN was identified *via* a yeast-2-hybrid screen and further confirmed by pull down assays

[295]. RNAi knockdown experiments have demonstrated the involvement TRN-SR2 in HIV-1 replication in both dividing and non-dividing cells. Interestingly TRN-SR2 knockdown has been shown to have little to no effect on MLV transduction [295, 296], suggesting a role of TRN-SR2 in HIV-1 nuclear import as HIV-1 is able to infect both dividing and non-dividing cells and is believed to gain access to chromatin *via* nuclear import whereas MLV gains access to chromatin during cell mitosis. Furthermore the reduction in HIV-1 replication observed by TRN-SR2 knockdown has been mapped by RT qPCR to be after reverse transcription but preceding integration [295]. The strongest evidence in support of TRN-SR2s role in HIV-1 nuclear import comes from a study, in which TRN-SR2 knockdown lead to a reduction in the nuclear verses cytoplasmic localisation of eGFP labelled PICs [295].

The involvement of TRN-SR2 in HIV-1 replication is now widely accepted, although the importance of the direct interaction between HIV-1 IN and TRN-SR2 is controversial. Numerous studies suggest that this interaction mediates the nuclear import of HIV-1, however recent studies indicate a functional interplay between TRN-SR2 and HIV-1 viral capsid (CA). There is now mounting evidence in support of the functional significance of TRN-SR2 interaction with the viral CA [297, 298]. The role of the direct interaction between IN and TRN-SR2 was first questioned by the results of a study using chimeras in which HIV-1 CA and IN are replaced by MLV counterparts. These experiments demonstrate that TRN-SR2s effects on HIV-1 replication are dependent on the viral CA and not IN [297, 299]. Further support for the importance of the viral CA came from studies using the mutant N74D [300], a HIV virus carrying a CA mutation which is unaffected by TRN-SR2 knockdown. In the same study N74D was shown to be unable to bind cleavage and polyadenylation specific factor 6 (CPSF6). CPSF6 is a pre-mRNA processing protein [301], which binds specifically to the N-terminal of HIV-1 CA. Its C-terminal domain contains a sequence similar to the RS domain found in SR proteins, and is required for localisation of CPFS6 to the nuclear compartment [300, 302]. This RS domain is thought to be an interaction site for TRN-SR2. Knockdown of TRN-SR2 led to an increase in cytoplasmic CPFS6 [303]. Full length CPSF6 is a nuclear protein, when overexpressed has no effect on HIV-1 infection. However, an N-terminal version of CPSF6 (1-358 amino acids) localises to the cytoplasm and overexpression reduces HIV-1 infection. A CPSF6 mutant lacking the RS domain inhibits HIV-1 replication but has no effect on MLV replication.

A study also showed that overexpression of a cytosolic full length CPSF6 inhibits HIV-1 infection during or prior to nuclear import. In support of the interaction of TRN-SR2 and CPFS6, a recent study showed that mutations within the TRN-SR2 CPFS6 recognition site impair CPSF6 binding and inhibit HIV-1 replication [303].

Recent studies point towards the ability of CPSF6 to inhibit HIV-1 replication, only when it accumulates in the cytoplasm; this accumulation of CPFS6 in the cytosol leads to premature engagement of the viral CA causing a delay in uncoating and nuclear import.

Zohn *et al.* have shown TRN-SR2 has an indirect effect on HIV-1 integration. Once the HIV-1 CA associated PICs enter the nucleus, TRN-SR2 removes the CA from the PIC to promote effective integration [304].

Larue *et al.* contested the ability of TRN-SR2 to directly bind to CA tubes, within the same study they also provide evidence that TRN-SR2 readily binds to functional intersomes in an *in vitro* model system. Using mass spectroscopy based protein footprinting and mutagenesis they have also identified the interacting amino acids to be within the CTD of HIV-1 IN and the C-terminal domain of TRN-SR2 [292]. These results were further strengthened by the identification of key amino acids in IN that are involved in the TRN-SR2 interacting interface, however 2 single point mutations (K266A and R269A) effects on HIV-1 replication were due to a block in reverse transcription [305]. The same group in further studies went on to identify a mutant HIV-1 IN with reduced affinity for TRN-SR2 which had no effect on reverse transcription activity (NL4-3 $IN^{R263A/K264A}$) but was defective for integration. Using an [306] eGFP-IN-labelled HIV fluorescence-based import assay which allows direct quantification of nuclear verses cytoplasmic PICs confirmed the block of integration by NL4-3 IN mutant to be at the nuclear import stage, providing evidence that the IN-TRN-SR2 direct interaction mediates nuclear import of HIV-1 PICs [306].

TRN-SR2 is not the only IN co-factor identified to be involved in nuclear import. Several other nuclear import factors and nucleoproteins have been shown to interact with IN these include Importin α1 [307-309], importin α3 [310, 311], importin 7 [312,

313], Nup62 [314] and Nup153 [300, 315, 316]. Importin α1 was shown to directly interact with HIV-1 IN through 2 nuclear localisation sequences and amino acids 211-219 of the CTD of HIV-1 IN [308]. This interaction was confirmed *via in vitro* binding studies [300, 310-312, 316, 317]. Knockdown of importin α3 demonstrated its requirement for HIV infection in a number of cell types [310]. This interaction was also attributed to the CTD of IN [310]. Importin 7 has also been implicated in HIV-1 nuclear import, however studies suggests it is not essential for HIV-1 replication but that it may be used by HIV-1 to maximise nuclear import. Nup62 has been shown to participate in several stages of HIV-1 replication, it was only recently identified as a direct binding partner of HIV-1 IN and confirmed *via* co-IP [314]. Knockdown of Nup 62 significantly inhibited the association of IN with chromatin thus inhibiting HIV-1 integration [314]. Nup153 interaction with HIV-1 IN was demonstrated to be through the C-terminal domain as overexpression of the C-terminal domain of Nup153 in cultured cells inhibited the nuclear import of HIV-1 IN [315].

DNA Dependant Protein Kinase (DNA-PK)

The integration of viral DNA creates a single stranded gapped intermediate in which the viral 5' ends are not joined to the host DNA this is most likely detected by the host cell as a major assault on the genomic DNA and it is generally accepted that cellular DNA repair mechanisms fill in and repair the gaps. The major mechanism of repair of DNA breaks in eukaryotic cells is the non-homologous end joining (NHEJ) pathway and is therefore an obvious candidate for the retroviral post-integration repair [318]. NHEJ repairs double stranded DNA breaks that occur during meiotic recombination and V(D)J recombination. This pathway is mediated by DNA-PK [319]. Heterodimers of KU70/86 bind double stranded DNA and recruit the catalytic subunit (DNA-PK_{CS}) to form the active DNA-PK.

The potential role of the NHEJ pathway in retroviral post-integration repair was first suggested by a study in which, retroviral infection of murine severe combined immunodeficient cells (*scid*) pre-B cells (NHEJ deficient cells) induced a high degree of apoptosis (80-90%) compared to wild type cells [319]. However a study in 2000 contested the role of NHEJ in post-integration repair. In contrast to previous studies their results suggest that NHEJ is not required for the post-integration repair at multiplicities of infection (MOI) <1 transducing unit

(TU)/cell, in NHEJ deficient cells [320]. Interestingly, transduction was observed to be more efficient in these cells [320]. However, a high MOI (>1TU/cell) increased apoptosis [320], suggesting the NHEJ pathway may play a prosurvival role. Further supporting evidence for this hypothesis, Li *et al.* [321] confirmed previous findings that higher tighter infections of NHEJ deficient mutants lead to an increase in cell death due to apoptosis. They also propose from their findings that the unintegrated double stranded viral DNA ends produced during reverse transcription promote apoptosis and the NHEJ pathway protects the unintegrated DNA from apoptosis by circularisation. This is believed to involve KU which has been shown to associate with the HIV-1 PIC [321]. In support of this a study has also shown that cells deficient in KU80 produced no LTR circles [322].

Although the majority of evidence points towards a protective role of the NHEJ pathway, a role in post-integration repair cannot be ruled out but seems highly unlikely as the NHEJ pathway is not known to repair single stranded gaps, only double stranded breaks.

However, a recent study suggests DNA-PK has the very opposite effect in $CD4^{+}$T cells [323]. They report that it is the viral integration step that promotes cell death in HIV-1 infected T cells, as demonstrated by the ability of the IN inhibitor raltegravier to prevent HIV-1 induced cell death in cell cultures and $CD4^{+}$ cells isolated from infected individuals [323]. Furthermore, a HIV-1 IN deficient mutant caused cell death of activated primary CD4 lymphocytes. The same study also report that the mechanism for activation of cell death during integration is the activation of DNA-PK. Evidence for this comes from treatment of HIV infected activated $CD4^{+}$ cells with inhibitors of p53 (a protein which complexes with DNA-PK to promote cell death) and DNA-PK_{CS} prevents cell death [323].

High-Mobility-Group Chromosomal Protein A1 (HMGA1)

HMGA1 is a non-histone protein which is involved in many cellular processes including regulation of inducible gene transcription, regulation of heterochromatin organisation as well as a potential oncogene role. It is a 107 amino acid protein which consists of 3 DNA binding domains (AT-hooks) with a RGRP (Arg-Gly-Arg-Pro) core motif, a novel cross linking domain located between the second and third AT-hook and a C-terminal tail.

HMGA1 preferentially binds to the minor groove of AT rich regions of double stranded DNA using its AT-hooks. It is predominantly found in the nucleus, especially in heterochromatin and preferentially binds with bent, supercoiled or distorted DNA structures.

HMGA1 was discovered by fractionation of uninfected cell extract that restored *in vitro* activity of salt stripped PICs [324], recombinant HMGA1 has been shown to be able to restore integration of salt stripped PICs. Early studies suggest that HMGA1 DNA binding brings the viral LTR ends closer together and unwinds the LTR termini, which in turn assists the binding of IN [325, 326]. However no direct stable interaction between HMGA1 and IN could be identified using co-IP assay hence HMGA1's role in integration requires further investigation.

As well as its role in integration HMGA1 has also been shown to play other roles in HIV-1 replication. It has been demonstrated to play a part in the specific splice site regulation of HIV-1. Most recent experimental data strongly suggests HMGA1 plays an important role in HIV-1 transcription [327]. Using DNase I footprinting, multiple high and low affinity HMGA1 biding sites have been identified within the HIV-1 LTR which overlap with several transcription factor binding sites including the site for activity protein-1 (AP-1) [328]. HMGA1 is able to enhance the binding of the inducible AP-1 factor, activating transcription factor-3 (ATF-3). This bound ATF-3 then recruits the chromatin remodelling complex hSW1/SNF facilitating transcriptional activation. Furthermore HMAG1 directly interacts with transactivating response element (TAR) of HIV-1 TAR is required for promotor transactivation by the viral transactivator of transcription (Tat). HMGA1 directly binds to TAR and inhibits Tat binding leading to a reduction in HIV-1 transcription, suggesting HMGA1 may also play a role in viral latency [329].

Allosteric Inhibition of HIV-1 Integrase Activity [330, 331]

Chicoric acid [222] and derivatives have previously been shown to possess useful anti-HIV activities [332-336]. A tetra-acetylated chicoric acid derivative was shown to be an IN inhibitor but also bind at the IN dimer interface [337, 338] disrupting the dynamic exchange of the IN subunits [339].

In 2001, Molteni *et al.* [340] reported a series of compounds that were typified by structures (Fig. **24**) (38-40). X-ray analysis of compounds (38) and (39) using the CCD of an IN mutant F185K (a second mutant, F185K/W131E was also employed but the structures were not well resolved) showed binding in a 5Å deep pocket at the dimer interface. The pocket has an overall negative charge and compound (38) binds *via* a strong charge-charge interaction between the carbonyl oxygen of Gln168 and the positively charged arsenic. Additional π-π interactions between Trp131 and Trp132 and one of the phenyl rings were also observed.

In vitro assays showed that some of the compounds exhibited inhibitory activity against IN, with compound (40) inhibiting in the low micromolar range.

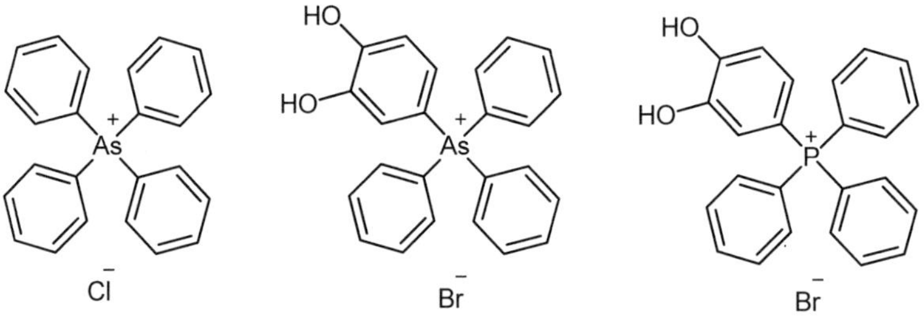

(38) (39) (40)

Figure 24: Early allosteric inhibitors that bound at the IN dimer interface.

Du *et al.* [341] provided further support to the concept of an allosteric binding site on IN in 2008 with the publication of a paper examining the activity of 1-pyrrolidineacetamide (N,N'-(methylene-di-4,1-phenylene) bis-1-pyrrolidineacetamide). A Surface Plasma Resonance (SPR) technology-based competitive inhibition assay showed that the compound had an IC_{50} 7.29 ± 0.68μM and could directly bind at the CCD. Cell culture assays showed that the 1-pyrrolidineacetamide inhibited replication of HIV-1 (III_B) with EC_{50} 17.05 μg/mL in C8166 cells. Molecular modelling simulations revealed that the compound interacted at the CCD dimer interface *via* interactions involving residues Thr174, Lys173 and Lys103. Site-directed mutagenesis studies in which the putative residues were replaced in turn with alanine confirmed the *in silico* model.

Wielens *et al.* [342] identified the same binding pocket that Du [341] and Kessl [339] had described in their respective studies. Using X-ray analysis of a mutated IN core domain complexed to sucrose the team identified a binding site that was 10Å from the LEDGF binding site. Located at the dimer interface and comprising residues E87, V88, I89, P90, E96, Y99, F100, K103 and K173 from both monomers, the study provided valuable structural information of the allosteric binding pocket.

Binding at the N-Terminal of IN

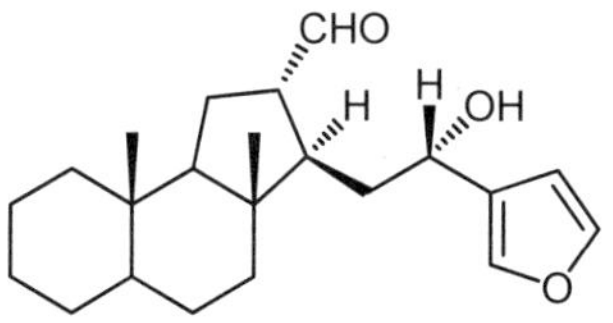

(41)

Figure 25: Hyrtiosal which is isolated from the marine sponge *Hyrtios erectus* and binds at the N-terminal domain *via* a hydrophobic interaction.

Hyrtiosal, (Fig. **25**; (41)) a natural product isolated from the marine sponge *Hyrtios erectus* was shown to inhibit HIV-1 IN [343]. The compound binds to IN at the N-terminal domain in a highly specific manner and molecular modelling studies suggested a largely hydrophobic interaction between the aliphatic carbon skeleton and residues Trp19, Lys34, Val37, Ala38 in monomer A and Ala38 and Ser39 in monomer B. Additional bonding interactions were also established between the ammonium group of Lys34 and the aldehyde of hyrtiosal and the hydroxyl groups of hyrtiosal and Ser17. An IC50 value of 9.60± 0.86μM was measured using an SPR technology-based competitive inhibition assay.

Inhibiting the LEDGF-IN Interaction [344-346]

As described previously LEDGF has been shown to be an important cellular protein that appears to be integral to the operational cycle of HIV-1 [264, 347] and IN mutants with alterations in the CCD fail to interact with LEDGF resulting in unsuccessful integration *in vivo*. *In vitro*, LEDGF has been shown to have a stimulatory effect [261, 348], whereas overexpression of LEDGF/p75 IBD appears to inhibit HIV replication by what has been hypothesised to be a shiftide mechanism [213, 349, 350].

The ability to disturb this LEDGF/p75 IN protein-protein interaction could well deliver a new class of drugs (Allosteric Integrase Inhibitors, ALLINIs) [330] for the treatment of HIV that are effective against INSTI resistant mutants.

The exact nature of all the components involved in the interaction between the PIC, LEDGF and chromosomal DNA are not known, however, there are three key domains of the LEDGF protein involved in the integration process; the PWWP domain made up from residues 1-91, the integrase binding domain (IBD) which is part of the C-terminal region and comprises residues 347-429 and a pair of 'AT-hook' motifs from residues 178-197 [351]. The primary interaction between LEDGF and IN is mediated by the IBD [176, 261, 263], although Maertens *et al.* [352] showed that the N-terminal domain of IN is also involved in binding LEDGF/p75.

The IBD was shown to be constituted from four long α-helices (α1, α2, α4 and α5) that are connected by hairpin turns; α1 is connected to α2, α4 is connected to α5 and α3 is connected to both α2 and α4. Additionally, a series of hydrophobic amino acid side chains are located on the hairpin turns and three of these residues have been identified as also being significant for binding (Ile-365, Phe-406 and Val-408), three so called 'hot-spot contacts'[353]. The hairpin loop connecting α1 and α2 contains an aspartic acid residue (Asp-366) which is vital for both the interaction of IN and LEDGF, but also appears to be a key part of LEDGF that is responsible for stimulating IN activity.

Important information regarding the nature of the protein-protein interaction involving IBD and the CCD of IN was published in 2005 [354]. The CCD-IBD interface was observed by X-ray analysis of a co-crystal of the CCD dimer with LEDGF. The interaction between the two protein faces is broadly hydrophobic with additional key residues that are involved in hydrogen bonding interactions. The CCD-dimer (A and B) contains a hydrophobic pocket into which the IBD protein inserts, with the main contact residues being Ile-365 and Asp-366.

Asp-366 (hydrogen bond acceptor) forms intermolecular hydrogen bonds with two amino-acids in the A unit of IN; Glu-170 and His-171 (hydrogen bond donors). Ile-365 interacts with five amino-acid residues of IN: Leu-102, Ala-128, Ala-129 and Trp-132 from B and Met-178 from A [354]

The Asp-366 residue of LEDGF appears to be particularly important for the IN-LEDGF interaction and work *in vitro* [354] has demonstrated that substitution of Asp-366 resulted in the abolition of the protein-protein interaction. Further mutagenesis studies have confirmed the importance of the LEDGF amino-acid side chains for key interactions [355, 356]. The IBD also mediates the interaction with HIV-2 IN [357].

Analysis of the X-ray crystal structure of a construct comprising LEDGF and HIV-2 revealed that residues Lys-401, Lys-402, Arg-404 and Arg-405 from IBD interacted *via* a series of hydrogen bonds with residues of the NTB domain of IN (Glu-6, Glu-10 and Glu-13) [47]. Molecular dynamics simulations also support the experimental evidence around the nature of the LEDGF/p75-IN interaction [358].

As delineated previously, the LEDGF/p75-IN interaction is largely mediated by the insertion of the IBD into the hydrophobic pocket formed at the IN dimer interface. This region of protein-protein binding [359] does appear to be amenable to targeting by small molecule inhibitors.

LEDGF/p75 – IN inhibitors [360]

The field has yet to settle on a single term to describe this group of compounds with various groups favouring different terms; lens epithelium-derived growth factor inhibitor, LEDGIN [361], Non-catalytic site integrase inhibitors, NCINI [362], IN-LEDGF allosteric inhibitors, INLAI [363] and allosteric integrase inhibitors ALLINI [330].

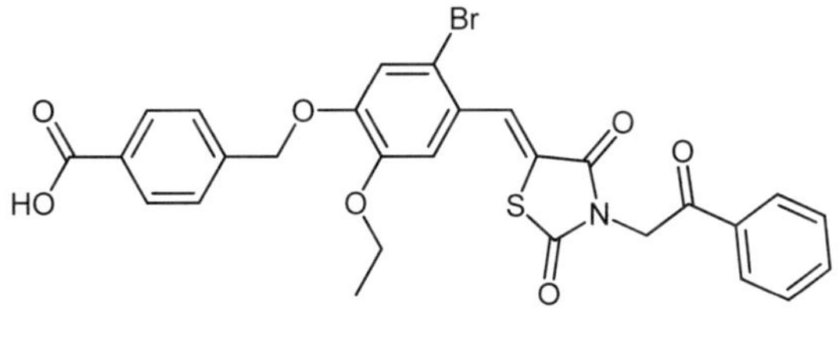

(42), D77

Figure 26: D77 was found to have significant inhibitory activity against the LEDGF-IN interaction.

Du *et al.* [364], evaluated D77 (Fig. **26**) which was purchased from a commercial source for antiviral activity using a range of techniques. Using a yeast two-hybrid system, D77 was found to have significant inhibitory activity against the LEDGF-

IN interaction whilst having no effect on the dimerization of IN. Further analysis using site-directed mutagenesis and Molecular orbital (MO) simulations identified that D77 interacted *via* hydrogen bonds, primarily *via* the carboxylic acid group with Thr174 from one dimer subunit and Gln95 from the other subunit. Additional residues in IN involved in binding were established; Trp131 and Thr125.

An *in silico* screening programme of a small molecule database identified 1,4-bis(5-(naphthalene-1-yl)thiophene-2-yl)naphthalene as having strong inhibitor activity against the LEDGF/p75-IN interaction and also affecting the nuclear translocation of IN. The compound bound at the hydrophobic pocket at the CCD dimer interface formed by residues Gln168, Ala169, Glu170 and Met 178 from subunit A and Thr93, Gln95, Thr125, Ala178, Trp131 and Trp137 of subunit B, with all interactions being hydrophobic in nature [365].

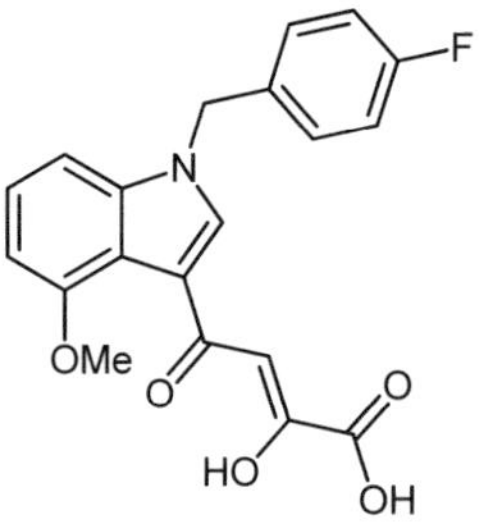

(43, CHI-1043)

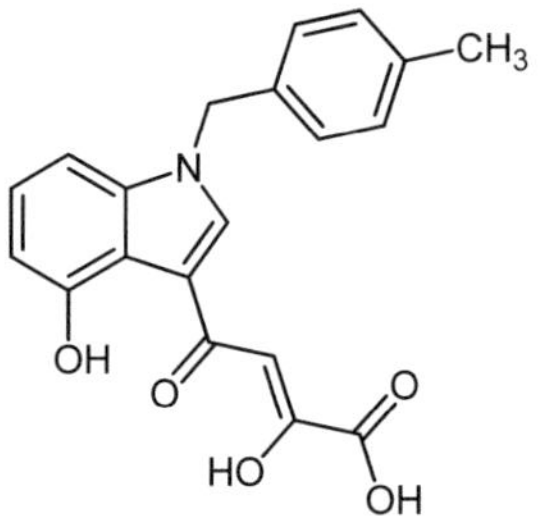

(44, CHIBA-3017)

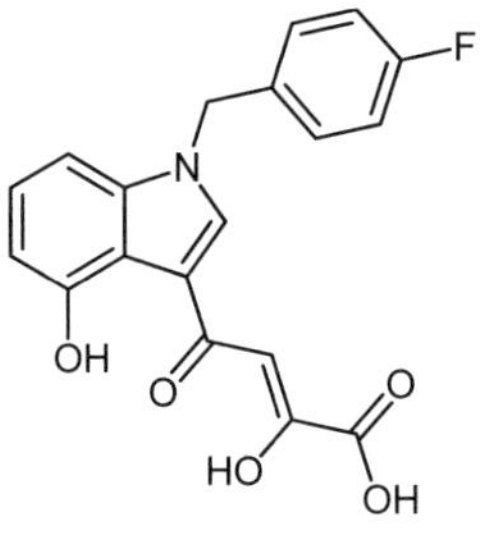

(45, CHIBA-3000)

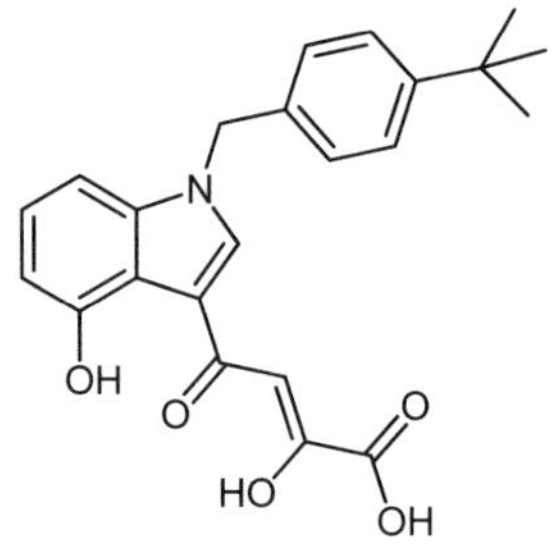

(46)

Figure 27: Indole based scaffold with activity against the LEDGF-IN interaction.

A series of substituted indoles characterised by CHIBA-3000, CHIBA-3017, CHI-1043 and (46) (Fig. **27**) [366-371] were reported to target the LEDGF-IN interaction.

The development of the compounds was driven by computational studies that identified key residues of the IBD; Il365, Asp366 and Phe406. The compounds bind through a series of hydrogen bonds and hydrophobic interactions [372]. The polar diketo acid moiety forms a series of hydrogen bonds with residues Glu170, His171, Thr174 and Gln95. The indole ring and substituted benzyl group present a hydrophobic region that interacts with the hydrophobic residue Trp131 and the *tert*-butyl group in the 4-position of the benzyl group of (46) gave a compound with good activity, $IC_{50} = 6.41 \mu M$ [371].

Many reports have been published outlining the utility of coumarin and related compounds as IN inhibitors [373, 374] and a coumarin derivative has been reported to inhibit the activity of IN possibly *via* binding at the IN dimer interface [375-377].

A series of compounds derived from benzo[d][1,3]dioxole-4-carboxylic acid were shown to bind to IN at two sites; the LEDGF/p75 binding site and a previously unreported site [378].

ALLINIs

The ALLINIs are a particularly interesting type of allosteric inhibitor and appear in infected cells to act during both early and late stages of replication, inhibiting both LEDGIN/p75 – IN binding and promoting aberrant IN multimerization with equal *in vitro* potency [379-386].

It has previously been demonstrated that the highly dynamic nature of the IN subunit interactions is critical for the correct assembly of the SSC [387, 388] and it is observed that *in vitro*, ALLINIs disrupt the formation of the stable SC [386]. In infected cells, ALLINIs interfere with a step at or prior to 3'-processing [362].

The ALLINIs are composed of a pharmacophore that comprises two binding domains; a hydrophobic unit composed of the quinoline and aryl substituent and a carboxylic acid that is hydrophilic. All members of this quinoline based family of compounds stabilize the interacting IN subunits *via* the carboxylic acid forming hydrogen bonds to one subunit, whilst the hydrophobic moieties interact with the second subunit *via* a hydrophobic interaction.

Work to understand and characterise all of the resistance mutations induced by ALLINIs is still ongoing, although a number of mutations have been observed, including Y99H, L102F, V126I, A128T, G134E, H171Q/T and T174I.

All of the resistance mutations are either amino-acid residues that interact with the compounds directly, or they are part of the surrounding pocket [362, 383, 389]. Recent work [390] employing a mutant virus expressing the A128T mutation has pointed to a possible role for ALLINI binding at the C-terminal domain resulting in aberrant multimerization.

HIV-2 IN is resistant to many of the members of this class of inhibitor [383].

A group at the University of Leuven have made many and varied contributions to the development of allosteric IN inhibitors [361]. Reports from the group outlined their work on the development of small molecule compounds that would ultimately lead to potent inhibitors of the IN-LEDGF/p75 interaction [379, 383] and a number of patents were filed covering other classes of LEDGIN [361].

NCINI (tBPQA)

tert-Butoxy-(4-phenyl-quinolin-3-yl)-acetic acids (tBPQA) reported as NCINIs and based around a substituted quinoline scaffold have been reported to be potent inhibitors of the LEDGF/p75 – IN interaction. A screening programme at Boehringer Ingelheim (BI) assessing members of an internal library against the 3'-processing reaction identified the forerunner to the tBPQA series [361]. The BI development group successfully explored the tBPQA pharmacophore and one candidate was progressed in to Phase I trials (Fig. **28**, No(47)) [391, 392]. The compounds were subsequently licensed to Gilead Sciences Inc. for further development [362].

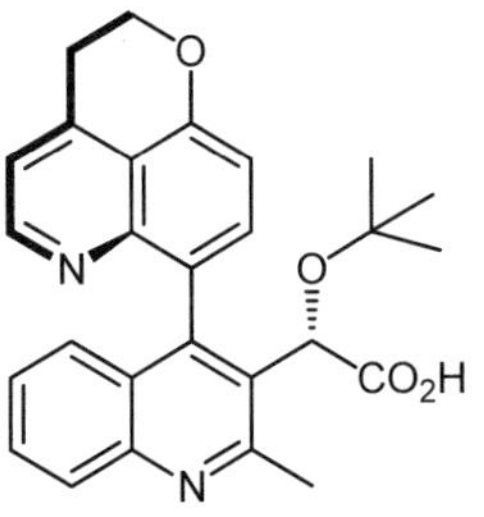

(47, BI 224436)

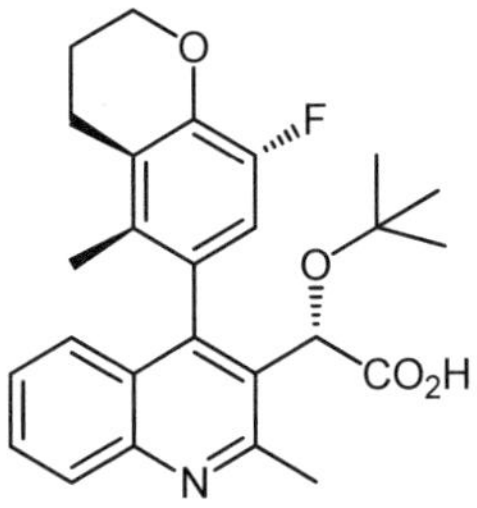

(48, GS-B)

Figure 28: Examples of the tBPQA class of allosteric inhibitors.

The Gilead team reported data on the mechanism of activity of tBPQAs represented by compounds like GS-B (Fig. **28**, (48)) [362]. Like other ALLINIs that utilise the quinoline scaffold, the compounds exert their effect through binding at the LEDGF pocket at the dimer interface. The polar carboxylic acid binds *via* two hydrogen bonds with residues Glu170, His171 and Thr174 and the hydrophobic quinoline and aryl moieties interact with Ala124, Thr125 and Trp131. The tBPQA binding induces a conformational change that reduces the flexibility of the IN dimer, hence the donor DNA is out of position in the active site of the enzyme. IC_{50} values ranging from 19 to 228nM were measured for the series using an IN-LEDGF interaction assay [393].

A group from Biodim Mutabilis [363] reported a series of compounds belonging to the aryl/heteroaryl-tertbutoxy-acetic acid family. One of the analogues, Mut 101 (Fig. **29**; 49) was described as an allosteric IN-LEDGF inhibitor that exerted an effect at the post-integration stage. The compounds inhibited the CCD-IBD interaction in addition to disrupting the interaction between IN and the full length LEDGF protein.

X-Ray analysis of Mut101 co-crystallised with the IN-CCD dimer showed that two molecules of Mut101 bound to the IN-CCD dimer, with Mut101 sitting in a pocket with hydrophobic residues on one side and two polar regions on two of the other faces; an acidic region and a region predominated by basic residues. The carboxylic acid of Mut101 forms three hydrogen bonds to the protein, one with Thr174 and two with His171 and Glu170.

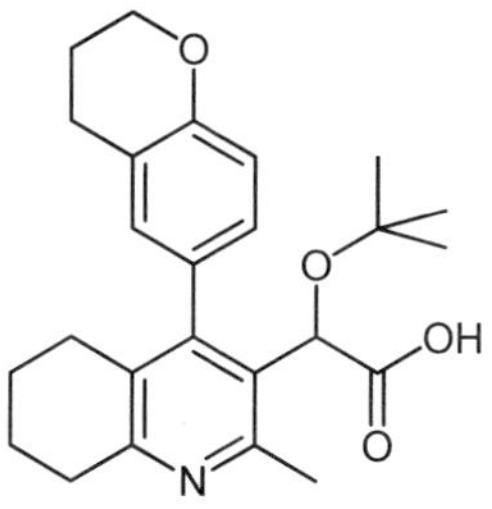

(49, Mut 101)

Figure 29: Mut 101disrupts both the CCD-IBD interaction and the interaction between IN and the full length LEDGF protein.

Analysis of the CCD-IN with Mut101 and without revealed two structural differences; both structural changes affect the catalytic site and explain the decrease in 3'-processing activity for the Mut101 bound form of IN. With the inhibitor bound structure, the alpha helices 115-122, 123-124 and 92-98 are structurally different with the loop containing Ile89, Pro90 and Ala91 being displaced. The second change is to the position of residues Gln95 and Glu170 in the Mut101 binding pocket where both residues are displaced. Mut101 binding induces a conformational change at the dimerization interface that in turn acts to stabilize the IN dimer.

In addition, size exclusion chromatography with IN that had been treated with Mut101 indicated that Mut101 binding may induce tetramer formation. A final particularly interesting feature of Mut101 is the promotion of post-integration defects. Further work to understand this post-integration block could well promote further development of this interesting allosteric IN-inhibitor.

In an effort to better understand the mechanistic detail of the mode of action of ALLINIs, a group examined the ALLINI pharmacophore and modified the hydrophobic region to generate a new class of related compounds, the MINI (selective multimeric IN inhibitors) (Fig. **30**, (51-52)) [385].

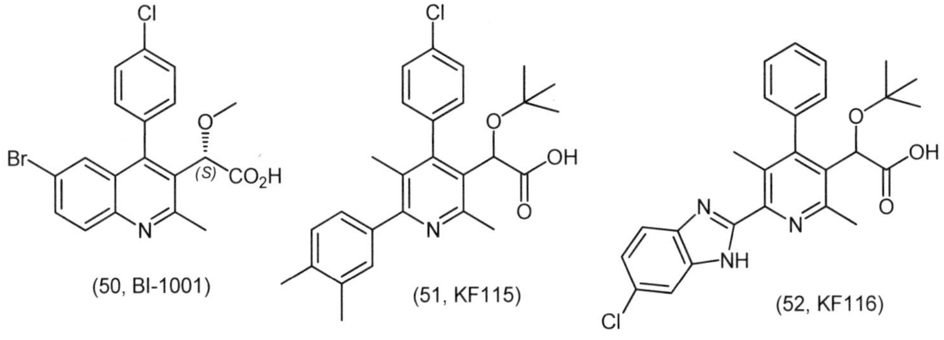

Figure 30: Original BI ALLINI lead and representative MINIs.

Using the ALLINI BI-1001, originally developed by BI as a lead, the group replaced the quinoline moiety with a substituted pyridine (Fig. **30**, (51, 52)). The team reasoned that by replacing the quinoline ring with a pyridine ring, the compounds would be able to interact with both subunits of the IN dimer to a greater degree than the existing ALLINIs.

The crystal structures of KF115 and KF116 bound to the HIV-1 IN CCD dimer revealed more extensive bonding interactions. For example, KF116 maintained the hydrogen bonding interactions with Glu170, His171 and Thr174 (subunit 2), but established additional interactions with subunit 1. The benzimidazole ring, which is orientated orthogonally to the pyridine ring, forms a hydrogen bond with residue Thr125 of subunit 1.

The additional bonding interactions of KF115 and KF116 with subunit 1 resulted in increased selectivity at modulating IN multimerization compared to LEDGF/p75binding,~ 50 fold and~ 60 fold for KF115 and KF116 respectively. There was also good correlation with antiviral potency; KF115 IC_{50} =~ 0.121μM and KF116~ 0.024μM. A particularly interesting property of KF116 was it maintained activity against the A128T mutant strain.

Work by De Luca [394] looked to identify possible new scaffolds targeting the IN-LEDGF/p75 interaction by using a structure-based *in silico* screen of a library of natural products, followed by *in vitro* testing in AlphaScreen assays. Two scaffolds were identified and one was progressed for further development as a new lead.

Resistance to HIV-1 Integrase Inhibitors [395]

The development of resistance to anti-HIV drugs by the HIV virus is a rapid phenomenon and is closely linked to the error-prone nature of HIV-1 RT and the lack of proof reading function [396, 397]. Patient compliance with medication regimes is also a factor in the development of resistance mutations and poor viral load suppression will enable the virus to develop such mutations [142, 398, 399]. In order to maintain the effectiveness of the HAART [400-402] therapy, it is often advisable to screen patients in order to select the most effective multi-drug HAART regime. Both genotypic [403] and phenotypic profiling have been reported [403, 404] in addition to a range of predictive modelling approaches [66, 405-407].

The extent of mutations reported for HIV-1 IN is extensive and has been reviewed previously [85, 141, 395, 408, 409]. The main resistance pathways against STIs involve the CCD of IN [102, 114, 161, 169, 410-413]. The three key acidic residues (D64, D116 and E152) are not affected by mutation, but a number of the amino acid residues that surround the active site are affected, with primary mutations including N155H, Q148K/R/H and Y143R/C [98, 414, 415].

The mutations to the residues around the catalytic triad are thought to either result in a conformational change to the catalytic site, or reduce the efficiency of viral DNA binding. The Q148H and N155H mutations induce conformational changes that increases the binding energy of the STI [410], whilst measurement of dissociation constants for IN-DNA complexes for raltegravir, elvitegravir and dolutegravir revealed that the mutations cause an increase in k_{off} for the STIs [408, 416].

3'-Processing

Many of the agents that have been evaluated to date have been shown to have an inhibitory activity against 3'-processing [330, 417] in addition to activity against the ST reaction but the field is still focused toward ST and allosteric inhibition of integrase.

Other Strategies to Inhibit IN

The nuclear import of proteins with molecular weights greater than 45kDa requires the use of a nuclear localisation signal (NLS) and associated nuclear pore complex (NPC) [418]. IN employs the nuclear import receptor, Impαβ to gain entry to the nucleus. Two compounds were identified *via* a high-throughput screening assay [419]; mifepristone specifically inhibited IN nuclear import and ivermectin which targets Impα/β-dependent transport of IN [419].

Non-Catalytic Activities of Integrase

Mutational studies of IN were the first indication that IN also performs a number of non-catalytic roles throughout the viral replication cycle and these functions are also thought to be critical for the viral replication cycle. Mutations with IN produce a vast array of phenotypic characteristics, IN mutations are divided into 2 groups depending on their effect of its catalytic activity; class I mutants have a direct effect on IN catalytic activity, whereas class II mutants disrupt virus replication but maintain a wild type level of catalytic activity. Class II mutants have been shown to affect reverse transcription, nuclear localisation and virus assembly and release.

IN mutants have been shown to block reverse transcription, leading to a loss of viral replication, IN and reverse transcriptase have been shown to both directly and indirectly interact with one another [201, 420-422]. The inhibition of reverse transcriptase *via* its interaction with IN is not directly related to its catalytic activity, as demonstrated by IN mutants that are defective of integration still actively synthesis viral DNA. The indirect IN interaction with reverse transcriptase may be due to a disruption of IN co-factor binding. However it has also been reported that a direct interaction between IN and reverse transcriptase can stimulate reverse transcription [423, 424].

IN has kayrophilic properties and several studies have identified potential IN NLS [425-429], however this signal is believed not to be a functional NLS, as IN fusion proteins which are >115kDa (corresponding to the size of an IN tetramer) do not localise to the nucleus [425]. More recent studies suggest that IN involvement in nuclear import is an indirect effect and is predominantly mediated *via* its interactions with cellular co-factors such as TRN-SR2 [295].

IN mutants have also been shown to cause defective HIV-1 virus assembly and release. The role of IN in virus partial assembly is further backed up by the ability of allosteric IN inhibitors to produce non-infectious virus particles. The mechanisms behind these defects remain largely unknown, although defective release is believed to involve the early activation of viral protease.

HIV-2 IN

HIV-2 is less widespread than HIV-1 being mostly confined to parts of Western Africa [430] and is less infective than HIV-1[431]. It does however present more of a problem for the clinician since it has a high degree of resistance to a number of the current anti-HIV drugs; it is resistant to all non-nucleotide reverse transcription inhibitors (NNRTIs) [432] and enfuvirtide, the fusion inhibitor [433]. It is also less sensitive to a number of the protease inhibitors [434]. The structure of HIV-2 IN has yet to be solved, however, phenotypic profiling of HIV-2 clinical isolates suggests that HIV-2 should have a similar susceptibility to IN inhibitors as HIV-1 and therefore offer the hope of treating individuals with HIV-2 [435].

ACKNOWLEDGEMENTS

The authors would like to thank the University of Sunderland for support.

CONFLICTS OF INTEREST

The authors confirm that this chapter contents have no conflict of interest.

REFERENCES

[1] Baltimore D. RNA-dependent DNA polymerase in virons of RNA tumor viruses. Nature 1970; 226: 1209-11.

[2] Tenim H, Mizutani S. RNA-dependent DNA polymerase in virons of Rous sarcoma virus. Nature 1970; 226: 1211-3.

[3] Hughes S, Shank P, Spector D, *et al.* Proviruses of avian sarcoma virus are terminally redundant, co-extensive with unintegrated linear DNA and integrated at many sites. Cell 1978; 15: 1397-410.

[4] Majors J, Varmus H. Nucleotide sequences at host-proviral junctions for mouse mammary tumour virus. Nature 1981; 289: 253-8.

[5] Grandgenett DP, Vora AC, Schiff RD. A 32,000-dalton nucleic acid-binding protein from avian retravirus cores possesses DNA endonulease activity. Virology 1978; 89: 119-32.

[6] Lightfoote M, Coligan J, Folks T, Fauci A, Martin M, Venkatesan S. Structural characterization of reverse transcriptase and endonuclease polypeptides of the acquired immunodeficiency syndrome retrovirus. J Virology 1986; 60: 771-5.

[7] Sherman P, Fyfe J. Human immunodeficiency virus integration protein expressed in *Escherichia coli* possesses selective DNA cleaving activity. Proc Natl Acad Sci USA 1990; 87: 5119-23.

[8] Dyda F, Hickman A, Jenkins T, Engelman A, Craigie R, Davies D. Crystal structure of the catalytic domain of HIV-1 integrase: similarity to other polynucleotidyl transferases. Science 1994; 266: 1981-6.

[9] Karageorgos L, Li P, Burrell C. Characterization of HIV replication complexes early after cell-to-cell infection. AIDS Res Hum Retroviruses 1993; 9(9): 817-23.

[10] Fassati A, Goff SP. Characterization of intracellular reverse transcription complexes of human immunodeficiency virus type 1. J Virol 2001; 75(8): 3626-35.

[11] Li M, Mizuuchi M, Burke T, Jr, Craigie R. Retroviral DNA integration: reaction pathway and critical intermediates. EMBO J 2006; 25: 1295-304.

[12] Wei SQ, Mizuuchi K, Craigie R. A large nucleoprotein assembly at the ends of the viral DNA mediates retroviral DNA integration. EMBO J 1997; 16(24): 7511-20.

[13] Wei SQ, Mizuuchi K, Craigie R. Footprints on the viral DNA ends in moloney murine leukemia virus preintegration complexes reflect a specific association with integrase. Proceedings of the National Academy of Sciences of the United States of America 1998; 95(18): 10535-40.

[14] Chen H, Wei SQ, Engelman A. Multiple Integrase Functions Are Required to Form the Native Structure of the Human Immunodeficiency Virus Type I Intasome. J Biol Chem 1999; 274: 17358-64.

[15] Chen H, Engelman A. Asymmetric processing of human immunodeficiency virus type 1 cDNA *in vivo*: implications for functional end coupling during the chemical steps of DNA transposition. Molecular and cellular biology 2001; 21(20): 6758-67.

[16] Bukrinsky M, Sharova N, Dempsey M, *et al.* Active nuclear import of human immunodeficency virus type 1 preintegration complexes. Proc Natl Acad Sci USA 1992; 89(14): 6580-4.

[17] Katz R, Greger J, Boimel P, Skalka A. Human immunodeficieny virus type 1 DNA nuclear import and integration are mitosis independent in cycling cells. J Virol 2003; 77(24): 13412-7.

[18] Rice P, Baker T. Comparative architecture of transposase and integrase complexes. Nat Struct Biol 2001; 8(5): 302-7.

[19] Nesmelova I, Hackett P. DDE transposases: Structural similarity and diversity. Adv Drug Deliv Rev 2010; 62(12): 1187-95.

[20] Nowotny M. Retroviral integrase superfamily: the structural perspective. EMBO reports 2009; 10: 144-51.

[21] Craig N. Unity in transposition reactions. Science 1995; 270(5234): 253-4.

[22] Curcio MJ, Derbyshire KM. The outs and ins of transposition: from mu to kangaroo. Nature reviews Molecular cell biology 2003; 4(11): 865-77.

[23] Davis D, Goryshin I, Reznikoff W, Rayment I. Three-dimensional structure of the Tn5 synaptic complex transposition intermediate. Science 2000; 289(5476): 77-85.

[24] Richardson J, Colloms S, Finnegan D, Wilkinshaw M. Molecular architecture of the Mos1 paired-end complex: the structural basis of DNA transposition in a eukaryote. Cell 2009; 138(6): 1096-108.

[25] Sakai J, Chalmers RM, Kleckner N. Identification and characterization of a pre-cleavage synaptic complex that is an early intermediate in Tn10 transposition. EMBO J 1995; 14(17): 4374-83.

[26] Li I, Krishnan L, P C, Engelman A. Structural biology of retroviral DNA integration. Virology 2011; 411(2): 194-205.

[27] Cai M, Zheng R, Caffrey M, Craigie R, Clore GM, Gronenborn AM. Solution structure of the N-terminal zinc binding domain of HIV-1 integrase. Nat Struct Biol 1997; 4(7): 567-77.

[28] Eijkelenboom AP, van den Ent FM, Vos A, Doreleijers JF, Hard K, Tullius TD, *et al.* The solution structure of the amino-terminal HHCC domain of HIV-2 integrase: a three-helix bundle stabilized by zinc. Current biology : CB 1997; 7(10): 739-46.

[29] Kulkosky J, Jones KS, Katz RA, Mack JP, Skalka AM. Residues critical for retroviral integrative recombination in a region that is highly conserved among retroviral/retrotransposon integrases and bacterial insertion sequence transposases. Molecular and cellular biology 1992; 12(5): 2331-8.

[30] Engelman A, Craigie R. Identification of conserved amino acid residues critical for human immunodeficiency virus type 1 integrase function *in vitro*. J Virol 1992; 66(11): 6361-9.
[31] Nowotny M, Gaidamakov SA, Crouch RJ, Yang W. Crystal structures of RNase H bound to an RNA/DNA hybrid: substrate specificity and metal-dependent catalysis. Cell 2005; 121(7): 1005-16.
[32] Eijkelenboom AP, Lutzke RA, Boelens R, Plasterk RH, Kaptein R, Hard K. The DNA-binding domain of HIV-1 integrase has an SH3-like fold. Nat Struct Biol 1995; 2(9): 807-10.
[33] Lodi PJ, Ernst JA, Kuszewski J, Hickman AB, Engelman A, Craigie R, *et al.* Solution structure of the DNA binding domain of HIV-1 integrase. Biochemistry 1995; 34(31): 9826-33.
[34] Craigie R. The molecular biology of HIV integrase. Future virology 2012; 7(7): 679-86.
[35] Engelman A, Mizuuchi M, Craigie R. HIV-1 DNA integration: mechanism of viral DNA cleavage and DNA strand transfer. Cell 1991; 67(6): 1211-21.
[36] Mizuuchi M. Polynucleotidyl transfer reactions in transpositional DNA recombination. J Biol Chem 1992; 267(30): 21273-6.
[37] Yang W, Lee J, Nowotny M. Making and breaking nucleic acids: Two Mg^{2+}- ion catalysis and substance specificity. Molecular Cell 2006; 22: 5-13.
[38] Hare S, Maertens G, P C. 3-processing and strand transfer catalysed by retroviral integrase in crystallo. EMBO J 2012; 31(13).
[39] Aiyar A, Hindmarsh P, Skalka AM, Leis J. Concerted integration of linear retroviral DNA by the avian sarcoma virus integrase *in vitro*: dependence on both long terminal repeat termini. J Virol 1996; 70(6): 3571-80.
[40] Sinha S, Grandgenett D. Recombinant human immunodeficiency virus type 1 integrase exhibits a capacity for full-site integration *in vitro* that is comparable to that of purified preintegration complexes from virus-infected cells. J Virol 2005; 79(13): 8208-16.
[41] Pandey K, Bera S, Grandgenett D. The HIV-1 integrase monomer induces a specific interaction with LTR DNA for concerted integration Biochemistry 2011; 50: 9788-96.
[42] Li M, Craigie R. Processing of viral DNA ends channels the HIV-1 integration reaction to concerted integration. J Biol Chem 2005; 280(32): 29334-9.
[43] Faure A, Calmels C, Desjobert C, *et al.* HIV-1 integrase crosslinked oligomers are active *in vitro*. Nucleic Acids Res 2005; 33(3): 977-86.
[44] Bera S, Pandey K, Vora A, Grandgenett D. Molecular interactions between HIV-1 integrase and the two viral DNA ends within the synaptic complex that mediates concerted integration. J Mol Biol 2009; 389: 183-98.
[45] Pandey K, Sinha S, Grandgenett D. Transcriptional coactivator LEDGF/p75 modulates human immunodeficiency virus type 1 integrase-mediated concerted integration. J Virol 2007; 81(8): 3969-79.
[46] Hare S, Gupta S, Valkov E, Engelman A, Cherepanov P. retroviral intasome assembly and inhibition of DNA strand transfer. Nature 2010; 464: 232-6.
[47] Hare S, Shun M, Gupta S, Valkov E, Engelman A, P C. A novel co-crystal structure affords the design of gain-of-function lentiviral integrase mutants in the presnece of modified PSIP1/LEDGF/p75. PLoS Pathog 2009; 5(1): e10000259.
[48] Guiot E, Carayon K, Delelis O, *et al.* Relationship between the oligomeric status of HIV-1 integrase on DNA and enzymatic activity. J Biol Chem 2006; 281(22): 22707-19.
[49] Chow S, Vincent K, Ellison V, Brown P. Reversal of integration and DNA splicing mediated by integrase of human immunodeficiency virus. Science 1992; 255(5045): 723-6.

[50] Gerton JL, Brown PO. The core domain of HIV-1 integrase recognizes key features of its DNA substrates. J Biol Chem 1997; 272(41): 25809-15.

[51] Laboulais C, Deprez E, Leh H, Mouscadet JF, Brochon JC, Le Bret M. HIV-1 integrase catalytic core: molecular dynamics and simulated fluorescence decays. Biophysical journal 2001; 81(1): 473-89.

[52] Asante-Appiah E, Skalka A. HIV-1 integrase: structural organization, conformational changes, and catalysis. Adv Virus Res 1999; 52: 351-69.

[53] Grobler J, Stillmock K, Binghua H, *et al.* Diketo acid inhibitor mechanism and HIV-1 integrase: Implications for metal binding in the active site of phosphotransferase enzymes. Proc Natl Acad Sci USA 2002; 99: 6661-6.

[54] Bujacz G, Alexandratost J, Wlodawer A, *et al.* Binding of different divalent cations to the active site of avian sarcoma virus integrase and their effects on enzymatic activity. J Biol Chem 1997; 272(29): 18161-8.

[55] Bushman F, Engelman A, Palmer I, Wingfield P, Craigie R. Domains of the integrase protein of human immunodeficiency virus type 1 responsible for polynucleotidyl transfer and zinc binding. Proc Natl Acad Sci USA 1993; 90: 3428-32.

[56] Valkov E, Gupta S, Hare S, *et al.* Functional and structural characterization of the integrase from the prototype foamy virus. Nucleic Acids Res 2009; 37: 243-55.

[57] Goldgur Y, Dyda F, Hickman A, *et al.* Three new structures of the core domain of HIV-1 integrase: an active site that binds magnesium. Proc Natl Acad Sci USA 1998; 95: 9150-4.

[58] Maignan S, Guilloteau J, Zhou-Li Q, Clement-Mella C, Mikol V. Crystal structures of the catalytic core domain of HIV-1 integrase free and complexed with its metal cofactor: high level of similarity of the active site with other viral integrases. J Mol Biol 1998; 282: 359-68.

[59] Maertens G, Hare S, Cherepanov P. The mechanism of retroviral integration through x-ray structures of its key intermediates. Nature 2010; 468: 326-9.

[60] Steitz T. DNA polymerases: structural diversity and common mechanisms. J Biol Chem 1999; 274: 17395-8.

[61] Beese L, Steitz T. Structural basis for the 3'-5' exonuclease activity of *Escherichia coli* DNA polymerase I: a two metal ion mechanism. EMBO J 1991; 10: 25-33.

[62] Vranken D, Weiss G. Introduction to bioorganic chemistry and chemical biology. 1st ed. New York: Garland Science; 2013.

[63] Gerton J, Herschlag D, Brown P. Stereospecificity of reactions catalysed by HIV-1 integrase. J Biol Chem 1999; 274(47): 33480-7.

[64] Li M, Jurado K, Lin LR, Engelman A, Craigie R. Engineered hyperactive integrase for concerted HIV-1 DNA integration. PLOS One 2014; 9(8): e105078.

[65] Gupta K, Curtis JE, Krueger S, Hwang Y, Cherepanov P, Bushman FD, *et al.* Solution conformations of prototype foamy virus integrase and its stable synaptic complex with U5 viral DNA. Structure 2012; 20(11): 1918-28.

[66] Johnson B, Metifiot M, Ferris A, Pommier Y, Hughes S. A homolgy model of HIV-1 integrase and anlysis of mutations designed to test the model. J Mol Biol 2013; 425: 2133-46.

[67] Wu X, Li Y, Crise B, Burgess SM, Munroe DJ. Weak palindromic consensus sequences are a common feature found at the integration target sites of many retroviruses. J Virol 2005; 79(8): 5211-4.

[68] Wu X, Li Y, Crise B, Burgess SM. Transcription start regions in the human genome are favored targets for MLV integration. Science 2003; 300(5626): 1749-51.
[69] Narezkina A, Taganov KD, Litwin S, Stoyanova R, Hayashi J, Seeger C, *et al.* Genome-wide analyses of avian sarcoma virus integration sites. J Virol 2004; 78(21): 11656-63.
[70] Engelman A, Cherepanov P. The lentiviral integrase binding protein LEDGF/p75 and HIV-1 replication. PLoS Pathog 2008; 4(3): e1000046.
[71] Poeschla EM. Integrase, LEDGF/p75 and HIV replication. Cellular and molecular life sciences : CMLS 2008; 65(9): 1403-24.
[72] Cherepanov P, Maertens G, Proost P, Devreese B, Van Beeumen J, Engelborghs Y, *et al.* HIV-1 integrase forms stable tetramers and associates with LEDGF/p75 protein in human cells. J Biol Chem 2003; 278(1): 372-81.
[73] Turlure F, Devroe E, Silver PA, Engelman A. Human cell proteins and human immunodeficiency virus DNA integration. Frontiers in bioscience : a journal and virtual library 2004; 9: 3187-208.
[74] Llano M, Vanegas M, Fregoso O, Saenz D, Chung S, Peretz M, *et al.* LEDGF/p75 determines cellular trafficking of diverse lentiviral but not murine oncoretroviral integrase proteins and is a component of functional lentiviral preintegration complexes. J Virol 2004; 78(17): 9524-37.
[75] Emiliani S, Mousnier A, Busschots K, Maroun M, Van Maele B, Tempe D, *et al.* Integrase mutants defective for interaction with LEDGF/p75 are impaired in chromosome tethering and HIV-1 replication. J Biol Chem 2005; 280(27): 25517-23.
[76] Busschots K, Vercammen J, Emiliani S, Benarous R, Engelborghs Y, Christ F, *et al.* The interaction of LEDGF/p75 with integrase is lentivirus-specific and promotes DNA binding. J Biol Chem 2005; 280(18): 17841-7.
[77] Ciuffi A, Llano M, Poeschla E, Hoffmann C, Leipzig J, Shinn P, *et al.* A role for LEDGF/p75 in targeting HIV DNA integration. Nat Med 2005; 11(12): 1287-9.
[78] Debyser Z, Cherepanov P, Maele B, De Clercq E, Witvrouw M. In search of authentic inhibitors of HIV-1 integration. Antiviral Chemistry & Chemotherapy 2002; 13: 1-15.
[79] Di Santo R. Inhibiting the HIV integration process: past, present, and the future. J Med Chem 2014; 57: 539-66.
[80] Marchand C, Maddali K, Metifiot M, Pommier Y. HIV-1 IN inhibitors: 2010 Update and perspectives. Curr Top Med Chem 2009; 9(11): 1016-37.
[81] Malet I, Calvez V, Marcelin A. The future of integrase inhibitors of HIV-1. Current Opinion in Virology 2012; 2: 580-7.
[82] Demeulemeester J, Christ F, Maeter M, Debyser Z. Fueling HIV-1 integrase drug design with structural insights. Drug Discovery Today: Technologies 2012; 9(3): e205-e12.
[83] Ramkumar K, Serrao E, Odde S, Neamati N. HIV-1 Integrase Inhibitors: 2007-2008 Update. Medicinal Research Reviews 2010; 30(6): 890-54.
[84] Nguyen B, Isaacs R, Teppler, *et al.* Raltegravir: the first HIV-1 integrase strand transfer inhibitor in the armamentarium. Ann NY Acad Sci 2011; 1222: 83-9.
[85] Lampiris H. Elvitegravir: a once-daily, boosted, HIV-1 integrase inhibitor. Expert Rev Anti Infect Ther 2012; 10(1): 13-20.
[86] Schrijvers R, Debyser Z. Combinational therapies for HIV: a focus on EVG/COBI/FTC/TDF. Expert Opin Pharmacother 2012; 13(13): 1969-83.
[87] Wu G, Abraham T, Saad N. Dolutegravir for the treatment of adult patients with HIV-1 infection. Expert Rev Anti Infect Ther 2014; 12(5): 535-44.

[88] Serrao E, Odde S, Ramkumar K, Neamati N. Raltegravir, elvitegravir, and metoogravir: the birth of "me-too" HIV-1 integrase inhibitors. Retrovirology 2009; 6(25).
[89] Maga G, Veljkovic N, Crespan E, *et al.* New *in silico* and conventional *in vitro* approaches to advance HIV drug discovery and design. Expert Opin Drug Discov 2013; 8(1): 83-92.
[90] Bhatt H, Patel P, Pannecouque C. Discovery of HIV-1 integrase inhibitors: pharmacophore mapping, virtual screening, molecular docking, synthesis, and biological evaluation. Chem Biol Drug Des 2014; 83: 154-66.
[91] Reddy K, Singh S. Combined ligand and structure-based approaches on HIV-1 integrase strand transfer inhibitors. Chemico-Biological Interactions 2014; 218: 71-81.
[92] Espeseth A, Felock P, Wolfe A, *et al.* HIV-1 integrase inhibitors that compete with the target DNA substrate define a unique strand transfer conformation for integrase. Proc Natl Acad Sci USA 2000; 97: 11244-9.
[93] Pandey K, Bera S, Zahm J, *et al.* Inhibition of human immunodeficiency virus type-1 concerted integration by strand transfer inhibitors which recognize a transient structural intermediate. J Virol 2007; 81: 12189-99.
[94] Dicker I, Samanta H, Li A, *et al.* Changes to the HIV long terminal repeat and to HIV integrase differentially impact HIV integrase assembly, activity, and the binding of strand trnasfer inhibitors. J Biol Chem 2008; 282: 31186-96.
[95] Johnson A, Santos W, Pais G, *et al.* Integration requires a specific interaction of the donor DNA terminal 5'-cytosine with glutamine 148 of the HIV-1 integrase flexible loop J Biol Chem 2006; 281: 461-7.
[96] Pandey K, Bera S, Vora A, Grandgenett D. Physical trapping of HIV-1 synaptic complex by different structural classes of integrase strand transfer inhibitors. Biochemistry 2010; 49: 8376-87.
[97] Pandey K, Bera S, Korolev S, *et al.* Rous sarcoma virus synaptic complex capable of concerted integration is kinetically trapped by human immunodeficiency virus integrase strand transfer inhibitors. J Biol Chem 2014; 289(28): 19648-58.
[98] Pommier Y, Johnson AA, Marchand C. Integrase inhibitors to treat HIV/AIDS. Nat Rev Drug Discov 2005; 4: 236-48.
[99] Pommier Y, Marchand C. Interfacial inhibitors: targeting macromolecular complexes. Nat Rev Drug Discov 2012; 11: 25-36.
[100] Bera S, Pandey K, Vora A, Grandgenett D. HIV-1 integrase strand transfer inhibitors stabilize an integrase-single blunt-ended DNA complex. J Mol Biol 2011; 410: 831-46.
[101] Langley D, Samanta H, Lin Z, *et al.* The terminal (catalytic) adenosine of HIV LTR controls the kinetics of binding and dissociation of HIV integrase strand transfer inhibitors. Biochemistry 2008; 47: 13481-8.
[102] Garvey E, Schwartz B, Gartland M, *et al.* Potent inhibitors of HIV-1 integrase display a two-step, slow binding inhibition mechanism which is absent in drug resistant T661/M154I mutant. Biochemistry 2009; 48: 1644-53.
[103] Kawasuji T, Fuji M, Yoshinaga T, Sato A, Fujiwara T, Kiyama R. A platform for designing HIV integrase inhibitors. Part 2. A two-metal binding model as a potential mechanism of HIV integrase inhibitors. Bioorg Med Chem 2006; 14: 8420-9.
[104] Hazuda D, Young S. Inhibitors of human immunodeficiency virus integration. In: De Clercq E, editor. Advances in antiviral drug design. 4. first ed. Amsterdam: Elsevier; 2004. p. 63-77.
[105] Egbertson M, Anthony N, Summa V. HIV Integrase Inhibitors: From Diketo acids to heterocyclic Templates: History of HIV Integrase Medicinal Chemistry at Merck West Point and Merck Rome (IRBM) Leading to Discovery of Raltegravir. In: Neamati N,

editor. HIV-1 Integrase - mechanism and inhibitor design. Wiley Series on Drug Discovery and Development. 1st ed. New Jersey: John Wiley & Sons; 2011. p. 197-230.

[106] Savarino A. A historical sketch of the discovery and development of HIV-1 integrase inhibitors. Expert Opin Investig Drugs 2006; 15(12): 1507-22.

[107] Hazuda D, Felock P, Witmer M, *et al.* Inhibitors of Strand Transfer That Prevent Integration and Inhibit HIV-1 Replication in Cells. Science 2000; 287(5453): 646-50.

[108] Kawasuji T, Yoshinaga T, Sato A, *et al.* A platform for designing HIV integrase inhibitors. Part 1: 2-Hydroxy-3-heteroaryl acrylic acid derivatives as novel HIV integrase inhibitor and modeling of hydrophilic and hydrophobic pharmacophores. Bioorg Med Chem 2006; 14: 8430-45.

[109] Selnick H, Hazuda D, Egbertson M, Guare J, Wai J, Young S, *et al.* inventorsPreparation of nitrogen-containing 4-heteroaryl-2,4-dioxobutyric acids useful as HIV integrase inhibitors1999.

[110] Marchand C, Zhang X, Pais G. Structural Determinants for HIV-1 Integrase Inhibition by β-Diketo Acids. J Biol Chem 2002; 277(15): 12596-603.

[111] Sykes P. A guidebook to mechanism in organic chemistry. 6th ed. Harlow, England: Longman; 1996. 416 p.

[112] Goldgur Y, Craigie R, Cohen G. Structure of the HIV-1 integrase catalytic domain complexed with an inhibitor: A platform for antiviral drug design. Proc Natl Acad Sci USA 1999; 96(23): 13040-3.

[113] Billich A. S-1360 Shionogi-GlaxoSmithKline. Curr Opin Investig Drugs 2003; 4: 206-9.

[114] Fikkert V, Van Maele B, Vercammen J, *et al.* Development of resistance against diketo derivatives of human immunodeficiency virus type 1 by progressive accumulation of integrase mutations. J Virol 2003; 77: 11459-70.

[115] Liao C, Nicklaus M. Tautomerism and Magnesium Chelation of HIV-1 Integrase Inhibitors: A Theoretical Study. ChemMedChem 2010; 5(7): 1053-66.

[116] Sechi M, Massimiliano D, Dallocchio R, *et al.* Design and Synthesis of Novel Indole β-Diketo Acid Derivatives as HIV-1 Integrase Inhibitors. J Med Chem 2004; 47(21): 5298-310.

[117] Sechi M, Bacchi A, Carcelli M, *et al.* From Ligand to Complexes: Inhibition of Human Immunodeficiency virus type 1 Integrase by β-Diketo Acid Metal Complexes. J Med Chem 2006; 49(14): 4248-60.

[118] Maurin C, Bailly F, Cotelle P. Improved preparation and structural investigation of 4-aryl-4-oxo-2-hydroxy-2-butenoic acids and methyl esters. Tetrahedron 2004; 60: 6479-86.

[119] Carcelli M, Rogolino D, Sechi M, *et al.* Antiretroviral activity of metal-chelating HIV-1 integrase inhibitors. European Journal of Medicinal Chemistry 2014; 83: 594-600.

[120] Clark D, Egbertson M, Embrey M, Fisher T, Guare J, Langford H, *et al.* inventors; Merck & Co. and Tularik, Inc, assignee. 1-(aromatic- or heteroaromatic-substituted)-3-(heteroaromatic substituted)-1,3-propanediones and uses thereof2001.

[121] Fujishita T, Sato A, Yoshinaga T, inventors; Fujishita, T,Sato, A, Yoshinaga, T, Shionogi & Co., Japan, assignee. Preparation of aromatic heterocycle compounds having HIV integrase inhibiting activities2000.

[122] Uenaka M, Kawata K, Nagai M, Endoh T, inventors; Uenaka, M, Kawata, K, Nagai, M, Endoh, T, Shionogi & Co., Japan, assignee. Novel processes for the preparation of substituted propenone derivatives.2000.

[123] Boulton J, McKillop A, editors. Pyridines and their Benzo Derivatives: (iii) Reactivity of Substituents. 1st ed. New York: Pergamon Press; 1984.
[124] Prachayasittikul V, Prachayasittikul S, Ruchirawat S, Prachayasittikul V. 8-Hydroxyquinolines: a review of their metal chelating properties and medicinal applications. Drug Design, Development and Therapy 2013; 7: 1157-78.
[125] Anthony N, Gomez R, Young S, Egbertson M, Wai J, Zhang X, *et al.* inventors; Merck & Co, assignee. Aza- and polyaza-naphthalenyl carboxamides useful as hiv integrase inhibitors2002.
[126] Hazuda D, Anthony N, Gomez R, *et al.* A naphthyridine carboxamide provides evidence for discordant resistance between mechanistically identical inhibitors of HIV-1 integrase. Proc Natl Acad Sci USA 2004; 101: 11233-8.
[127] Cotelle P. New hexahydrodiazocino-napthyridine triones as HIV-1 integrase inhibitors: W02008048538 A1. Expert Opin Ther Patents 2009; 19(1): 87-93.
[128] Johns B, Svolto A. Advances in two metal-metal chelation inhibitors of HIV integrase. Expert Opin Ther Patents 2008; 18(11): 1225-37.
[129] Garvey E, Johns B, Gartland M, *et al.* The naphthyridinone GSK364735 is a novel, potent human immunodeficiency virus type 1 integrase inhibitor and antiretroviral. Antimicrob Agents Chemother 2008; 52(3): 901-8.
[130] Johns B, Weatherfield J, Allen S, *et al.* The use of oxadiazole and triazole substituted naphthyridines as HIV-1 integrase inhibitors. Part 1: establishing the pharmacophore. Bioorg Med Chem Lett 2009; 19(6): 1802-6.
[131] Johns B, Weatherfield J, Allen S, *et al.* 1,3,4-oxadiazole substituted naphthyridines as HIV-1 integrase inhibitors. Part 2: SAR of the C5 position. Bioorg Med Chem Lett 2009; 19(6): 1807-10.
[132] Pace P, Nizi E, Pacini B, *et al.* The monoethyl ester of meconic acid is an active site inhibitor of HCV NS5B RNA-dependent RNA polymerase. Bioorg Med Chem Lett 2004; 14(12): 3257-61.
[133] Summa V, Petrocchi A, Pace P, *et al.* Discovery of a,g-diketo acids as potent selective and reversible inhibitors of hepatitis C virus NS5b RNA-dependent RNA polymerase. J Med Chem 2004; 47(1): 14-7.
[134] Guare J, Wai J, Gomez R, *et al.* A series of 5-aminosubstituted 4-fluorobenzyl-8-hydroxy-[1,6]naphthyridine-7-carboxamide HIV-1 integrase inhibitors. Bioorg Med Chem Lett 2006; 16: 2900-4.
[135] Pendri A, Meanwell N, Peese K, Walker M. New first and second generation inhibitors of human immunodeficieny virus-1 integrase. Expert Opin Ther Patents 2011; 21(8): 1173-89.
[136] Summa V, Petrocchi A, Matassa V, *et al.* 4,5-Dihydroxypyrimidine carboxamides and N-alkyl-5-hydroxypyrimidine carboxamides are potent, selective HIV integrase inhibitors with good pharmacokinetic profiles in preclinical species. J Med Chem 2006; 49: 6646-9.
[137] Pace P, Di Francesco M, Gardelli C, *et al.* Dihydroxypyrimidine-4-carboxamides as novel potent and selective HIV integrase inhibitors. J Med Chem 2007; 50: 2225-39.
[138] Gardelli C, Nizi E, Muraglia E, *et al.* Discovery and synthesis of HIV integrase inhibitors: Development of potent and orally bioavailable N-methyl pyrimidones. J Med Chem 2007; 50: 4953-75.
[139] Summa V, Petrocchi A, Scarpelli R, *et al.* Discovery of ISENTRESSTM a potent, selective orally bioavailable HIV-integrase inhibitor for the treatment of HIV-AIDS infection. J Med Chem 2008; 51(18): 5843-55.

[140] Shafer R. Rationale and Uses of a Public HIV Drug-Resistance Database. Journal of Infectious Diseases 2006; 198(Suppl 1): S51-8.

[141] Ceccherini-Silberstein F, Malet I, D'Arrigo R, Antinori A, Marcelin A, Perno C-F. Characterization and structural Analysis of HIV-1 Integrase Conservation. AIDS Rev 2009; 11: 17-29.

[142] Blanco J-L, Varghese V, Rhee S-Y, Gatell J, Shafer R. HIV-1 integrase inhibitor resistance and its clinical implications. Journal of Infectious Diseases 2011; 203: 1204-14.

[143] Grinsztejn B, Nguyen B, Katlama C, *et al.* Safety and efficacy of the HIV-1 integrase inhibitor raltegravir (MK-0518) in treatment-experiecned patients with multidrug-resistant virus: a phase II randomised controlled trial. Lancet 2007; 369: 1261-9.

[144] Zhang D, Debnath B, Yu S, *et al.* Design and discovery of 5-hydroxy-6-oxo-1,6-dihydropyrimidine-4-carboxamide inhibitors of HIV-1 integrase. Bioorganic & Medicinal Chemistry 2014.

[145] Yu S, Sanchez T, Liu Y, Yin Y, Neamati N, Zhao G. Design and synthesis of novel pyrimidone analogues as HIV-1 integrase inhibitors. Bioorg Med Chem Lett 2013; 23: 6134-7.

[146] Di Francesco M, Pace P, Fiore F, *et al.* Development of 2-tbutyl-N-methyl pyrimidones as potent inhibitors of HIV integrase. Bioorg Med Chem Lett 2008; 18(8): 2709-13.

[147] Wang Z, Tang J, Salomon C, Dreis C, Vince R. Pharmacophore and structure-activity relationships of integrase inhibition within a dual inhibitor scaffold of HIV reverse transcriptase and integrase. Bioorg Med Chem Lett 2010; 18: 4202-11.

[148] Ferrara M, Fiore F, Summa V, Gardelli C. Development of 2-pyrrolidinyl-N-methyl pyrimidones as potent and orally bioavailable HIV integrase inhibitors. Bioorg Med Chem Lett 2010; 20: 5031-4.

[149] Tang J, Maddali K, Metifiot Y, *et al.* 3-Hydroxypyrimidine-2,4-diones as an inhibitor scaffold of HIV integrase. J Med Chem 2011; 54: 2282-92.

[150] Tang J, Maddali K, Dreis C, *et al.* 6-Benzoyl-3-hydroxypyrimidine-2,4-diones as dual inhibitors of HIV reverse transcriptase and integrase. Bioorg Med Chem Lett 2011; 21: 2400-2.

[151] Lea G, Vandegraaffa D, Rhodesa E, *et al.* Discovery of potent HIV integrase inhibitors active against raltegravir resitant viruses. Bioorg Med Chem Lett 2010; 20: 5013-8.

[152] Tang J, Kasthuraiah M, Dreis C, *et al.* N-3 hydroxylation of pyrimidine-2,4-diones yields dual inhibitors of HIV reverse transcriptase and integrase. ACS Med Chem Lett 2010; 2: 63-7.

[153] Seo B, Uchil V, Okello M, *et al.* Discovery of a potent HIV integrase inhibitor that leads to a prodrug with significant anti-HIV activity. ACS Med Chem Lett 2011; 2: 877-81.

[154] Okello M, Mishra S, Nishonov M, Nair V. Notable difference in anti-HIV activity of integrase inhibitors as a consequence of geometric and enantiometric configurations. Bioorg Med Chem Lett 2013; 23: 4112-6.

[155] Shinkai H, Sato M, Matsuzaki Y. Elvitegravir: novel quinolone HIV-1 integrase strand transfer inhibitor. In: Neamati N, editor. HIV-1 Integrase: mechanism and inhibitor design. Wiley series on drug discovery and development. 1st ed. New Jersey: John Wiley & Sons; 2011. p. 231-8.

[156] Marchand C, Johnson AA, Karki R, *et al.* Metal-dependent inhibition of HIV-1 integrase by β-diketo acids and resistance of the soluble double mutant (F185K/C280S). Mol Pharmacol 2003; 64: 600-9.

[157] Oversteegen L, Shah M, Rovini H. HIV combination products. Nature reviews drug discovery 2007; 6: 951-2.

[158] Larson K, Wang K, Delille C, Otofokun I, Acosta E. Pharmacokinetic enhancers in HIV therapeutics. Clin Pharmacokin [Internet]. 2014 16th September.

[159] Zhao X, Smith S, Metifiot M, *et al.* 4-Amino-1-hydroxy-2-oxo-1,8-naphthyridine-containing compounds having high antiviral potency against cells harboring raltegravir-resistant integrase mutants. J Med Chem 2014; 57: 1573-82.

[160] Zhao X, Smith S, Metifiot M, *et al.* 4-Amino-1-hydroxy-2-oxo-1,8-naphthyridine-containing compounds having high potency against raltegravir-resistant integrase mutants of HIV-1. J Med Chem 2014; 57: 5190-202.

[161] Metifiot M, Johnson B, Smith S, *et al.* MK-0536 inhibits HIV-1 integrases resistant to raltegravir. Antimicrob Agents Chemother 2011; 55(11): 5127-33.

[162] Desai M, Meanwell N, editors. Successful Strategies for the Discovery of Antiviral Drugs. 1st ed: Royal Society of Chemistry; 2013.

[163] Kobayashi M, Yoshinaga T, Seki C, *et al. In Vitro* Antiretroviral Properties of S/GSK1349572, a Next-Generation HIV Integrase Inhibitor. Antimicrob Agents Chemother 2011; 55(2): 813-21.

[164] Egbertson M, Moritz J, Melamed J, *et al.* A potent and orally active HIV-1 integrase inhibitor. Bioorg Med Chem Lett 2007; 17(5): 1392-8.

[165] Boros E, Edwards S, Foster M, *et al.* Synthesis and Antiviral Activity of 7-Benzyl-4-hydroxy-1,5-naphthyridin-2(1H)-one HIV Integrase Inhibitors. J Med Chem 2009; 52(9): 2754-61.

[166] Krishnan L, Li X, Naraharisetty L, Hare S, Cherepanov P, Engelman A. Structure-based modeling of the functional HIV-1 intasome and its inhibition. Proc Natl Acad Sci USA 2010; 107(36): 15910-5.

[167] Agrawal A, DeSoto J, Fullagar J, *et al.* Probing chelation motifs in HIV integrase inhibitors. Proc Natl Acad Sci USA 2012; 109(7): 2251-6.

[168] Kawasuji T, Johns B, Yoshida T, *et al.* Carbamoyl Pyridone HIV-1 Integrase Inhibitors. 1. Molecular Design and Establishment of an Advanced Two-Metal Binding Pharmacophore. J Med Chem 2012; 55(20): 8735-44.

[169] Marinello J, Marchand C, Mott B, Bain A, Thomas C, Pommier Y. Comparison of raltegravir and elvitegravir on HIV-1 integrase catalytic reactions and on a series of drug-resistant integrase mutants. Biochemistry 2008; 47(36): 9345-54.

[170] Jarmy G, Heinelein M, Weissbrich B, Jassoy C, Rethwilm A. Phenotypic analysis of the sensitivity of HIV-1 to inhibitors of the reverse transcriptase, protease, and integrase using a self-inactivating virus vector system. J Med Virol 2001; 64(3): 223-31.

[171] Min S, Sloan L, DeJesus E, *et al.* Antiviral activity, safety, and pharmacokinetics/pharmacodynamics of dolutegravir as 10-day monotherapy in HIV-1-infected adults. AIDS Res Hum Retroviruses 2011; 25(14): 1737-45.

[172] Dolgin E. Long-acting HIV drugs advanced to overcome adherence challenge. Nature Medicine 2014; 20(4): 323-4.

[173] Spreen W, Margolis D, Pottage Jr J. Long-acting injectable antiretrovirals for HIV treatment and prevention. Curr Opin HIV AIDS 2013; 8: 565-71.

[174] Study to evaluate the safety tolerability and acceptability of long acting injections of the human immunodeficiency virus (HIV) integrase inhibitor, GSK1265744, in HIV uninfected men (ECLAIR) [Internet]. US. National Institutes of Health. 2014 [cited 25 August 2014].

[175] Fardis M, Jin H, Chen X, *et al.* Conformationally constrained tricyclic HIV integrase inhibitors. In: Neamati N, editor. HIV-1 intgerase: Mechanism and Inhibitor design. Wiley series on drug discovery and development. 1st ed. New Jersey: John Wiley & Sons; 2011. p. 239-54.
[176] Cherepanov P, Ambrosio A, Rahman S, Ellenberger T, Engelman A. Structural basis for the recognition between HIV-1 integrase and transcriptional cofactor p75. Proc Natl Acad Sci USA 2005; 102(48): 17308-13.
[177] Abdel-Magid A. HIV integrase inhibitors for treatment of HIV infections and AIDS. ACS Med Chem Lett 2014; 5: 102-3.
[178] Zhao X, Semenova E, Vu B, *et al.* 2,3-Dihydro-6,7-dihydroxy-1H-isoindol-1-one based HIV-1 integrase inhibitors. J Med Chem 2008; 51: 251-9.
[179] Zhao X, Maddali K, Vu B, *et al.* Examination of halogen substituent effects on HIV-1 integrase inhibitors derived from 2,3-dihydro-6,7-dihydroxy-1H-isoindol-1-ones and 4,5-dihydroxy-1H-isoindole-1,3(2H)-diones. Bioorg Med Chem Lett 2009; 19: 2714-7.
[180] Mathieu M, Maddali K, Johnson B, *et al.* Activities, crystal structure, and molecular dynamics of dihydro-1H-isoindole derivatives, inhibitors of HIV-1 integrase. ACS Chem Biol 2013; 8: 209-17.
[181] Plewe M, Butler S, Dress K, *et al.* Azaindole hydroxamic acids are potent HIV-1 integrase inhibitors. J Med Chem 2009; 52: 7211-9.
[182] Langer T, Hoffmann R, editors. Pharmacophores and pharmacophore searches. 1st ed. Weinheim, Germany: Wiley-VCH; 2006.
[183] Dayam R, Al-Mawsawi L, Zawahir Z, Witvrouw M, Debyser Z, Neamati N. Quinolone 3-carboxylic acid pharmacophore: design of second generation HIV-1 integrase inhibitors. J Med Chem 2008; 51: 1136-44.
[184] Tintori C, Manetti N, Veljkovic N, *et al.* Novel Virtual Screening Protocol Based on the Combined Use of Molecular Modeling and Electron-Ion Interaction Potential Techniques To Design HIV-1 Integrase Inhibitors. J Chem Inf Model 2007; 47: 1536-44.
[185] Tintori C, Corradi V, Magnani M, Manetti F, Botta M. Targets Looking for Drugs: A Multistep Computational Protocol for the Development of Structure-Based Pharmacophores and Their Applications for Hit Discovery. J Chem Inf Model 2008; 48: 2166-79.
[186] Mugnaini C, Rajamaki S, Tintori C, *et al.* Toward novel HIV-1 integrase binding inhibitors: Molecular modeling, synthesis, and biological studies. Bioorg Med Chem Lett 2007; 17: 5370-3.
[187] Rinaldi M, Tintori C, Franchi L, *et al.* A versatile and practical synthesis toward the development of novel HIV-1 integrase inhibitors. ChemMedChem 2011; 6: 343-52.
[188] Mouscadet J-F, Deprez E, Desmaele D, D'Angelo J. Development of Styrylquinoline Integrase Inhibitors. In: Neamati N, editor. HIV-1 Integrase - mechanism and inhibitor design. Wiley Series on Drug Discovery and Development. 1st ed. New Jersey: John Wiley & Sons; 2011. p. 325-39.
[189] Mouscadet JF, Desmaele D. Chemistry and structure-activity relationship of the styrylquinoline-type HIV integrase inhibitors. Molecules 2010; 15(5): 3048-78.
[190] Deprez E, Barbe S, Kolaski M, *et al.* Mechanism of HIV-1 integrase inhibition by styrylquinoline derivatives *in vitro*. Mol Pharmacol 2004; 65: 85-98.
[191] Bonnenfant S, Thomas C, Vita C, *et al.* Styrylquinolines, Integrase Inhibitors Acting Prior to Integration: a New Mechanism of Action for Anti-Integrase Agents. Journal of Virology 2004; 78(11): 5728-36.

[192] Ma X, Zhang X, Tan J, Chen W, *et al.* Exploring binding mode for styrylquinoline HIV-1 integrase inhibitors using comparative molecualr field analysis and docking studies. Acta Pharmacol Sin 2004; 25: 950-8.

[193] Courcot B, Fraisse F, Becker P, *et al.* Crystal and Electronic Structures of Magnesium (II), Copper (II), and Mixed Magnesium (II)- Copper (II) Complexes of the Quinoline Half of Styrylquinoline-Type HIV-1 Integrase Inhibitors. J Phys Chem B 2007; 111: 6042-50.

[194] Mekouar K, Mouscadet JF, Desmaele D, *et al.* Styrylquinoline derivatives: A new class of potent HIV-1 integrase inhibitors that block HIV-1 replication in CEM cells. J Med Chem 1998; 41: 2846-57.

[195] Zouhiri F, Danet M, Benard C, *et al.* HIV-1 replication inhibitors of the styrylquinoline class: Introduction of an additional carboxyl group at the C-5 position of the quinoline. Tetrahedron Lett 2005; 46: 2201-5.

[196] Lutzke R, Eppens N, Weber P, Houghten R, Plasterk R. Identification of a hexapeptide inhibitor of the human immunodeficiency virus integrase protein by using a combinatorial chemical library. Proc Natl Acad Sci USA 1995; 92: 11456-60.

[197] Rochford S, Ford J, Ovenden S, *et al.* A novel aspochalasin with HIV-1 integrase inhibitory activity from *Aspergillus flavipes* J Antibiot (Tokyo) 2005; 58: 279-83.

[198] Singh S, Ondeyka J, Schleif W, *et al.* Integramide A and B, two novel non-ribosomal linear peptides containing nine Calpha-methyl amino acids produced by fungal fermentations that are inhibitors of HIV-1 integrase. Org Lett 2002; 4: 1431-4.

[199] Gleenberg I, Herschhorn A, Hizi A. inhibition of the activities of reverse transcriptase and integrase of human immunodeficiency virus type-1 by peptides derived from the homolgous viral protein R (Vpr). J Mol Biol 2007; 369: 1230-43.

[200] Gleenberg I, Avidan O, Goldgur Y, Herschhorn A, Hizi A. Peptides derived from reverse transcriptase of human immunodeficiency virus type 1 as novel inhibitors of the viral integrase. J Biol Chem 2005; 280: 21987-96.

[201] Tasara T, Maga G, Hottiger M, Hubscher U. HIV-1 reverse transcriptase and integrase enzymes physically interact and inhibit each other. FEBS Letters 2001; 507: 39-44.

[202] Bischerour J, Tauc P, Leh H, De Rocquigny H, Roques B, Mouscadet JF. C-Terminal domain of Vpr stimulates HIV-1 IN-mediated homologous strand transfer of mini-viral DNA. Nucleic Acids Res 2003; 31: 2694-702.

[203] Suzuki S, Urano E, Hashimoto C, *et al.* Peptide HIV-1 integrase inhibitors from HIV-1 gene products. J Med Chem 2010; 53: 5356-60.

[204] Moody I, Verde S, Overstreet C, Robinson WJ, Weiss G. *In vitro* evolution of an HIV integrase binding protein from a library of C-terminal domain γS-crystallin variants. Bioorg Med Chem Lett 2012; 22: 5584-9.

[205] Zawahir Z, Neamati N. Inhibition of HIV-1 integrase activity by synthetic peptides derived from the HIV-1 HXB2 Pol region of the viral genome. Bioorg Med Chem Lett 2006; 16(19): 5199-202.

[206] Li HY, Zawahir Z, Song LD, Long YQ, Neamati N. Sequence-based design and discovery of peptide inhibitors of HIV-1 integrase: insight into the binding mode of the enzyme. Journal of medicinal chemistry 2006; 49(15): 4477-86.

[207] Long YQ, Huang SX, Zawahir Z, Xu ZL, Li H, Sanchez TW, *et al.* Design of cell-permeable stapled peptides as HIV-1 integrase inhibitors. Journal of medicinal chemistry 2013; 56(13): 5601-12.

[208] Henchey LK, Jochim AL, Arora PS. Contemporary strategies for the stabilization of peptides in the alpha-helical conformation. Current opinion in chemical biology 2008; 12(6): 692-7.

[209] Maes M, Loyter A, Friedler A. Peptides that inhibit HIV-1 integrase by blocking its protein-protein interactions. FEBS 2012; 279: 2795-809.

[210] Benyammini H, Friedler A. Using peptides to study protein-protein interactions. Future Med Chem 2010; 2: 989-1003.

[211] Hayouka Z, Levin A, Maes M, *et al.* Mechanism of action of the HIV-1 integrase inhibitory peptide LEDGF 361-370. Biochemical and Biophysical Research Communications 2010; 394: 260-5.

[212] Zhao L, Chmielewski J. Integrase dimerization and activity with crosslinked interfacial peptides. Bioorganic & Medicinal Chemistry 2013; 21: 4041-4.

[213] Hayouka Z, Rosenbluh J, Levin A, *et al.* Inhibiting HIV-1 integrase by shifting its oligomerization equilibrium. Proc Natl Acad Sci USA 2007; 104: 8316-21.

[214] Rhodes D, Peat T, Vandegraaff N, *et al.* Crystal structures of novel allosteric peptide inhibitors of HIV integrase identify new interactions at the LEDGF binding site. ChemBioChem 2011; 12: 2311-5.

[215] Desimmie B, Humbert M, Lescrinier E, *et al.* Inhibition of HIV replication by cyclic peptides targeting LEDGF/p75. Mol Ther 2012; 20(11): 2064-75.

[216] Cavalluzzo C, Christ F, Voet A, *et al.* Identification of small peptides inhibiting the integrase-LEDGF/p75 interaction through targeting the cellular co-factor. JPept Sci 2013; 19: 651-8.

[217] Nair V, Chi G. Nucleotide-based inhibitors of HIV integrase. In: Neamati N, editor. HIV-1 integrase - mechanism and inhibitor design. Wiley Series on Drug Discovery and Development. 1st ed. New Jersey: John Wiley & Sons; 2011. p. 379-88.

[218] Ojwang J, Buckheit R, Pommier Y, *et al.* T30177, An oligonucleotide stabilized by an intramolecular guanosine octet, is a potent inhibitor of laboratory strains and clinical isolates of human immunodeficiency virus type 1. Antimicrob Agents Chemother 1995; 39: 2426-35.

[219] Singh I, Bodiwala H. Recent advances in anti-HIV natural products. Nat Prod Rep 2010; 27: 1781-800.

[220] Singh S, Pelaez F, Hazuda D, Lingham R. Discovery of natural product inhibitors of HIV-1 integrase at Merck. Drugs Future 2005; 30(3): 277-99.

[221] Matsumoto T, Hidaka K, Nakayama T, Fukui K. The synthesis and configuration of fukiic acid derivatives. Chem Lett 1972: 1-4.

[222] Williams C, Goldstone F, Greenham J. Flavonoids, cinnamic acids and coumarins from different tissues and medicinal preparations of *Taraxacum officinale* Phytochemistry 1996; 42: 121-7.

[223] Queffelec C, Bailly F, Mbemba G, *et al.* The total synthesis of fukiic acid, an HIV-1 integrase inhibitor. European Journal of Medicinal Chemistry 2008; 43: 2268-71.

[224] Lee SU, Shin C-G, Lee C-K, Lee Y. Caffeoylglycolic acid and caffeoylamino acid derivatives, halfmers of L-chicoric acid, as new HIV-1 integrase inhibitors. European Journal of Medicinal Chemistry 2007; 42: 1309-15.

[225] Bodiwala H, Sabde S, Gupta P, *et al.* Design and synthesis of caffeoyl-anilides as *portmanteau* inhibitors of HIV-1 integrase and CCR5. Bioorg Med Chem 2011; 19: 1256-63.

[226] Reddy M, Rao M, Rhodes D, *et al.* Lamellarin α 20-sulfate, an inhibitor of HIV-1 integrase active against HIV-1 virus in cell culture. J Med Chem 1999; 42: 1901-7.

[227] Jayasuriya H, Guan Z, Polishook J, *et al.* Isolation, Structure, and HIV-1 Integrase Inhibitory Activity of Cytosporic Acid, a Fungal Metabolite Produced by a Cytospora sp. J Nat Prod 2003; 66: 551-3.

[228] Singh S, Ondeyka J, Schleif W, Felock P, Hazuda D. Chemistry and Structure–Activity Relationship of HIV-1 Integrase Inhibitor Integracide B and Related Natural Products. J Nat Prod 2003; 66(10): 1338-44.

[229] Vidal V, Potterat O, Louvel S, *et al.* Library-Based Discovery and Characterization of Daphnane Diterpenes as Potent and Selective HIV Inhibitors in Daphne gnidium. J Nat Prod 2012; 75(3): 414-9.

[230] Pawar R, Das T, Mishra S, *et al.* Synthesis, anti-HIV activity, integrase enzyme inhibition and molecualr modeling of catechol, hydroquinone and quinol labdane anlogs. Bioorg Med Chem Lett 2014; 24: 302-7.

[231] Semenova E, Johnson AA, Marchand C, Davis D, Yarchoan R, Pommier Y. Preferential inhibition of the magnesium-dependent strand transfer reaction of HIV-1 integrase by α-hydroxytropolones. Mol Pharmacol 2006; 69: 1454-60.

[232] Didierjean J, Isel C, Querre F, *et al.* Inhibition of human immunodeficiency virus type 1 reverse transcriptase, RNase H and integrase activities by hydroxytropolones. Antimicrob Agents Chemother 2005; 49: 4884-94.

[233] Neamati N, Hong H, Sunder S, Milne G, Pommier Y. Potent inhibitors of human immunodeficiency virus type 1 integrase: identification of a novel four-point pharmacophore and tetracyclines as novel inhibitors. Mol Pharmacol 1997; 52: 1041-55.

[234] Patil S, Kamath S, Sanchez T, Neamati N, Schianazi R, Buolamwini J. Synthesis and biological evaluation of novel 5(H)-phenanthridin-6-ones, 5(H)-phenanthridin-6-one diketo acid, and polycyclic aromatic diketo acid analogs as new HIV-1 integrase inhibitors. Bioorg Med Chem 2007; 15: 1212-28.

[235] Sharma H, Sanchez T, Neamati N, *et al.* Synthesis, docking, and biological studies of phenanthrene β–diketo acids as novel HIV-1 integrase inhibitors. Bioorg Med Chem Lett 2013; 23: 6164-51.

[236] Greaves T, Drummond C. Protic Ionic Liquids: Properties and Applications. Chem Rev 2008; 108(1): 206-37.

[237] Maddali K, Kumar V, Marchand C, Pommier Y, Malhotra S. Biological evaluation of imidazolium- and ammonium-based salts as HIV-1 integrase inhibitors. Med Chem Commun 2011; 2: 143-50.

[238] Neamati N, Mazumder A, Sunder S, *et al.* Highly potent synthetic polyamides, bisdistamycins, and lexitropsins as inhibitors of human immunodeficiency virus type 1 integrase. Mol Pharmacol 1998; 54: 280-90.

[239] Bushman F, Lewinski M, Ciuffi A, Barr S, Leipzig J, Hannenhalli S, *et al.* Genome-wide analysis of retroviral DNA integration. Nature reviews Microbiology 2005; 3(11): 848-58.

[240] Van Maele B, Busschots K, Vandekerckhove L, Christ F, Debyser Z. Cellular co-factors of HIV-1 integration. Trends Biochem Sci 2006; 31(2): 98-105.

[241] Taltynov O, Desimmie B, Demeulemeester J, Christ F, Debyser Z. Cellular cofactors of lentiviral integrase: from target validation to drug discovery. Mol Biol Int 2012: 2012: 863405.

[242] Suzuki Y, Craigie R. The road to chromatin - nuclear entry of retroviruses. Nature reviews Microbiology 2007; 5(3): 187-96.

[243] Ge H, Yuanzheng S, Roeder R. Isolation of cDNAs encoding novel transcription coactivators p52 and p75 reveals an alternate regulatory mechanism of transcriptional activation. EMBO J 1998; 17(22): 6723-9.

[244] Yokoyama A, Cleary ML. Menin critically links MLL proteins with LEDGF on cancer-associated target genes. Cancer cell 2008; 14(1): 36-46.

[245] Bartholomeeusen K, Christ F, Hendrix J, Rain JC, Emiliani S, Benarous R, *et al.* Lens epithelium-derived growth factor/p75 interacts with the transposase-derived DDE domain of PogZ. J Biol Chem 2009; 284(17): 11467-77.

[246] Maertens GN, Cherepanov P, Engelman A. Transcriptional co-activator p75 binds and tethers the Myc-interacting protein JPO2 to chromatin. J Cell Sci 2006; 119(Pt 12): 2563-71.

[247] Bartholomeeusen K, De Rijck J, Busschots K, Desender L, Gijsbers R, Emiliani S, *et al.* Differential interaction of HIV-1 integrase and JPO2 with the C terminus of LEDGF/p75. J Mol Biol 2007; 372(2): 407-21.

[248] Shinohara T, Singh DP, Fatma N. LEDGF, a survival factor, activates stress-related genes. Progress in retinal and eye research 2002; 21(3): 341-58.

[249] Fatma N, Singh DP, Shinohara T, Chylack LT, Jr. Transcriptional regulation of the antioxidant protein 2 gene, a thiol-specific antioxidant, by lens epithelium-derived growth factor to protect cells from oxidative stress. J Biol Chem 2001; 276(52): 48899-907.

[250] Fatma N, Kubo E, Chylack LT, Jr., Shinohara T, Akagi Y, Singh DP. LEDGF regulation of alcohol and aldehyde dehydrogenases in lens epithelial cells: stimulation of retinoic acid production and protection from ethanol toxicity. Am J Physiol 2004; 287(2): C508-C16.

[251] Shin JH, Piao CS, Lim CM, Lee JK. LEDGF binding to stress response element increases alphaB-crystallin expression in astrocytes with oxidative stress. Neuroscience letters 2008; 435(2): 131-6.

[252] Kubo E, Fatma N, Sharma P, Shinohara T, Chylack LT, Jr., Akagi Y, *et al.* Transactivation of involucrin, a marker of differentiation in keratinocytes, by lens epithelium-derived growth factor (LEDGF). J Mol Biol 2002; 320(5): 1053-63.

[253] Takamura Y, Fatma N, Kubo E, Singh DP. Regulation of heavy subunit chain of gamma-glutamylcysteine synthetase by tumor necrosis factor-alpha in lens epithelial cells: role of LEDGF/p75. American journal of physiology Cell physiology 2006; 290(2): C554-66.

[254] Matsui H, Lin LR, Singh DP, Shinohara T, Reddy VN. Lens epithelium-derived growth factor: increased survival and decreased DNA breakage of human RPE cells induced by oxidative stress. Investigative ophthalmology & visual science 2001; 42(12): 2935-41.

[255] Singh DP, Kubo E, Takamura Y, Shinohara T, Kumar A, Chylack LT, Jr., *et al.* DNA binding domains and nuclear localization signal of LEDGF: contribution of two helix-turn-helix (HTH)-like domains and a stretch of 58 amino acids of the N-terminal to the trans-activation potential of LEDGF. J Mol Biol 2006; 355(3): 379-94.

[256] Brown-Bryan TA, Leoh LS, Ganapathy V, Pacheco FJ, Mediavilla-Varela M, Filippova M, *et al.* Alternative splicing and caspase-mediated cleavage generate antagonistic variants of the stress oncoprotein LEDGF/p75. Molecular cancer research : MCR 2008; 6(8): 1293-307.

[257] Ochs RL, Muro Y, Si Y, Ge H, Chan EK, Tan EM. Autoantibodies to DFS 70 kd/transcription coactivator p75 in atopic dermatitis and other conditions. The Journal of allergy and clinical immunology 2000; 105(6 Pt 1): 1211-20.

[258] Dietz F, Franken S, Yoshida K, Nakamura H, Kappler J, Gieselmann V. The family of hepatoma-derived growth factor proteins: characterization of a new member HRP-4 and classification of its subfamilies. Biochem J 2002; 366(Pt 2): 491-500.
[259] Stec I, Nagl SB, van Ommen GJ, den Dunnen JT. The PWWP domain: a potential protein-protein interaction domain in nuclear proteins influencing differentiation? FEBS Lett 2000; 473(1): 1-5.
[260] Maertens G, Cherepanov P, Debyser Z, Engelborghs Y, Engelman A. Identification and characterization of a functional nuclear localization signal in the HIV-1 integrase interactor LEDGF/p75. J Biol Chem 2004; 279(32): 33421-9.
[261] Cherepanov P, Devroe E, Silver PA, A E. Identification of an Evolutionarily Conserved Domain in Human Lens Epithelium-derived Growth Factor/Transcriptional Co-activator p75 (LEDGF/p75) That Binds HIV-1 Integrase. J Biol Chem 2004; 279(47): 48883-92.
[262] Llano M, Vanegas M, Hutchins N, Thompson D, Delgado S, Poeschla EM. Identification and characterization of the chromatin-binding domains of the HIV-1 integrase interactor LEDGF/p75. J Mol Biol 2006; 360(4): 760-73.
[263] Vanegas M, Llano M, Delgado S, Thompson D, Peretz M, Poeschla E. Identification of the LEDGF/p75 HIV-1 integrase-interaction domain and NLS reveals NLS-independent chromatin tethering. J Cell Sci 2005; 118(8): 1733-43.
[264] Vandegraaff N, Devroe E, Turlure F, Silver P, Engelman A. Biochemical and genetic analyses of integrase-interacting proteins lens epithelium-derived growth factor (LEDGF)/p75 and hepatoma-derived growth factor related protein 2 (HRP2) in preintegration complex function and HIV-1 replication. Virology 2006; 346: 415-26.
[265] Cherepanov P, Sun ZY, Rahman S, Maertens G, Wagner G, Engelman A. Solution structure of the HIV-1 integrase-binding domain in LEDGF/p75. Nat Struct Mol Biol 2005; 12(6): 526-32.
[266] Cherepanov P. LEDGF/p75 interacts with divergent lentiviral integrases and modulates their enzymatic activity *in vitro*. Nucleic Acids Res 2007; 35(1): 113-24.
[267] Carlson M, Laurent BC. The SNF/SWI family of global transcriptional activators. Curr Opin Cell Biol 1994; 6(3): 396-402.
[268] Morozov A, Yung E, Kalpana GV. Structure-function analysis of integrase interactor 1/hSNF5L1 reveals differential properties of two repeat motifs present in the highly conserved region. Proceedings of the National Academy of Sciences of the United States of America 1998; 95(3): 1120-5.
[269] Das S, Cano J, Kalpana GV. Multimerization and DNA binding properties of INI1/hSNF5 and its functional significance. J Biol Chem 2009; 284(30): 19903-14.
[270] Kalpana GV, Marmon S, Wang W, Crabtree GR, Goff SP. Binding and stimulation of HIV-1 integrase by a human homolog of yeast transcription factor SNF5. Science 1994; 266(5193): 2002-6.
[271] Yung E, Sorin M, Pal A, Craig E, Morozov A, Delattre O, *et al.* Inhibition of HIV-1 virion production by a transdominant mutant of integrase interactor 1. Nat Med 2001; 7(8): 920-6.
[272] Maroun M, Delelis O, Coadou G, Bader T, Segeral E, Mbemba G, *et al.* Inhibition of early steps of HIV-1 replication by SNF5/Ini1. J Biol Chem 2006; 281(32): 22736-43.
[273] Sorin M, Yung E, Wu X, Kalpana GV. HIV-1 replication in cell lines harboring INI1/hSNF5 mutations. Retrovirology 2006; 3: 56.
[274] Maillot B, Levy N, Eiler S, Crucifix C, Granger F, Richert L, *et al.* Structural and functional role of INI1 and LEDGF in the HIV-1 preintegration complex. PLoS One 2013; 8(4): e60734.

[275] Agbottah E, Deng L, Dannenberg LO, Pumfery A, Kashanchi F. Effect of SWI/SNF chromatin remodeling complex on HIV-1 Tat activated transcription. Retrovirology 2006; 3: 48.
[276] Ariumi Y, Serhan F, Turelli P, Telenti A, Trono D. The integrase interactor 1 (INI1) proteins facilitate Tat-mediated human immunodeficiency virus type 1 transcription. Retrovirology 2006; 3: 47.
[277] Mahmoudi T, Parra M, Vries RG, Kauder SE, Verrijzer CP, Ott M, *et al.* The SWI/SNF chromatin-remodeling complex is a cofactor for Tat transactivation of the HIV promoter. J Biol Chem 2006; 281(29): 19960-8.
[278] Treand C, du Chene I, Bres V, Kiernan R, Benarous R, Benkirane M, *et al.* Requirement for SWI/SNF chromatin-remodeling complex in Tat-mediated activation of the HIV-1 promoter. EMBO J 2006; 25(8): 1690-9.
[279] Easley R, Carpio L, Dannenberg L, Choi S, Alani D, Van Duyne R, *et al.* Transcription through the HIV-1 nucleosomes: effects of the PBAF complex in Tat activated transcription. Virology 2010; 405(2): 322-33.
[280] Jacque JM, Stevenson M. The inner-nuclear-envelope protein emerin regulates HIV-1 infectivity. Nature 2006; 441(7093): 641-5.
[281] Cai M, Huang Y, Zheng R, Wei SQ, Ghirlando R, Lee MS, *et al.* Solution structure of the cellular factor BAF responsible for protecting retroviral DNA from autointegration. Nat Struct Biol 1998; 5(10): 903-9.
[282] Zheng R, Ghirlando R, Lee MS, Mizuuchi K, Krause M, Craigie R. Barrier-to-autointegration factor (BAF) bridges DNA in a discrete, higher-order nucleoprotein complex. Proceedings of the National Academy of Sciences of the United States of America 2000; 97(16): 8997-9002.
[283] Lee MS, Craigie R. Protection of retroviral DNA from autointegration: involvement of a cellular factor. Proceedings of the National Academy of Sciences of the United States of America 1994; 91(21): 9823-7.
[284] Furukawa K. LAP2 binding protein 1 (L2BP1/BAF) is a candidate mediator of LAP2-chromatin interaction. J Cell Sci 1999; 112 (Pt 15): 2485-92.
[285] Suzuki Y, Yang H, Craigie R. LAP2alpha and BAF collaborate to organize the Moloney murine leukemia virus preintegration complex. EMBO J 2004; 23(23): 4670-8.
[286] Shun MC, Daigle JE, Vandegraaff N, Engelman A. Wild-type levels of human immunodeficiency virus type 1 infectivity in the absence of cellular emerin protein. J Virol 2007; 81(1): 166-72.
[287] Lai MC, Lin RI, Huang SY, Tsai CW, Tarn WY. A human importin-beta family protein, transportin-SR2, interacts with the phosphorylated RS domain of SR proteins. J Biol Chem 2000; 275(11): 7950-7.
[288] Kataoka N, Bachorik JL, Dreyfuss G. Transportin-SR, a nuclear import receptor for SR proteins. The Journal of cell biology 1999; 145(6): 1145-52.
[289] Lai MC, Lin RI, Tarn WY. Transportin-SR2 mediates nuclear import of phosphorylated SR proteins. Proceedings of the National Academy of Sciences of the United States of America 2001; 98(18): 10154-9.
[290] Lai MC, Kuo HW, Chang WC, Tarn WY. A novel splicing regulator shares a nuclear import pathway with SR proteins. EMBO J 2003; 22(6): 1359-69.
[291] Anguissola S, McCormack WJ, Morrin MA, Higgins WJ, Fox DM, Worrall DM. Pigment epithelium-derived factor (PEDF) interacts with transportin SR2, and active nuclear import is facilitated by a novel nuclear localization motif. PLoS One 2011; 6(10): e26234.

[292] Larue R, Gupta K, Wuensch C, Shkriabai N, Kessl JJ, Danhart E, *et al.* Interaction of the HIV-1 intasome with transportin 3 protein (TNPO3 or TRN-SR2). J Biol Chem 2012; 287(41): 34044-58.

[293] Bono F, Cook AG, Grunwald M, Ebert J, Conti E. Nuclear import mechanism of the EJC component Mago-Y14 revealed by structural studies of importin 13. Mol Cell 2010; 37(2): 211-22.

[294] Imasaki T, Shimizu T, Hashimoto H, Hidaka Y, Kose S, Imamoto N, *et al.* Structural basis for substrate recognition and dissociation by human transportin 1. Mol Cell 2007; 28(1): 57-67.

[295] Christ F, Thys W, De Rijck J, Gijsbers R, Albanese A, Arosio D, *et al.* Transportin-SR2 imports HIV into the nucleus. Current biology : CB 2008; 18(16): 1192-202.

[296] Brass AL, Dykxhoorn DM, Benita Y, Yan N, Engelman A, Xavier RJ, *et al.* Identification of host proteins required for HIV infection through a functional genomic screen. Science 2008; 319(5865): 921-6.

[297] Krishnan L, Matreyek KA, Oztop I, Lee K, Tipper CH, Li X, *et al.* The requirement for cellular transportin 3 (TNPO3 or TRN-SR2) during infection maps to human immunodeficiency virus type 1 capsid and not integrase. J Virol 2010; 84(1): 397-406.

[298] Valle-Casuso JC, Di Nunzio F, Yang Y, Reszka N, Lienlaf M, Arhel N, *et al.* TNPO3 is required for HIV-1 replication after nuclear import but prior to integration and binds the HIV-1 core. J Virol 2012; 86(10): 5931-6.

[299] Thys W, De Houwer S, Demeulemeester J, Taltynov O, Vancraenenbroeck R, Gerard M, *et al.* Interplay between HIV entry and transportin-SR2 dependency. Retrovirology 2011; 8: 7.

[300] Lee K, Ambrose Z, Martin TD, Oztop I, Mulky A, Julias JG, *et al.* Flexible use of nuclear import pathways by HIV-1. Cell host & microbe 2010; 7(3): 221-33.

[301] Ruegsegger U, Beyer K, Keller W. Purification and characterization of human cleavage factor Im involved in the 3' end processing of messenger RNA precursors. J Biol Chem 1996; 271(11): 6107-13.

[302] Cardinale S, Cisterna B, Bonetti P, Aringhieri C, Biggiogera M, Barabino SM. Subnuclear localization and dynamics of the Pre-mRNA 3' end processing factor mammalian cleavage factor I 68-kDa subunit. Molecular biology of the cell 2007; 18(4): 1282-92.

[303] Maertens GN, Cook NJ, Wang W, Hare S, Gupta SS, Oztop I, *et al.* Structural basis for nuclear import of splicing factors by human Transportin 3. Proceedings of the National Academy of Sciences of the United States of America 2014; 111(7): 2728-33.

[304] Zhou Z, Barry de Longchamps N, Schmitt A, Zerbib M, Vacher-Lavenu MC, Bomsel M, *et al.* HIV-1 efficient entry in inner foreskin is mediated by elevated CCL5/RANTES that recruits T cells and fuels conjugate formation with Langerhans cells. PLoS Pathog 2011; 7(6): e1002100.

[305] De Houwer S, Demeulemeester J, Thys W, Taltynov O, Zmajkovicova K, Christ F, *et al.* Identification of residues in the C-terminal domain of HIV-1 integrase that mediate binding to the transportin-SR2 protein. J Biol Chem 2012; 287(41): 34059-68.

[306] De Houwer S, Demeulemeester J, Thys W, Rocha S, Dirix L, Gijsbers R, *et al.* The HIV-1 Integrase Mutant R263A/K264A Is 2-fold Defective for TRN-SR2 Binding and Viral Nuclear Import. J Biol Chem 2014; 289(36): 25351-61.

[307] Gallay P, Stitt V, Mundy C, Oettinger M, Trono D. Role of the karyopherin pathway in human immunodeficiency virus type 1 nuclear import. J Virol 1996; 70(2): 1027-32.

[308] Gallay P, Hope T, Chin D, Trono D. HIV-1 infection of nondividing cells through the recognition of integrase by the importin/karyopherin pathway. Proceedings of the National Academy of Sciences of the United States of America 1997; 94(18): 9825-30.
[309] Haffar OK, Popov S, Dubrovsky L, Agostini I, Tang H, Pushkarsky T, *et al.* Two nuclear localization signals in the HIV-1 matrix protein regulate nuclear import of the HIV-1 pre-integration complex. J Mol Biol 2000; 299(2): 359-68.
[310] Ao Z, Danappa Jayappa K, Wang B, Zheng Y, Kung S, Rassart E, *et al.* Importin alpha3 interacts with HIV-1 integrase and contributes to HIV-1 nuclear import and replication. J Virol 2010; 84(17): 8650-63.
[311] Jayappa KD, Ao Z, Yang M, Wang J, Yao X. Identification of critical motifs within HIV-1 integrase required for importin alpha3 interaction and viral cDNA nuclear import. J Mol Biol 2011; 410(5): 847-62.
[312] Fassati A, Gorlich D, Harrison I, Zaytseva L, Mingot JM. Nuclear import of HIV-1 intracellular reverse transcription complexes is mediated by importin 7. EMBO J 2003; 22(14): 3675-85.
[313] Ao Z, Huang G, Yao H, Xu Z, Labine M, Cochrane AW, *et al.* Interaction of human immunodeficiency virus type 1 integrase with cellular nuclear import receptor importin 7 and its impact on viral replication. J Biol Chem 2007; 282(18): 13456-67.
[314] Ao Z, Jayappa KD, Wang B, Zheng Y, Wang X, Peng J, *et al.* Contribution of host nucleoporin 62 in HIV-1 integrase chromatin association and viral DNA integration. J Biol Chem 2012; 287(13): 10544-55.
[315] Woodward CL, Prakobwanakit S, Mosessian S, Chow SA. Integrase interacts with nucleoporin NUP153 to mediate the nuclear import of human immunodeficiency virus type 1. J Virol 2009; 83(13): 6522-33.
[316] Matreyek KA, Engelman A. The requirement for nucleoporin NUP153 during human immunodeficiency virus type 1 infection is determined by the viral capsid. J Virol 2011; 85(15): 7818-27.
[317] Armon-Omer A, Graessmann A, Loyter A. A synthetic peptide bearing the HIV-1 integrase 161-173 amino acid residues mediates active nuclear import and binding to importin alpha: characterization of a functional nuclear localization signal. J Mol Biol 2004; 336(5): 1117-28.
[318] Jeggo PA. DNA breakage and repair. Advances in genetics 1998; 38: 185-218.
[319] Daniel R, Katz RA, Skalka AM. A role for DNA-PK in retroviral DNA integration. Science 1999; 284(5414): 644-7.
[320] Baekelandt V, Claeys A, Cherepanov P, De Clercq E, De Strooper B, Nuttin B, *et al.* DNA-Dependent protein kinase is not required for efficient lentivirus integration. J Virol 2000; 74(23): 11278-85.
[321] Li L, Olvera JM, Yoder KE, Mitchell RS, Butler SL, Lieber M, *et al.* Role of the non-homologous DNA end joining pathway in the early steps of retroviral infection. EMBO J 2001; 20(12): 3272-81.
[322] Jeanson L, Subra F, Vaganay S, Hervy M, Marangoni E, Bourhis J, *et al.* Effect of Ku80 depletion on the preintegrative steps of HIV-1 replication in human cells. Virology 2002; 300(1): 100-8.
[323] Cooper A, Garcia M, Petrovas C, Yamamoto T, Koup RA, Nabel GJ. HIV-1 causes CD4 cell death through DNA-dependent protein kinase during viral integration. Nature 2013; 498(7454): 376-9.

[324] Farnet CM, Bushman FD. HIV-1 cDNA integration: requirement of HMG I(Y) protein for function of preintegration complexes *in vitro*. Cell 1997; 88(4): 483-92.
[325] Hindmarsh P, Ridky T, Reeves R, Andrake M, Skalka AM, Leis J. HMG protein family members stimulate human immunodeficiency virus type 1 and avian sarcoma virus concerted DNA integration *in vitro*. J Virol 1999; 73(4): 2994-3003.
[326] Li L, Yoder K, Hansen MS, Olvera J, Miller MD, Bushman FD. Retroviral cDNA integration: stimulation by HMG I family proteins. J Virol 2000; 74(23): 10965-74.
[327] Henderson A, Bunce M, Siddon N, Reeves R, Tremethick DJ. High-mobility-group protein I can modulate binding of transcription factors to the U5 region of the human immunodeficiency virus type 1 proviral promoter. J Virol 2000; 74(22): 10523-34.
[328] Van Lint C, Emiliani S, Ott M, Verdin E. Transcriptional activation and chromatin remodeling of the HIV-1 promoter in response to histone acetylation. EMBO J 1996; 15(5): 1112-20.
[329] Eilebrecht S, Wilhelm E, Benecke BJ, Bell B, Benecke AG. HMGA1 directly interacts with TAR to modulate basal and Tat-dependent HIV transcription. RNA biology 2013; 10(3): 436-44.
[330] Engelman A, Kessl J, Kvaratskhelia M. Allosteric inhibition of HIV-1 integrase activity. Curr Opin Chem Biol 2013; 17(3): 339-45.
[331] Al-Mawsawi L, Neamati N. Allosteric inhibitor development targeting HIV-1 integrase. ChemMedChem 2011; 6: 228-41.
[332] Robinson WJ. L-chicoric acid, an inhibitor of human immunodeficiency virus type 1 (HIV-1) integrase, improves on the *in vitro* anti-HIV effect of zidovudine plus prtoease inhibitor (AG1350). Antivir Res 1998; 39: 101-11.
[333] Robinson WJ, Cordeiro M, Abdel-Malek S, *et al.* Dicaffeoylquinic acid inhibitors of human immunodeficiency virus integrase: inhibition of the core catalytic domain of human immunodeficiency virus integrase. Mol Pharmacol 1996; 50: 846-55.
[334] McDougall B, King P, Wu B, *et al.* Diacaffeoylquinic and diaffeoyltartaric acids as selective inhibitors of human immunodeficiency virus type 1 integrase. Antimicrob Agents Chemother 1998; 42: 140-6.
[335] Mahmood N, Moore P, De Tommasi N, *et al.* Inhibition of HIV infection by caffeoylquinic acid derivatives. Antimicrob Agents Chemother 1993; 4: 235-40.
[336] Pluymers W, Neamati N, Pannecouque C, *et al.* Viral entry as the primary target for the anti-HIV activity of chicoric acid and its tetra-acetyl esters. Mol Pharmacol 2000; 58: 641-8.
[337] Lin Z, Neamati N, Zhao H, *et al.* Chicoric acid analogues as HIV-1 integrase inhibitors. J Med Chem 1999; 42(8): 1401-14.
[338] Shkriabai N, Sachindra S, Hess S, *et al.* Identification of an inhibitor-binding site to HIV-1 integrase with affinity acetylation and mass spectrometry. Proc Natl Acad Sci USA 2004; 101(18): 6894-9.
[339] Kessl J, Eidahl J, Shkriabai N, *et al.* An allosteric mechanism for inhibiting HIV-1 integrase with a small molecule Mol Pharmacol 2009; 76: 824-32.
[340] Molteni V, Greenwald J, Rhodes D, *et al.* Identification of a small-molecule binding site at the dimer interface of the HIV integrase catalytic domain. Acta Crystallographica Section D 2001; D57: 536-44.
[341] Du L, Zhao Y-x, Yang L-m, *et al.* Symmetrical 1-pyrrolidineacetamide showing anti-HIV activity through a new binding site on HIV-1 integrase. Acta Pharmacol Sin 2008; 29(10): 1261-7.

[342] Wielens J, Headey S, Jeevarajah D, *et al.* Crystal structure of the HIV-1 integrase core domain in complex with sucrose reveals details of an allosteric inhibitory binding site. FEBS Letters 2010; 584: 1455-62.
[343] Du L, Shen L, Yu Z, *et al.* Hyrtiosal, from the marine sponge *Hyrtios erectus,* inhibits HIV-1 integrase binding to viral DNA by a new inhibitor binding site. ChemMedChem 2008; 3: 173-80.
[344] Debyser Z, Desimmie B, Taltynov O, Demeulemeester J, Christ F. Validation of host factors of HIV integration as novel drug targets for anti-HIV therapy. Med Chem Commun 2014; 5: 314-20.
[345] Tavassoli A. Targeting the protein-protein interactions of the HIV lifecycle. Chem Soc Rev 2011; 40: 1337-46.
[346] Jurando K, Engelman A. Multimodal mechanism of action of allosteric HIV-1 integrase inhibitors. Expert reviews in molcular medicine 2013; 15: e14.
[347] Llano M, Saenz D, Meehan A, *et al.* An Essential Role for LEDGF/p75 in HIV Integration. Science 2006; 314: 461-4.
[348] P C. LEDGF/p75 interacts with divergent lentiviral integrases and modulates their enzymatic activity *in vitro*. Nucleic Acids Res 2007; 35(11): 113-24.
[349] Hayouka Z, Rosenbluh J, Levin A, Maes M, Loyter A, Friedler A. Peptides derived from HIV-1 Rev inhibit HIV-1 integrase in a shiftide mechanism. Biopolymers 2008; 90: 481-7.
[350] Armon-Omer A, Levin A, Hayouka Z, *et al.* Correlation between shiftide activity and HIV-1 integrase inhibition by a peptide selected from a combinatorial library. J Mol Biol 2008; 276: 971-82.
[351] Hare S, Cherepanov P. The interaction between Lentiviral integrase and LEDGF: structural and functional insights. Viruses 2009; 1: 780-801.
[352] Maertens G, P C, Pluymers W, *et al.* LEDGF/p75 is essential for nuclear and chromosomal targeting of HIV-1 integrase in human cells. J Biol Chem 2003; 278: 33528-39.
[353] London N, Raveh B, Schueler-Furman O. Druggable protein-protein interactions - from hot spots to hot segments. Curr Opin Chem Biol 2013; 17: 952-9.
[354] P C, Sun Z-YJ, Rahman S, Maertens G, Wagner G, Engelman A. Solution structure of the HIV-1 integrase-binding domain of LEDGF/p75. Nature structural & Molecular biology 2005; 12(6): 526-32.
[355] Rahman S, Lu R, Vandegraaff N, P C, Engelman A. Structure-based mutagenesis of the integrase-LEDGF/p75 interface uncouples a strict correlation between *in vitro* protein binding and HIV-1 fitness. Virology 2007; 357(1): 79-90.
[356] Busschots K, Voet A, De Maeyer M, *et al.* Identification of the LEDGF/p75 Binding Site in HIV-1 Integrase. Journal of Molecular Biology 2007; 365(5): 1480-92.
[357] Hare S, Di Nunzio F, Labeja A, Wang J, Engelman A, P C. Structural basis for functional tetramerization of lentiviral integrase. PLoS Pathog 2009; 5(7): e10000515.
[358] Tintori C, Veljkovic N, Veljkovic V, Botta M. Computational studies of the interaction between the HIV-1 integrase tetramer and the cofactor LEDGF/p75: insights from molecular dynamics simultaions and informational spectrum method. Proteins 2010; 78: 3396-408.
[359] Milroy L-G, Grossmann T, Hennig S, Brunsveld L, Ottmann C. Modulators of protein-protein interactions. Chem Rev 2014; 114: 4695-748.
[360] Christ F, Debyser Z. The LEDGF/p75 integrase interaction, a novel target for anti-HIV therapy. Virology 2013; 435: 102-9.

[361] Demeulemeester J, Chaltin P, Marchand A, De Maeyer M, Debyser Z, Christ F. LEDGINs, non-catlytic site inhibitors of HIV-1 integrase: a patent review (2006-2014). Expert Opin Ther Patents 2014; 24(6): 1-24.

[362] Tsiang M, Jones G, Niedziela-Majka A, *et al.* New class of HIV-1 integrase (IN) inhibitors with a dual mode of action. J Biol Chem 2012; 287(25): 21189-203.

[363] Le Rouzic E, Bonnard D, Chasset S, *et al.* Dual inhibition of HIV-1 replication by integrase-LEDGF allosertic inhibitors is predominant at the post-integration stage. Retrovirology 2013; 10: 144.

[364] Du L, Zhao Y, Chen J, *et al.* D77, one benzoic acid derivative, functions as a novel anti-HIV-1 inhibitor targeting the interaction between integrase and cellular LEDGF/p75. Biochemical and Biophysical Research Communications 2008; 375: 139-44.

[365] Gu W-G, Ip DT-M, Liu S, *et al.* 1,4-bis(5-(naphthalen-1-yl)thiophen-2-yl)naphthalene, a small molecule, functions as a novel anti-HIV-1 inhibitor targeting the interaction between integrase and cellular Lens epithelium-derived growth factor. Chemico-Biological Interactions 2014.

[366] De Luca, Barreca M, Ferro S, *et al.* Pharmacophore-Based Discovery of Small-Molecule Inhibitors of Protein–Protein Interactions between HIV-1 Integrase and Cellular Cofactor LEDGF/p75. ChemMedChem 2009; 4(8): 1311-6.

[367] De Luca L, Ferro S, Gitto R, *et al.* Small molecules targeting the interaction between HIV-1 integrase and LEDGF/p75 cofactor. Bioorg Med Chem Lett 2010; 18: 7515-21.

[368] De Luca L, Ferro S, Morreale F, *et al.* Inhibitors of the interactions between HIV-1 IN and the cofactor LEDGF/p75. ChemMedChem 2011; 6: 1184-91.

[369] De Luca L, Ferro S, Morreale F, *et al.* Fragment hopping approach directed at design of HIV IN-LEDGF/p75 interaction inhibitors. J Enzyme Inhib Med Chem 2013; 28(5): 1002-9.

[370] De Luca L, Gitto R, Christ F, *et al.* 4-[1-(4-Fluorobenzyl)-4-hydroxy-1H-indol-3-yl]-2-hydroxy-4-oxobut-2-enoic acid as a prototype to develop dual inhibitors of HIV-1 integration process. Antivir Res 2011; 92: 102-7.

[371] Ferro S, De Luca L, Morreale F, *et al.* Synthesis and biological evaluation of novel antiviral agents as protein-protein interaction inhibitors. J Enzyme Inhib Med Chem 2014; 29(2): 237-42.

[372] De Luca L, Morreale F, Chimirri A. Insight into the fundamental interactions between LEDGF binding site inhibitors and integrase combining docking and molecular dynamics simulations. J Chem Inf Model 2012; 52: 3245-54.

[373] Zhao H, Neamati N, Hong H, Mazumder A, Wang S, Sunder S, *et al.* Coumarin-based inhibitors of HIV integrase. Journal of medicinal chemistry 1997; 40(2): 242-9.

[374] Burke TR, Jr., Fesen MR, Mazumder A, Wang J, Carothers AM, Grunberger D, *et al.* Hydroxylated aromatic inhibitors of HIV-1 integrase. Journal of medicinal chemistry 1995; 38(21): 4171-8.

[375] Mazumder A, Wang S, Neamati N, Nicklaus M, Sunder S, Chen J, *et al.* Antiretroviral agents as inhibitors of both human immunodeficiency virus type 1 integrase and protease. Journal of medicinal chemistry 1996; 39(13): 2472-81.

[376] Mazumder A, Neamati N, Sunder S, Schulz J, Pertz H, Eich E, *et al.* Curcumin analogs with altered potencies against HIV-1 integrase as probes for biochemical mechanisms of drug action. Journal of medicinal chemistry 1997; 40(19): 3057-63.

[377] Al-Mawsawi LQ, Fikkert V, Dayam R, Witvrouw M, Burke TR, Jr., Borchers CH, *et al.* Discovery of a small-molecule HIV-1 integrase inhibitor-binding site. Proceedings of the National Academy of Sciences of the United States of America 2006; 103(26): 10080-5.

[378] Peat TS, Rhodes DI, Vandegraaff N, Le G, Smith JA, Clark LJ, *et al.* Small molecule inhibitors of the LEDGF site of human immunodeficiency virus integrase identified by fragment screening and structure based design. PLoS One 2012; 7(7): e40147.

[379] Christ F, Voet A, Marchand A, *et al.* Rational design of small-molecule inhibitors of the LEDGF/p75-integrase interaction and HIV replication. Nat Chem Biol 2010; 6: 442-8.

[380] Jurando K, Wang H, Slaughter A, *et al.* Allosteric integrase inhibitor potency is determined through the inhibition of HIV-1 particle maturation. Proc Natl Acad Sci USA 2013; 110(21): 8690-5.

[381] Desimmie B, Schrijvers R, Demeulemeester J, *et al.* LEDGINs inhibit late stage HIV-1 replication by modulating integrase multimerization in the virons. Retrovirology 2013; 10(57): 1-16.

[382] Balakrishnan M, Yant S, Tsai L, *et al.* Non-catalytic site HIV-1 integrase inhibitors disrupt core maturation and induce a reverse transcription block in target cells. PLOS One 2013; 8(9): e74163.

[383] Christ F, Shaw S, Demeulemeester J, *et al.* Small-molecule inhibitors of the LEDGF/p75 binding site of integrase block HIV replication and modulate integrase multimerization. Antimicrob Agents Chemother 2012; 56: 4365-74.

[384] Gupta K, Brady T, Dyer B, *et al.* Allosteric inhibition of human immunodeficiency virus integrase: late block during viral replication and abnormal multimerization involving specific protein domains. J Biol Chem 2014; 289: 20477-88.

[385] Sharma A, Slaughter A, Jena N, *et al.* A new class of multimerization selective inhibitors of HIV-1 integrase. PLoS Pathog 2014; 10: e1004171.

[386] Kessl J, Jena N, Koh Y, *et al.* Multimode, cooperative mechanism of action of allosteric HIV-1 integrase inhibitors. J Biol Chem 2012; 287(20): 16801-11.

[387] McKee C, Kessl J, Shkriabai N, Dar M, Engelman A, Kvaratskhelia M. Dynamic Modulation of HIV-1 Integrase Structure and Function by Cellular Lens Epithelium-derived Growth Factor (LEDGF) Protein. J Biol Chem 2008; 283: 31802-12.

[388] Kessl J, Li M, Ignatov M, *et al.* FRET analysis reveals distinct conformations of IN tetramers in the presence of viral DNA or LEDGF/p75. Nucleic Acids Res 2011; 39(20): 9009-22.

[389] Feng L, Sharma A, Slaughter A, *et al.* The A128T resistance mutation reveals aberrant protein multimerization as the primary mechanism of action of allosteric HIV-1 integrase inhibitors. J Biol Chem 2013; 288(22): 15813-20.

[390] Shkriabai N, Venkatasubramanian D, Slaughter A, *et al.* A Critical Role of the C-terminal Segment for Allosteric Inhibitor-induced Aberrant Multimerization of HIV-1 Integrase. J Biol Chem 2014; 289: 26430-40.

[391] Fader L, Malenfant E, Parisien M, *et al.* Discovery of BI 224436, a noncatalytic site integrase inhibitor (NCINI) of HIV-1. ACS Med Chem Lett 2014; 5: 422-7.

[392] Fenwick C, Amad M, Bailey M, *et al.* Preclinical profile of BI 224436, a novel HIV-1 non-catalytic-site integrase inhibitor. Antimicrob Agents Chemother 2014; 58(6): 3233-44.

[393] Tsiang M, Jones G, Hung M, *et al.* Affinities between the binding partners of the HIV-1 integrase dimer-lens epithelium-derived growth factor (IN dimer-LEDGF) complex. J Biol Chem 2009; 284: 33580-99.

[394] De Luca L, Morreale F, Christ F, Debyser Z, Ferro S, Gitto R. New scaffolds of natural origin as Integrase-LEDGF/p75 interaction inhibitors: virtual screening and activity assays. European Journal of Medicinal Chemistry 2013; 68: 405-11.

[395] Hombrouck A, Clayton R, Voet A, Witvrouw M, Debyser Z. Resistance to inhibitors of HIV-1 integrase. In: Neamati N, editor. HIV-1 integrase: mechanism and inhibitor design. Wiley Series on drug discovery and development. 1st ed. New Jersey, USA: John Wiley & Sons; 2011. p. 477-98.

[396] Mansky L, Tenim H. Lower *in vivo* mutation rate of human immunodeficiency virus type 1 than that predicted from the fidelity of purified reverse transcriptase. J Virol 1995; 69(8): 5087-94.

[397] Coffin JM. HIV population dynamics *in vivo*: implications for genetic variation, pathogenesis, and therapy. Science 1995; 267(5197): 483-9.

[398] Bangsberg D, Hecht F, Charlebosis E, *et al.* Adherence to protease inhibitors, HIV-1 viral load, and development of drug resistance in an indigent population. AIDS 2000; 14(4): 357-66.

[399] Haubrich R, Little S, Currier J, *et al.* The value of patient-reported adherence to antiretroviral therapy in predicting virologic and immunologic response. California Collaborative Treatment Group. AIDS 1999; 13(9): 1099-107.

[400] Gulick R, Mellors J, Havlir D, *et al.* Treatment with indinavir, zidovudine, and lamivudine in adults with human immunodeficency virus infection and prior antiretroviral therapy. The New England Journal of Medicine 1997; 337: 734-9.

[401] Hammer S, Squires K, Hughes M, *et al.* A controlled trial of two nucleoside analogues plus indinavir in persons with human immunodeficiency virus infection and CD4 cell counts of 200 per cubic millimeter or less. AIDS Clinical Trials Group 320 Study team. The New England Journal of Medicine 1997; 337: 725-33.

[402] British HIV Association guidelines for the treatment of HIV-1 positive adults with antiretroviral therapy 2012. HIV Medicine 2014; 15(suppl 1): 1-85.

[403] Cortez K, Maldarelli F. Clinical management of HIV drug resistance. Viruses 2011; 3(4): 347-78.

[404] Prosperi M, De Luca A. Computational models for prediction of response to antiretroviral therapies. AIDS Rev 2012; 14(2): 145-53.

[405] Xue W, Jin X, Ning L, Wang M, Liu H, Yao X. Exploring the molecular mechanism of cross-resistance to HIV-1 integrase strand transfer inhibitors by molecular dynamics simulation and residue interaction network analysis. J Chem Inf Model 2012; 53: 210-22.

[406] Chen Q, Buolamwini J, Smith J. Impact of resistance mutations on inhibitor binding to HIV-1 integrase. J Chem Inf Model 2013; 53(12): 3297-307.

[407] Masso M, Chuang G, Hao K, Jain S, Vaisman I. Structure-based predictors of resistance to the HIV-1 integrase inhibitor elvitegravir. Antiviral Research 2014; 106: 5-12.

[408] Mesplede T, Quashie P, Wainberg M. Resitance to HIV integrase inhibitors. Curr Opin HIV AIDS 2012; 7: 401-8.

[409] Geretti A, Armenia D, Ceccherini-Silberstein F. Emerging patterns and implications of HIV-1 integrase inhibitor resistance. Curr Opin Infect Dis 2012; 25: 677-86.

[410] Hare S, Vos A, Clayton R, Thuring J, Cummings M, P C. Molecular mechanisms of retroviral integrase inhibition and the evolution of viral resistance. Proc Natl Acad Sci USA 2010; 107(46): 20057-62.

[411] Hare S, Smith J, Metifiot M, *et al.* Structural and functional analyses of the second-generation integrase strand transfer inhibitor doultegravir (S/GSK1349572). Mol Pharmacol 2011; 80(4): 565-72.

[412] Metifiot M, Maddali K, Naumova A, Zhang X, Marchand C, Pommier Y. Biochemical and pharmacological analyses of HIV-1 integrase flexible loop mutants resitant to raltegravir. Biochemistry 2010; 49: 3715-22.

[413] Dicker I, Terry B, Lin Z, *et al.* Biochemical analysis of HIV-1 integrase variants resistant to strand transfer inhibitors. J Biol Chem 2008; 283(35): 23599-609.

[414] Mouscadet JF, Delelis O, Marcelin A, Tchertanov L. Resistance to HIV-1 integrase inhibitors: A structural perspective. Drug Resistance Updates 2010; 13(4-5): 139-50.

[415] Weber J, Rose J, Vazquez A, *et al.* Resitance mutations outside the integrase coding region have an effect on human immunodeficiency virus replicative fitness but do not affect its susceptibility to integrase strand transfer inhibitors. PLOS One 2013; 8(6): e65631.

[416] Hightower K, Wang R, Deanda F. Doultegravir (S/GSK1349572) exhibits significantly slower dissociation than raltegravir and elvitegravir from wild-type and integrase inhibitor-resistant HIV-1 integrase-DNA complexes. Antimicrob Agents Chemother 2011; 55: 4552-9.

[417] Busschots K, De Rijck J, Christ F, Debyser Z. In search of small molecules blocking interactions between HIV proteins and intracellular cofactors. Mol BioSyst 2009; 5: 21-31.

[418] Hatch E, Hetzer M. Breaching the nuclear envelope in development and disease. JCell Biol 2014; 205(2): 133-41.

[419] Wagstaff K, Sivakumaran H, Heaton S, Harrich D, Jans D. Ivermectin is a specific inhibitor of importin α/β–mediated nuclear import able to inhibit replication of HIV-1 and dengue virus. Biochem J 2012; 443: 851-6.

[420] Herschhorn A, Oz-Gleenberg I, Hizi A. Quantitative analysis of the interactions between HIV-1 integrase and retroviral reverse transcriptases. Biochem J 2008; 412(1): 163-70.

[421] Wilkinson TA, Januszyk K, Phillips ML, Tekeste SS, Zhang M, Miller JT, *et al.* Identifying and characterizing a functional HIV-1 reverse transcriptase-binding site on integrase. J Biol Chem 2009; 284(12): 7931-9.

[422] Wu X, Liu H, Xiao H, Conway JA, Hehl E, Kalpana GV, *et al.* Human immunodeficiency virus type 1 integrase protein promotes reverse transcription through specific interactions with the nucleoprotein reverse transcription complex. J Virol 1999; 73(3): 2126-35.

[423] Dobard CW, Briones MS, Chow SA. Molecular mechanisms by which human immunodeficiency virus type 1 integrase stimulates the early steps of reverse transcription. J Virol 2007; 81(18): 10037-46.

[424] Zhu K, Dobard C, Chow SA. Requirement for integrase during reverse transcription of human immunodeficiency virus type 1 and the effect of cysteine mutations of integrase on its interactions with reverse transcriptase. J Virol 2004; 78(10): 5045-55.

[425] Devroe E, Engelman A, Silver PA. Intracellular transport of human immunodeficiency virus type 1 integrase. J Cell Sci 2003; 116(Pt 21): 4401-8.

[426] Petit C, Schwartz O, Mammano F. Oligomerization within virions and subcellular localization of human immunodeficiency virus type 1 integrase. J Virol 1999; 73(6): 5079-88.

[427] Tsurutani N, Kubo M, Maeda Y, Ohashi T, Yamamoto N, Kannagi M, *et al.* Identification of critical amino acid residues in human immunodeficiency virus type 1 IN required for efficient proviral DNA formation at steps prior to integration in dividing and nondividing cells. J Virol 2000; 74(10): 4795-806.

[428] Cherepanov P, Pluymers W, Claeys A, Proost P, De Clercq E, Debyser Z. High-level expression of active HIV-1 integrase from a synthetic gene in human cells. FASEB J 2000; 14(10): 1389-99.

[429] Pluymers W, Cherepanov P, Schols D, De Clercq E, Debyser Z. Nuclear localization of human immunodeficiency virus type 1 integrase expressed as a fusion protein with green fluorescent protein. Virology 1999; 258(2): 327-32.

[430] de Sila T, Cotton M, Rowland-Jones S. HIV-2: The forgotten AIDS virus. Trends Microbiol 2008; 16: 588-95.

[431] Popper S, Sarr A, Gueye-Ndiaye A, Mboup S, Essex M, Kanki P. Low plasma human immunodeficiency virus type 2 viral load is independent of proviral load: Low virus production *in vivo*. J Virol 2000; 74: 1554-7.

[432] Azijn H, Tirry I, Vingerhoets J, *et al.* TMC278, a next generation nonnucleoside reverse transcriptase inhibitor (NNRTI), active against wild-type and NNRTI-resistant HIV-1. Antimicrob Agents Chemother 2010; 54: 718-27.

[433] Poveda E, Rodes B, Toro C, Soriano V. Are fusion inhibitors active against all HIV variants? AIDS Res Hum Retroviruses 2004; 20: 347-8.

[434] Rodes B, Sheldon J, Toro C, Jimenez V, Alvarez M, Soriano V. Susceptibility to protease inhibitors in HIV-2 primary isolates from patients failing antiretroviral therapy. J Antimicrob Chemother 2006; 57: 709-13.

[435] Perez-Bercoff D, Triqueneaux P, Lambert C, *et al.* Polymorphisms of HIV-2 integrase and selection of resistance to raltegravir. Retrovirology 2010; 7: 98.

CHAPTER 7

Nephrotoxicity Associated with HAART

Siddhartha Yedla, Parikshit T. Hameer and Naheed Ansari*

Division of Nephrology, Department of Medicine, Jacobi Medical Center, Albert Einstein College of Medicine, Bronx New York 10461, USA

Abstract: The introduction of highly active antiretroviral therapy (HAART) in 1990s radically changed the course and management of HIV infection. Although there have been substantial reductions in morbidity and mortality of HIV- virus Infected patients, the antiretroviral medications have been associated with various toxicities, including those affecting the kidney. The prevalence of acute and chronic kidney disease has been increasing among HIV-infected patients in the United States and kidney disease has emerged as a key predictor of mortality [1-3]. The toxicities associated with the long term use of this treatment have now become a major issue and researchers have focused on understanding the cellular mechanisms underlying these drug-induced adverse effects [4]. Nephrotoxicity from antiretroviral drugs may manifest as tubular necrosis, kidney stones, acute and chronic kidney diseases. The objective of this article is to review the potential adverse effects of HAART on the kidney, with emphasis on specific antiretroviral agents that have been associated with direct kidney injury and associated metabolic disorders. Kidney injury caused by HAART is typically reversible with early detection and discontinuation of the offending agent. Nephrologists should be aware of the potential toxicity of these agents to avoid delays in diagnosis and treatment [5].

Keywords: Chronic kidney disease, diabetes mellitus, highly active antiretroviral therapy (HAART), HIV infection, hyperlipidemia, lactic acidosis, lipodystrophy syndrome, nephrolithiasis, nephrotoxicity, renal insufficiency, tubulopathies.

INTRODUCTION

The introduction of HAART therapy for the treatment of HIV infection over the last decade has resulted in a significant reduction in the morbidity and mortality resulting from AIDS and HIV-related disease. Over time use of antiretroviral

***Corresponding author Naheed Ansari:** Division of Nephrology, Department of Medicine, Jacobi Medical Center, Albert Einstein College of Medicine, Bronx New York 10461, USA; Tel: 718-918-3176; Fax: 718-918-8364; E-mail: Naheed.Ansari@nbhn.net

(ARV) therapy has changed from single drug to combination multidrug regimens that were able to suppress viral multiplication in most HIV-infected patients. As a result, HIV infection has transformed into a chronic manageable disease requiring long-term ARV treatment.

In spite of the evident benefits of antiretroviral therapy and suppressed viral replication, antiretroviral drugs can induce a reversible or irreversible renal damage. The kidney plays a major role in the metabolism and excretion of antiretroviral drugs and this makes it vulnerable to several types of injuries, including acute kidney injury (AKI), tubulopathies, chronic kidney disease (CKD), and end-stage renal disease requiring renal replacement therapy. A variety of other systemic adverse effects other than nephrotoxicity have also been recognized, including lipodystrophy syndrome, hyperlipidemia, lactic acidosis, osteopenia and osteoporosis, and hyperglycemia. This chapter reviews various classes of HAART and the effects of drugs on the kidney.

Antiretroviral Drug Classes

There are five major types of drugs used to treat HIV/AIDS (Table **1**)

1) Nucleoside (and nucleotide) reverse transcriptase inhibitors (NRTIs)
2) Non-nucleoside reverse transcriptase inhibitors (NNRTIs)
3) Protease inhibitors (PIs)
4) Entry inhibitors (Fusion Inhibitors and CCR-5 Antagonists)
5) Integrase Inhibitors

Table 1: Shows various classes of anti-retroviral drugs used in treatment of HIV infection

Class	Drugs
Nucleoside (and nucleotide) reverse transcriptase inhibitors (NRTIs)	Tenofovir (TDF), Emtricitabine (FTC), Lamivudine (3TC), Abacavir (ABC), Stavudine (d4T), Zidovudine (ZDV), Didanosine (ddI).

Table 1: contd...

Non-nucleoside reverse transcriptase inhibitors (NNRTIs)	Efavirenz (EFV), Nevirapine (NVP), Etravirine (ETV), Rilpivirine (RPV).
Protease inhibitors (PIs)	Saquinavir (SQV), Ritonavir (RTV), Lopinavir (LPV) Indinavir (IDV), Nelfinavir (NFV), Atazanavir (ATV), Fosamprenavir (FPV), Darunavir (DRV).
Entry inhibitors (Fusion Inhibitors and CCR-5 Antagonists)	Enfuvirtide (T-20), Maraviroc (MVC),
Integrase Inhibitors	Raltegravir (RAL), Elvitegravir (EVG). Dolutegravir (DTG)

Standard HAART therapy typically consists of three or more HIV drugs, most commonly two NRTIs in combination with a non-nucleoside reverse transcriptase inhibitor (NNRTI), protease inhibitor or, most recently, integrase inhibitor.

Types of Regimens

Preferred regimens for non-pregnant patients approved by FDA are given below.

NNRTI Based Regimen

Efavirenz/Tenofovir/Emtricitabine

PI-Based Regimens

1) Atazanavir/Ritonavir + Tenofovir/Emtricitabine
2) Darunavir/Ritonavir + Tenofovir/Emtricitabine

Integrase Inhibitor Based Regimen (INSTI)

1) Dolutegravir + Tenofovir/emtricitabine
2) Elvitegravir + Cobicistat + Tenofovir/emtricitabine (STRIBILD)
3) Raltegravir + Tenofovir/emtricitabine

4) Dolutegravir + Abacavir/Lamivudine

Note

*Efavirenz is teratogenic. Consider non efavirenz containing regimen in women who are planning to become pregnant or are sexually active and not using effective contraception.

*Tenofovir should be used with caution in patients with renal insufficiency.

HIV Life Cycle and Current Drug Targets

HIV virus infects cells of the immune system, mainly CD4 lymphocytes. When a CD4 cell is infected with HIV, the virus goes through several steps to replicate itself into active infectious virions.

Extracellular virions enter their target cell through a complex three-step process, that include attachment to the CD4 receptor, binding to the CCR5 or CXCR4 coreceptors, membrane fusion and release of capsid into the cell. After entry into the cell the nucleocapsid gets uncoated and releases its viral genes and enzymes into host cell. The HIV reverse transcriptase enzyme converts transcription of HIV single stranded RNA into double stranded HIV DNA also known as provirus. The provirus enters into the host cell nucleus and integrates with the host chromosomal DNA. The provirus uses host cell RNA polymerase to create copies of the HIV genomic material, and also messenger RNA (mRNA) which will be used to make HIV proteins. The HIV protease enzyme cleaves polypeptide chains, allowing the virus to mature and bud from the cell surface.

Current antiretroviral drugs used to target these steps in the HIV life cycle are shown in Fig. (**1**).

CCR5 antagonist (Maraviroc) prevents entry by binding to the chemokine coreceptor on the host CD4+ cell. Fusion inhibitor (Enfuvirtide) prevents entry by binding to glycoprotein on the viral envelope.

NRTIs and NNRTIs compete with host nucleotides to serve as the substrate for reverse transcriptase chain elongation resulting in chain termination and cessation of viral replication.

The integrase inhibitors prevent incorporation of HIV provirus DNA into host cell chromosomal DNA thus preventing the lifelong infection.

Protease inhibitors bind to protease enzyme, and prevent the formation of precursor proteins thus making the virions incomplete and noninfectious [69].

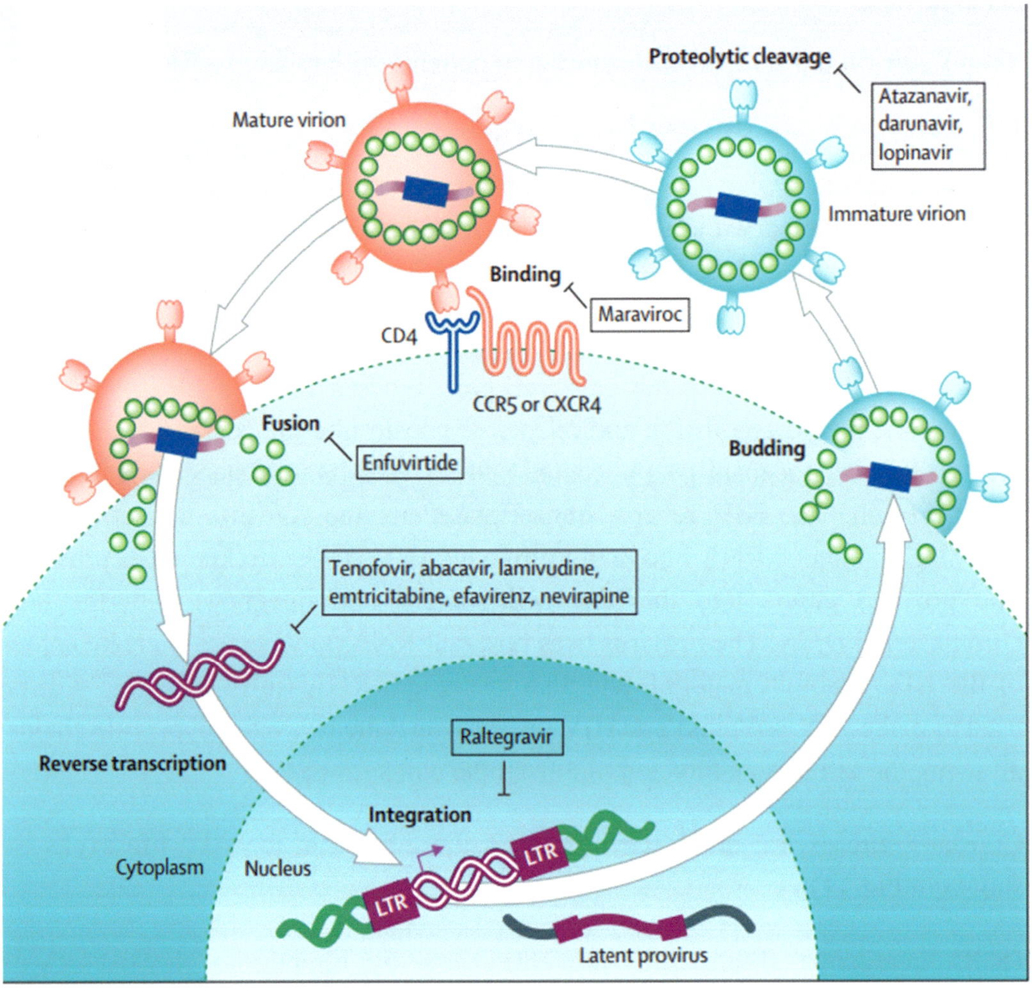

Figure 1: HIV life cycle and antiretroviral drug targets [71].

Protease Inhibitors

Protease inhibitors function as competitive inhibitors that directly bind and inactivate the HIV protease enzyme, which is necessary for assembly and maturation of virions. In general, the PIs are primarily metabolized in the liver and thus do not exhibit profound nephrotoxicity.

However with the exception of the newer agents (tipranavir and darunavir), all of the PIs have been associated with urolithiasis. Indinavir which is no more used in clinical practice has been most often associated with renal toxic effects, including crystalluria, nephrolithiasis, dysuria, hematuria, renal colic, papillary necrosis, renal atrophy, acute interstitial nephritis, and acute and chronic renal failure [6, 7] (Table **2**). Indinavir crystals exhibit birefringence and appear as tapered or flat rectangular plates with wide variations in size (Fig. **2**) [8].

The incidence of complications among indinavir-treated patients in studies was about 8 to 10 cases per 100 treatment-years and the risk factors include low body weight, higher doses, warm environmental temperatures, [9] underlying kidney disease, hepatitis C coinfection, and concomitant use of trimethoprim-sulfamethoxazole [10-13]. Urologic symptoms and elevations in serum creatinine are usually reversible and normalize within weeks after the discontinuation of indinavir, although irreversible renal damage has been described in few cases [7, 14].

Protease inhibitors must be boosted by low dose ritonavir (100 or 200 mg), a potent inhibitor of cytochrome P450 3A4 (CYP3A4) and CYP2D6. It can cause significant increase in serum drug concentration levels of other protease inhibitors (PIs) thus allowing a reduction in pill burden, dosing frequency, and food restriction. In rare cases atazanavir can be used non-boosted.

Atazanavir is a newer PI, with good potency and favorable side effects. The renal profile of atazanavir was found to be safe in various cohort studies and randomized controlled studies. Since its use has increased recently, several case reports of atazanavir associated nephrolithiasis were reported over a four year period of study [15, 16] (Table **2**). Risk factors for urine crystallization include low water intake, high urinary, and a prior history of urinary stones may have a greater risk of urine crystallization. Atazanavir or atazanavir/tenofovir therapy has also been associated with isolated cases of interstitial nephritis and acute renal failure, but discontinuation of the therapy resulted in a rapid reversal of renal function [17, 18].

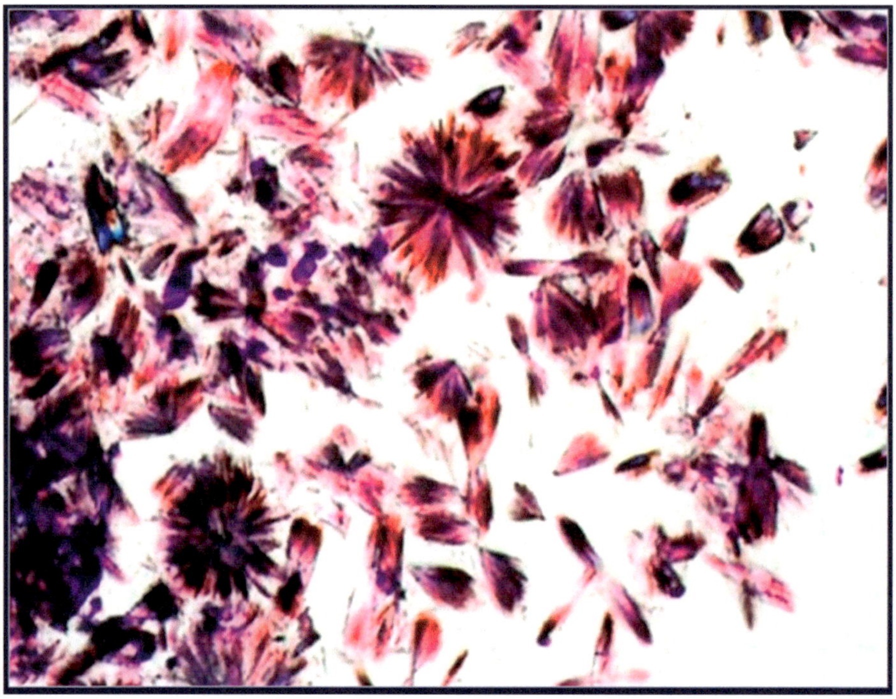

Figure 2: Microscopic appearance of Indinavir crystals in urine sediment [72].

NRTI'S (Nucleoside/Nucleotide Reverse Transcriptase Inhibitors)

NRTIs are the backbone of current combination antiretroviral therapy. Both nucleoside and nucleotide reverse transcriptase inhibitors (NRTIs) are a class of antiretroviral drugs whose chemical structure constitutes a modified version of a natural nucleoside. These drugs after intracellular phosphorylation inhibit the viral reverse transcriptase by competitive substrate insertion into DNA strands, thus halting viral DNA synthesis. The NRTI class includes seven agents, zidovudine, lamivudine, emtricitabine, abacavir, didanosine, stavudine, and tenofovir. The only nucleotide analog currently approved for the treatment of HIV infection is tenofovir.

The NRTIs are primarily excreted by the kidneys except abacavir, and require dose adjustment in patients with compromised renal function. Renal elimination is mediated by both glomerular filtration and tubular secretion. NRTIs uptake into proximal tubular epithelial cells occurs through human organic anion transporters (hOATs) and organic cation transporters on the basolateral membrane [5].

Mitochondrial toxicity is a more common adverse effect of NRTIs, particularly didanosine and stavudine. Typical manifestations include hyperlactatemia, pancreatitis, and hepatic steatosis [19]. Lactic acidosis is a relatively frequent adverse event. It can be found in up to 20% to 30% of patients treated with NRTIs, more often seen in patients on long term HAART treatment.

Mitochondrial toxicity is caused by the inhibition of mitochondrial DNA polymerase gamma by the nucleoside analogues as they have strong affinity for the DNA polymerase enzymes. As a result there is a decreased expression of the mitochondrial DNA (mt DNA), resulting in decreased number of mitochondria and eventually leading to loss of oxidative phosphorylation function. The clinical signs and symptoms depend on the target organ damage, some common side effects include myopathy, neuropathy, hepatic steatosis and lactic acidemia. Potentially fatal side effects such as lactic acidosis and pancreatitis are rare [20]. Treatment includes stopping of the offending agent and substituting with alternative drug with less mitochondrial toxicity (lamivudine, emtricitabine, tenofovir). For symptomatic patients close monitoring with supportive therapy in a hospital setting is recommended. In case of intractable lactic acidosis, hemodialysis is the treatment of option.

Cidofovir is a nucleotide analogue with potent activity against CMV retinitis in AIDS patients [30]. Nephrotoxic effects are mostly related to renal proximal tubular cell dysfunction and are dose dependent. Cidofovir nephrotoxicity leads to decreased renal function, proximal tubular dysfunction and rarely chronic interstitial nephritis [21-23]. Renal dysfunction is usually reversible after discontinuation of the drug. It should be avoided in patients who are on other nephrotoxic drugs (Aminoglycosides, NSAIDS, and Amphotericin-B). Serum Creatinine and urine protein levels should be monitored 48 hours before each dose.

Adefovir is a nucleotide analog of adenosine monophosphate, used in the treatment of HIV patients coinfected with HBV. Adefovir is added to the existing HIV regimen for the treatment of coinfection. Renal tubular dysfunction was observed in few studies. Patients having baseline renal insufficiency, hypertension and diabetes mellitus are more prone for renal injury. It can also be used as a monotherapy in lamivudine resistant HBV infection [24-27].

Tenofovir

Tenofovir disoproxil fumarate is the only nucleotide reverse transcriptase inhibitor (NtRTI) analog presently used and approved by the US Food and Drug Administration (FDA) for the treatment of HIV infection. It is structurally similar to adefovir and cidofovir [28].

Several risk factors have been identified in developing tenofovir associated renal toxicity. They include older age, black race, low body weight, various comorbidities (hypertension, diabetes mellitus, chronic hepatitis C), pre-existing renal dysfunction, concomitant use of nephrotoxic drugs or some antiretroviral agents (such as ritonavir-boosted PIs and didanosine), and advanced HIV disease [29-33].

The proximal tubular cell is the main target of tenofovir toxicity due to its complement of cell membrane transporters that favor tenofovir accumulation. Tenofovir is taken up into proximal tubular epithelial cells through basolateral membrane human organic anion transporters (hOAT), and it is secreted into the tubular lumen across the apical membrane by multidrug resistance-associated proteins transporters (MRP) (Fig. **3**) [3].

There are several reports that have found evidence of potential tenofovir nephrotoxicity [34-36]. The renal complications include both glomerular damage (with resultant reduced GFR) and proximal tubular dysfunction which include (proteinuria, calcium and phosphorus dysregulation, Fanconi syndrome, reduced bone mineral density, and diabetes insipidus). These may present as acute kidney injury or chronic kidney disease [37, 38]. The most common renal biopsy finding is proximal tubular injury, ranging from diffuse, mild to severe. The light microscopic findings in Tenofovir nephrotoxicity resemble changes seen in other forms of toxic acute tubular necrosis which include luminal ectasia, irregular luminal contours, prominent nucleoli, and loss of brush border. A distinctive finding from other forms of toxic ATN is prominent eosinophilic intracytoplasmic inclusions in proximal tubular epithelial cells (Fig. **4**).

The major ultrastructural findings include acute proximal tubular degenerative changes and in some proximal tubular epithelia, the number of mitochondria is markedly reduced, consistent with mitochrondrial depletion. Mitochondria vary widely in size and shape, ranging from small and rounded to markedly enlarged and swollen with irregular contours. Many of the enlarged mitochondria display prominent clumping, loss, and disorientation of cristae (Fig. **5**).

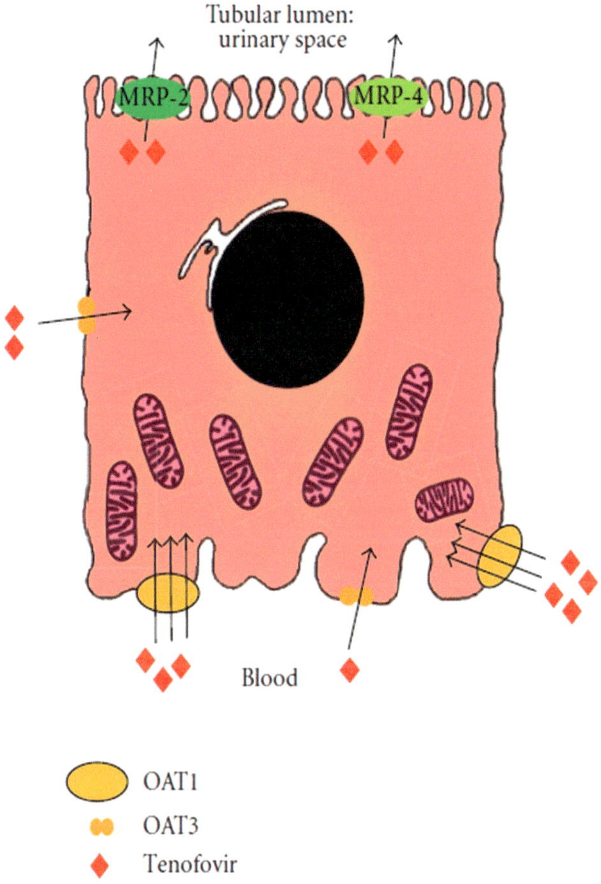

Figure 3: Tenofovir handling by proximal tubular cells. Tenofovir secretion by proximal tubular cells: OAT1 is the main transporter uptaking tenofovir into the proximal tubular cell, although OAT3 also collaborates. Once inside this mitochondria-rich cell type, tenofovir must be extruded into the tubular lumen by MRP-2 and MRP-4. Blocking tenofovir uptake by OAT1 may protect tubular cells by keeping intracellular tenofovir level low. Thus, probenecid is routinely used to prevent cidofovir nephrotoxicity since cidofovir is also transported into tubular cells by OAT1. There is less experience preventing tenofovir nephrotoxicity. A decreased GFR will increase plasma tenofovir levels and proximal tubular cell uptake through OAT1. Blocking tenofovir extrusion by MRP-2 and MRP-4 by pharmacological interference may also boost tenofovir nephrotoxicity. OAT: organic acid transporter; MRP: multidrug resistance protein [73].

The main clinical manifestations of tenofovir toxicity are proximal tubulopathy resulting in proteinuria, hypokalemia, glycosuria, hypophosphatemia due to phosphaturia, and aminoaciduria. In some cases, tenofovir-associated nephropathy manifests as partial or complete Fanconi syndrome, [39-45] (Table **2**). Fanconi syndrome is a generalized proximal tubulopathy. Other manifestations of proximal tubulopathy include osteomalacia and decreased bone mass due to phosphate wasting and/or calcitriol deficiency, since calcitriol is synthesized by mitochondria in proximal tubules [46-49].

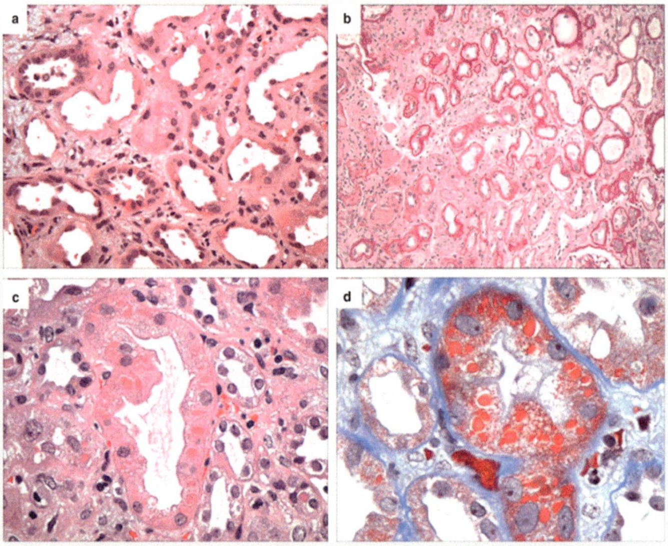

Figure 4: Tenofovir nephrotoxicity. (**a**) Proximal tubules exhibit diffuse and severe acute degenerative changes including luminal ectasia, cytoplasmic simplification, irregular luminal contours, loss of brush border, and focal apoptosis with epithelial desquamation, with adjacent interstitial edema. These findings are similar to toxic acute tubular necrosis (hematoxylin and eosin). (**b**) A low-power field showing tubular simplification and interstitial fibrosis. These light microscopic findings are consistent with an acute and chronic tubulointerstitial nephropathy (periodic acid-Schiff,). (**c**) A characteristic feature of TDF nephrotoxicity is eosinophilic intracytoplasmic inclusions within proximal tubular epithelial cells (hematoxylin and eosin). (**d**) The proximal tubular inclusions stain red with trichrome stain [34].

Concomitant use of ritonavir (alone or in combination with lopinavir or other PI) raises plasma concentrations of tenofovir and may increase the risk for renal dysfunction. Therefore proper dosing for the level of GFR should be maintained and close monitoring of patients who are taking this combination of medications is recommended.

Treatment of tenofovir associated AKI mandates discontinuation of tenofovir. Course of renal disease is variable after cessation of tenofovir. It takes around weeks to months for improvement renal function after discontinuing the drug [50, 51]. Early recognition and withdrawal of the drug are keys to avoid irreversible tubular damage. Due to the potential risk of nephrotoxicity, biannual monitoring of renal function in HIV patients receiving tenofovir with GFR <90mL/min, is recommended by HIV/IDSA association in their new guidelines [41, 52].

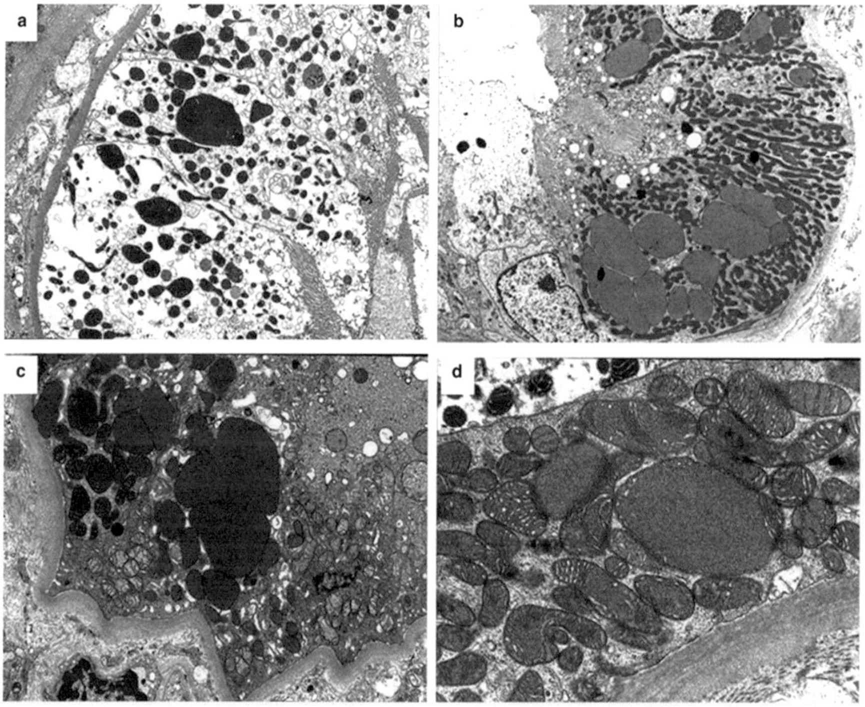

Figure 5: (**a**) A low-magnification field demonstrates the wide range in size and shape of mitochrondria within proximal tubular epithelial cells (**b**) Markedly enlarged mitochondria are interspersed with normal-sized mitochrondria in proximal tubular cells. One cell is undergoing degeneration with shedding of cytoplasmic fragments into the tubular lumen. (**c**) At higher magnification, the enlarged mitochrondria are largely devoid of cristae. In contrast, cristae are easily identified in adjacent, normal-sized mitochondria (**d**) Abnormalities in the number and distribution of mitochondrial cristae are best appreciated at high magnification. In this field, there is focal loss of cristae, as well as clustering of residual cristae at the peripheral mitochrondrial membrane [34].

Tenofovir alafenamide fumarate (TAF) is a new prodrug of TDF, currently undergoing clinical rails. TAF is largely delivered as TAF to lymphocytes and macrophages, then metabolized intracellularly to tenofovir and phosphorylated to the active tenofovir DP. Randomized (phase 1 and phase 2) clinical trials showed efficacy and safety profile of TAF over TDF, as part of a regimen containing FTC, EVG and COBI in ART-naive patients. TAF attained higher antiviral activity, higher intracellular concentrations, and smaller rise in serum creatinine levels and lower decline in the glomerular function compared to TDF. TAF exposure was associated with significantly smaller changes in estimated creatinine clearance, renal tubular proteinuria, and bone mineral density [53-54].

NNRTIs

The non-nucleoside reverse transcriptase inhibitors (NNRTIs) inhibit HIV replication by binding to viral reverse transcriptase and blocking its function. These drugs are very effective in decreasing the HIV viremia and raising the CD 4 counts. The NNRTIs include delavirdine, nevirapine, efavirenz, etravirine and rilpivirine. NNRTIs exhibit minimal nephrotoxicity because they are primarily metabolized by the liver (hepatic cytochrome P450 system) and do not undergo active renal secretion. Clinical evidence of NNRTI-mediated renal toxicity is very limited. Nevaripine is associated with AKI in pregnant patient in a study [55]. Efavirenz is associated with urolithiasis in couple of case reports [56, 57] and is contraindicated in patients as it is associated with cranial malformations in animal studies.

Entry Inhibitors

Fusion Inhibitors

Fusion inhibitors are class of antiretrovirals that binds to the components of HIV virus envelope to prevent fusion of the virus with the host cell membrane. Enfuvirtide is the first drug approved in this class. In a study (TORO trial) conducted over 328 patients, one case of membranoproliferative glomerulonephritis has been reported. Other than this, it has not been associated with nephrotoxicity.

CCR-5 Antagonists

CCR5 antagonists function by blocking the entry of HIV virus into the host cell. Maraviroc is the only drug in this class that has been approved for use in HIV patients. Clinical trials have shown that maraviroc does not have significant nephrotoxic effects.

Integrase Inhibitors

These comprise new class of HIV medications. Integrase inhibitors block the action of integrase, a viral enzyme required for incorporation of viral DNA into host cell genome, thus stopping the replication of the virus. Raltegravir is the first drug in this class to be approved by FDA in 2007 for use in treatment-naive and treatment-experienced HIV-infected patients.

Elvitegravir is subsequently approved in 2012 as a part of a combination regimen that incorporates tenofovir,emtricitabine, boosted by cobicistat into a single tablet (EVG/COBI/FTC/TDF). Cobicistat (COBI) is a potent cytochrome P450 3A (CYP3A) inhibitor and pharmacokinetic booster to increases the serum drug level of Elvitegravir [58]. Cobicistat inhibits tubular secretion of creatinine resulting in mild increase in serum creatinine concentration, however these elevations do not appear to have affected any change in glomerular filtration rate (GFR). The changes in serum creatinine after starting fixed-dose regimen need to be carefully monitored as the tenofovir component of the combination regimen can occasionally cause significant renal injury. Any increase of serum creatinine more than 0.4 mg/dL should not be attributed to the effect of cobicistat alone and should prompt a more thorough evaluation for acute kidney injury [58]. Raltegravir and Elvitegravir are currently preferred drugs in the INSTI class. However both of these drugs have cross resistance and low genetic barrier for drug resistance.

Dolutegravir is the new second generation Integrase inhibitor that has been approved by the FDA in 2013. Various randomized clinical trials had shown several beneficial effects of dolutegravir over other integrase inhibitors in treatment naive patients and treatment experienced subjects. It has shown significant virologic suppression and good tolerability. Dolutegravir causes rise in serum creatinine level due to the reversible inhibition of tubular creatinine secretion without affecting the glomerular filtration rate. The rise in creatinine level occurs within the first 4 weeks of treatment with dolutegravir or cobistat and they remain stable through 48 weeks. The prolonged intracellular half-life and its high genetic barrier to drug resistance are favorable factors compared to other INSTI drugs [59].

Given their potency, efficacy, and safety, integrase inhibitors represent an important advancement in HIV-1 therapy. In various clinical trials conducted for evaluating integrase inhibitors, no evidence of nephrotoxicity has been reported [60-63].

Table 2: Summary of nephrotoxic effects of HAART [74]

Class	Drugs	Adverse effects	Frequency
Protease inhibitors	Indinavir	Crystalluria, nephrolithiasis, dysuria, acute interstitial nephritis with crystalline casts in tubules, and papillary necrosis.	Frequent
	Ritonavir	Acute renal failure.	Rare
	Atazanavir	Acute interstitial nephritis.	Very rare
	Saquinavir	Renal calculi	Very rare
Nucleotide reverse transcriptase inhibitors	Adefovir	Acute tubular toxicity, and partial Fanconi syndrome	Frequent
	Tenofovir	Acute tubular toxicity, partial Fanconi syndrome, and nephrogenic diabetes insipidus.	Acute tubular toxicity(Frequent), Fanconi syndrome(Rare)
Nucleoside reverse transcriptase inhibitors	Abacavir	Acute interstitial nephritis.	Very rare
	Didanosine	Nephrogenic diabetes insipidus, Fanconi syndrome	
	Lamivudine Stavudine	Renal tubular acidosis.	Very rare

Metabolic Side Effects of HAART Therapy

Glucose Metabolism

The prevalence of insulin resistance, glucose intolerance and diabetes has risen significantly since the introduction of ART. In a study (INITIO Trail) conducted on 881 HIV-infected patients over three years who were started on antiretroviral therapy, the incidence of metabolic syndrome was found to be 8 to 12 cases per100 person years [64].

Dyslipidemias

Both HIV infection and HAART therapy have been associated with dyslipidemias. These are characterized by increased levels of VLDL, LDL, and lipoprotein, and reduced levels of HDL [5, 65].

The pathophysiology of dyslipidemia in HIV patients is not yet fully understood. It has not yet been established that, if the dyslipidemia occurs by a direct consequence of ART or by the interaction of various factors, such as the anti-retroviral therapy, genetic predisposition, or other factors such as host response to HIV infection [66].

Cardiovascular Events

The usage of antiretroviral therapy improved life expectancy and a reduction in the incidence of opportunistic infections in HIV patients. However, due to the prevalence of diabetes mellitus, dyslipidemia and lipodystrophy, increased premature cardiovascular diseases have been described. This predisposition to atherosclerosis could result from HIV infection or from metabolic changes resulting from the use of antiretroviral therapy or from both [67, 68].

Chronic Kidney Disease

HAART treated patients may develop chronic kidney disease. Patients with partial recovery of renal function after an episode of AKI are more vulnerable in developing chronic kidney disease. Long-term therapy with indinavir or cidofovir may cause chronic renal impairment. Renal atrophy has also been has been associated with long-term treatment with indinavir [22, 69, 70]. NNTRIs and most of the protease inhibitors and integrase inhibitors can be used in these patients (Except Indinavir, Cidofovir and Atazanavir).

CONCLUSION

Antiretroviral therapies have been associated with significant side effects including nephrotoxicity and metabolic disorders. Antiretroviral therapy can cause renal dysfunction directly by inducing acute tubular necrosis, acute interstitial nephritis, crystal nephropathy and renal tubular disorders or indirectly *via* drug interactions. Regular monitoring of renal function should be advocated in HIV patients receiving antiretroviral therapy especially if the regimen includes nephrotoxic agents. Early identification of risk factors, systematic screening for chronic causes of CKD, and proper referrals for kidney disease management are beneficial in patient care.

ACKNOWLEDGEMENTS

Declared none.

CONFLICT OF INTEREST

The authors confirm that this chapter contents have no conflict of interest.

REFERENCES

[1] Schwartz EJ, Szczech LA, Ross MJ, Klotman ME, Winston JA, Klotman PE. Highly active antiretroviral therapy and the epidemic of HIV+ end-stage renal disease. J Am Soc Nephrol 2005; 16: 2412-20.

[2] Wyatt CM, Arons RR, Klotman PE, Klotman ME. Acute renal failure in hospitalized patients with HIV: risk factors and impact on in-hospital mortality. AIDS 2006; 20: 561-5.

[3] Selik RM, Byers RH Jr, Dworkin MS. Trends in diseases reported on US death certificates that mentioned HIV infection, 1987-1999. J Acquir Immune Defic Syndr 2002; 29: 378-87.

[4] Apostolova N. Blas-Garcia A. Esplugues JV. Mitochondrial toxicity in HAART: an overview of *in vitro* evidence. Curr Pharm Des 2011; 17(20): 2130-44.

[5] Jennifer J and Wyatt CM. Antiretroviral Medications: Adverse Effects on the Kidney. Adv Chronic Kidney Dis 2010; 17(1): 72-82.

[6] Roling J, Schmid H, Fischereder M, Draenert R, Goebel FD. HIV-associated renal diseases and highly active antiretroviral therapy-induced nephropathy. Clin Infect Dis 2006; 42: 1488-95.

[7] Daugas E, Rougier JP, Hill G. HAART-related nephropathies in HIV-infected patients. Kidney Int 2005; 67: 393-403.

[8] Gagnon R, Tecimer S, Watters A, *et al.* Prospective study of urinalysis abnormalities in HIV-positive individuals treated with indinavir. Am J Kidney Dis 2000; 36: 507-15.

[9] Fux CA, Simcock M, Wolbers M, *et al.* Tenofovir use is associated with a reduction in calculated glomerular filtration rates in the Swiss HIV Cohort Study. Antivir Ther 2007; 12: 1165-73.

[10] Dieleman JP, Sturkenboom MC, Jambroes M, *et al.* Risk factors for urological symptoms in a cohort of users of the HIV protease inhibitor indinavir sulfate: the ATHENA cohort. Arch Intern Med 2002; 162: 1493-501.

[11] De Araujo M, Seguro AC. Trimethoprim-sulfamethoxazole (TMP/SMX) potentiates indinavir nephrotoxicity. Antivir Ther 2002; 7: 181-4.

[12] Herman JS, Ives NJ, Nelson M, Gazzard BG, Easterbrook PJ. Incidence and risk factors for the development of indinavir-associated renal complications. J Antimicrob Chemother 2001; 48: 355-60.

[13] Casado JL, Moreno A, Sabido R, *et al.* A clinical study of the combination of 100 mg ritonavir plus 800 mg indi navir as salvage therapy: infl uence of increased plasma drug levels in the rate of response. HIV Clin Trials 2000; 1: 13-9.

[14] Angel-Moreno-Maroto A, Suarez-Castellano L, Hernandez-Cabrera M, Perez-Arellano JL. Severe efavirenz induced hypersensitivity syndrome with acute renal failure. J Infect 2006; 52: 39-40.

[15] Nadler RB, Rubenstein JN, Eggener SE, *et al.* The etiology of urolithiasis in HIV infected patients. J Urol 2003; 169: 475.
[16] Chan-Tack KM, Truffa MM, Struble KA, Birnkrant DB. Atazanavir-associated nephrolithiasis: cases from the US Food and Drug Administration's Adverse Event Reporting System. AIDS 2007; 21: 1215.
[17] Brewster UC, Perazella MA. Acute interstitial nephritis associated with atazanavir, a new protease inhibitor. Am J Kidney Dis 2004; 44: 81-4.
[18] Schmid S, Opravil M, Moddel M, *et al.* Acute interstitial nephritis of HIV-positive patients under atazanavir and tenofovir therapy in a retrospective analysis of kidney biopsies. Virchows Arch 2007; 450: 665-70.
[19] John M, Mallal S: Hyperlactatemia syndromes in people with HIV infection. Curr Opin Infect Dis 2002; 15: 23-9.
[20] Boubaker K, Flepp M, Sudre P, *et al.* Hyperlactatemia and antiretroviral therapy: the Swiss HIV cohort Study. Clin Infect Dis 2001; 33: 1931-7.
[21] Vittecoq D, Dumitrescu L, Beaufils H, Deray G: Fanconi syndrome associated with cidofovir therapy. Antimicrob Agents Chemother 1997; 41: 1846.
[22] Vandercam B, Moreau M, Goffin E, Marot JC, Cosyns JP, Jadoul M. Cidofovir-induced end-stage renal failure. Clin Infect Dis 1999; 29: 948-9.
[23] Izzedine H, Launay-Vacher V, Deray G. Antiviral Drug-Induced Nephrotoxicity. Am J Kidney Dis 2005; 45: 804-17.
[24] Benhamou Y, Thibault V, Vig P, *et al.* Safety and efficacy of adefovir dipivoxil in patients infected with lamivudine-resistant hepatitis B and HIV-1. J Hepatol 2006; 44: 62.
[25] Ha NB, Ha NB, Garcia RT, Trinh HN, Vu AA, Nguyen HA, Nguyen KK, Levitt BS, Nguyen MH. Renal dysfunction in chronic hepatitis B patients treated with adefovir dipivoxil. Hepatology 2009; 50: 727-34.
[26] Gara N, Zhao X, Collins MT, *et al.* Renal tubular dysfunction during long-term adefovir or tenofovir therapy in chronic hepatitis B. Aliment Pharmacol Ther 2012; 35: 1317.
[27] Benhamou Y, Bochet M, Thibault V, *et al.* Safety and efficacy of adefovir dipivoxil in patients co-infected with HIV-1 and lamivudine-resistant hepatitis B virus: an open-label pilot study. Lancet 2001; 358: 718.
[28] Gallant JE, Deresinski S. Tenofovir disoproxil fumarate, Clin Infect Dis 2003; 37(7): 944-50.
[29] Kalayjian RC. Renal issues in HIV infection. Curr HIV/AIDS Rep. 2011; 8: 164-71.
[30] Fernandez-Fernandez B, Montoya-Ferrer A, Sanz AB*, et al.* Tenofovir nephrotoxicity: 2011 update. AIDS Res Treat 2011; 354908.
[31] Hall AM, Hendry BM, Nitsch D, Connolly JO. Tenofovir associated kidney toxicity in HIV-infected patients: a review of the evidence. Am J Kidney Dis 2011; 57: 773-80.
[32] Horberg M, Tang B, Towner W, *et al.* Impact of tenofovir on renal function in HIV-infected, antiretroviral-naïve patients. J Acquir Immune Defic Syndr 2010; 53: 62-9.
[33] Calza L, Trapani F, Tedeschi S*, et al.* Tenofovir-induced renal toxicity in 324 HIV-infected, antiretroviral-naïve patients. Scand J Infect Dis 2011; 43: 656-60.
[34] Herlitz LC, Mohan S, Stokes MB, Radhakrishnan J, D'Agati VD, Markowitz GS. Tenofovir nephrotoxicity: acute tubular necrosis with distinctive clinical, pathological, and mitochondrial abnormalities. Kidney Int 2010; 78(11): 1171-7.
[35] Côté HC, Magil AB, Harris M *et al.* Exploring mitochondrial nephrotoxicity as a potential mechanism of kidney dysfunction among HIV-infected patients on highly active antiretroviral therapy. Antivir Ther 2006; 11(1): 79-86.

[36] Coca S, Perazella MA. Rapid communication: acute renal failure associated with tenofovir: evidence of drug induced nephrotoxicity. Am J Med Sci 2002. 324; (6): 342-4.

[37] Calza L. Renal Toxicity Associated with Antiretroviral Therapy. HIV Clin Trials 2012; 13(4): 189-211.

[38] Izzedine H, Harris M, Perazella MA. The nephrotoxic effects of HAART. Nat Rev Nephrol 2009; 5: 563-73.

[39] Izzedine H, Isnard-Bagnis C, Hulot JS, *et al.* Renal safety of tenofovir in HIV treatment-experienced patients. AIDS, 2004; 18 (7): 1074-6.

[40] Pozniak AL, Gallant JE, DeJesus E *et al.* Tenofovir disoproxil fumarate, emtricitabine, and efavirenz *versus* fixeddose zidovudine/lamivudine and efavirenz in antiretroviralnaive patients: virologic, immunologic, and morphologic changes—a 96-week analysis. J Acquir Immune Defic Syndr 2006; 43(5): 535-40.

[41] Cooper RD, Wiebe N, Smith N, Keiser P, Naicker S, Tonelli M. Systematic review and meta-analysis: renal safety of tenofovir disoproxil fumarate in HIV-infected patients. Clin Infect Dis 2010; 51: 496-505.

[42] Irizarry-Alvarado JM, Dwyer JP, Brumble LM, Alvarez S, Mendez JC. Proximal tlibular dysfunction associated with tenofovir and didanosine causing fanconi syndrome and diabetes insipidus: a report of 3 cases. AIDS Read 2009; 19(3): 114-21.

[43] Peyrière H, Reynes J, Rouanet I *et al.* Renal tubular dysfunction associated with tenofovir therapy: report of 7 cases. J Acquir Immune Defic Syndr 2004; 35(3): 269-73.

[44] Zimmermann AE, Pizzoferrato T, Bedford J, Morris A, Hoffman R, Braden G. Tenofovir-associated acute and chronic kidney disease: a case of multiple drug interactions. Clin Infect Dis 2006; 42 (2) 283-90.

[45] Gupta SK. Tenofovir-associated fanconi syndrome: review of the FDA adverse event reporting system. AIDS Patient Care STDS 2008; 22 (2): 99-103.

[46] Perrot S, Aslangul E, Szwebel T, Caillat-Vigneron N, Le Jeunne C. Bone pain due to fractures revealing osteomalacia related to tenofovir-induced proximal renal tubular dysfunction in a human immunodeficiency virus-infected patient. J Clin Rheumatol 2009; 15(2): 72-4.

[47] Parsonage MJ, Wilkins EG, Snowden N, Issa BG, Savage MW. The development of hypophosphataemic osteomalacia with myopathy in two patients with HIV infection receiving tenofovir therapy. HIV Med 2005; 6(5): 341-6.

[48] Van Rompay KK, Brignolo LL, Meyer DJ *et al.* Biological effects of short-term or prolonged administration of 9-[2-(Phosphonomethoxy) Propyl] Adenine (Tenofovir) to newborn and infant rhesus macaques. Antimicrob Agents Chemother 2004; 48(5): 1469-87.

[49] Castillo AB, Tarantal AF, Watnik MR, Martin RB. Tenofovir treatment at 30 mg/kg/day can inhibit cortical bone mineralization in growing rhesus monkeys (Macaca mulatta). J Orthop Res 2002; 20(6): 1185-9.

[50] de la Prada FJ, Prados AM, Tugores A, Uriol M, Saus C, Morey A. Acute renal failure and proximal renal tubular dysfunction in a patient with acquired immunodeficiency syndrome treated with tenofovir. Nefrologia. 2006; 26: 626-30.

[51] Karras A, Lafaurie M, Furco A *et al.* Tenofovir-related nephrotoxicity in human immunodeficiency virus-infected patients: three cases of renal failure, fanconi syndrome, and nephrogenic diabetes insipidus. Clin Infect Dis 2003; 36: 1070-3.

[52] Gupta SK, Eustace JA, Winston JA *et al.* Guidelines for the management of chronic kidney disease in HIV-infected patients: recommendations of the HIV medicine association of the infectious diseases society of America. Clin Infect Dis 2005; 40: 1559-85.

[53] Ruane P, De Jesus E, Berger D, *et al.* Antiviral activity, safety, and pharmacokinetics/pharmacodynamics of tenofovir alafenamide as 10-daymonotherapy in HIV-1-positive adults. J Acquir Immune Defic Syndr 2013; 63: 449-55.

[54] Zolopa A, Ortiz R, Sax P, *et al.*Comparative study of tenofovir alafenamide *vs* tenofovir disoproxil fumarate, each with elvitegravir, cobicistat, and emtricitabine, for HIV treatment [abstract 99LB]. 20th Conference on Retroviruses and Opportunistic Infections; 3-6 March 2013; Atlanta, GA, USA.

[55] Knudtson E, Para M, Boswell H, *et al.* Drug rash with eosinophilia and systemic symptoms syndrome and renal toxicity with a nevirapine-containing regimen in a pregnant patient with human immunodeficiency virus. Obstet Gynecol 2003; 101: 1094-7.

[56] Wirth GJ, Teuscher J, Graf JD, *et al.* Efavirenz induced urolithiasis. Urol Res 2006; 34: 288-9.

[57] Izzedine H, Valantin MA, Daudon M, *et al.* Efavirenz urolithiasis. AIDS 2007; 21: 1992.

[58] German P, Liu HC, Szwarcberg J *et al.* Effect of Cobicistat on Glomerular Filtration Rate in Subjects With Normal and Impaired Renal Function. J Acquir Immune Defic Syndr 2012; 61: 32-40.

[59] Boyd M. Dolutegravir—A promising antiretroviral in development. Lancet Infect Dis 2012; 12(2): 90-1.

[60] Steigbigel R, Cooper D, Kumar P, *et al.* Raltegravir with optimized background therapy for resistant HIV-1 infection. N Engl J Med 2008; 359: 339-54.

[61] DeJesus E, Berger D, Markowitz M, *et al.* Antiviral activity, pharmacokinetics, and dose response of the HIV-1 integ rase inhibitor GS-9137 (JTK-303) in treatment-naive and treatment-experienced patients. J Acquir Immune Defic Syndr 2006; 43: 1-5.

[62] Zolopa AR, Mullen M, Berger D, *et al.* The HIV integrase inhibitor GS-9137 has potent antiretroviral activity in treatment-experienced patients [Oral Presentation 143LB]. Paper presented at: 14th Conference on Retroviruses and Opportunistic Infections.2007; 25-28.

[63] Zolopa AR, Lampiris H, Blick G, *et al.* The HIV Integrase Inhibitor Elvitegravir (EVG/r) Has Potent and Durable Antiretroviral Activity in Treatment- Experienced Patients with Active Optimized Background Therapy (OBT) [Oral Presentation]. Paper presented at 47th Annual Interscience Conference on Antimicrobial Agents and Chemotherapy (ICAAC). 2007: 17-20.

[64] Wand H, Calmy A, Carey DL, *et al.* Metabolic syndrome, cardiovascular disease and type 2 diabetes mellitus after initiation of antiretroviral therapy in HIV infection. AIDS 2007; 21: 2445.

[65] Mouser V. Atherosclerosis and HIV in the highly active antiretroviral therapy era: towards an epidemic of cardiovascular disease? AIDS 2003; 17 (1): 65-9.

[66] Masiá-Canuto M, Morell EB, Rodero FG. Alteraciones lipídicas y riesgo cardiovascular asociado a la terapia antirretroviral. Enferm Infecc Microbiol Clin 2006; 24 (10): 637-48.

[67] Rerkpattanapipat P, Wongpraparut N, Jacobs LE, Kotler MN. Cardiac manifestations of acquired immunodeficiency syndrome. Arch Intern Med 2000; 160 (5): 602-8.

[68] Milei J, Grana D, Fernández Alonso G, Matturri L. Cardiac involvement in acquired immunodeficiency syndrome: a review to push action. Clin Cardiol 1998; 21: 465-72.

[69] Hanabusa H, Tagami H, Hataya H: Renal atrophy associated with long-term treatment with indinavir. N Engl J Med 1999; 340: 392-3.

[70] Carr A, Cooper DA. Adverse effects of antiretroviral therapy. Lancet 2000; 356: 1423-30.

[71] Volberding PA, Deeks SG. Antiretroviral therapy and management of HIV infection. Lancet 2010; 376(9734): 49-62.

[72] Kopp JB, Miller KD, Mican JM, *et al.* Microscopic finding of Indinavir crystals in urinary sedimentCrystalluria and urinary tract abnormalities associated with Indinavir. Ann Intern Med 1997; 127: 119-25.

[73] Fernandez-Fernandez B, Montoya-Ferrer A, Sanz AB. Tenofovir Nephrotoxicity: 2011 Update. Hindawi Publishing Corporation AIDS Research and Treatment. 2011; Article ID 354908, 11 pages, 2011. doi: 10.1155/2011/354908.

[74] Said SM, Nasr SH, Samsa R, Markowitz GS, D'Agati VD. Nephrotoxicity of antiretroviral therapy in an HIV-infected patient. Kidney Int 2007; 71: 1071-5.

Subject Index

A

B

C

D

E

F

T

U

V

X

Made in the USA
Monee, IL
08 May 2026

49715033R00178